Workbook for Lippincott's Textbook
for Nursing Assistants

Third Edition

PAMELA J. CARTER, RN, BSN, MEd, CNOR
Program Coordinator/Instructor
School of Health Professions
Davis Applied Technology College
Kaysville, Utah

 Wolters Kluwer | Lippincott Williams & Wilkins
Health
Philadelphia · Baltimore · New York · London
Buenos Aires · Hong Kong · Sydney · Tokyo

Acquisitions Editor: Elizabeth Nieginski
Product Manager: Eric Van Osten
Vendor Manager: Cynthia Rudy
Director of Nursing Production: Helen Ewan
Designer: Holly McLaughlin
Manufacturing Coordinator: Karin Duffield
Production Services / Compositor: Aptara, Inc.

3rd edition

9 8 7 6 5 4 3 2

ISBN-13: 978-1-60547-636-0
ISBN-10: 1-60547-636-6

Care has been taken to confirm the accuracy of the information presented and to describe generally accepted practices. However, the author, editors, and publisher are not responsible for errors or omissions or for any consequences from application of the information in this book and make no warranty, expressed or implied, with respect to the currency, completeness, or accuracy of the contents of the publication. Application of this information in a particular situation remains the professional responsibility of the practitioner; the clinical treatments described and recommended may not be considered absolute and universal recommendations.

The author, editors, and publisher have exerted every effort to ensure that drug selection and dosage set forth in this text are in accordance with the current recommendations and practice at the time of publication. However, in view of ongoing research, changes in government regulations, and the constant flow of information relating to drug therapy and drug reactions, the reader is urged to check the package insert for each drug for any change in indications and dosage and for added warnings and precautions. This is particularly important when the recommended agent is a new or infrequently employed drug.

Some drugs and medical devices presented in this publication have Food and Drug Administration (FDA) clearance for limited use in restricted research settings. It is the responsibility of the health care provider to ascertain the FDA status of each drug or device planned for use in his or her clinical practice.

To purchase additional copies of this book, call our customer service department at (800) 638-3030 or fax orders to (301) 223-2320. International customers should call (301) 223-2300. Visit Lippincott Williams & Wilkins on the Internet: http://www.lww.com. Lippincott Williams & Wilkins customer service representatives are available from 8:30 a.m. to 6:00 p.m. EST.

LWW.COM

Preface

Workbook for Lippincott's Textbook for Nursing Assistants, developed alongside the textbook with the aid of an instructional design team, is designed to help students internalize and apply the important concepts and facts presented in the textbook. Students will benefit from first reading the assignment in the textbook and then completing the corresponding workbook assignment. This approach allows students to review and reinforce the information that they have just read. In addition, after working on the workbook assignment, students who are having difficulty understanding the information presented in the textbook will know what type of questions they need to ask in class the following day. This ability to recognize areas of difficulty helps students to better utilize instruction time.

A UNIQUE ORGANIZATION

The organization of each chapter in the workbook follows the same organization as the corresponding chapter in *Lippincott's Textbook for Nursing Assistants.* This unique organization enhances flexibility with regard to assignments—it is easy to assign all, or just part of, a workbook chapter, according to the needs of your particular curriculum. In addition, this unique organization allows students to identify particular areas of difficulty where more clarification and review is needed. **Key Learning Points,** derived from the learning objectives in the textbook, are given for each sub-topic within the chapter and help the student to easily identify the concepts that are being reviewed and reinforced.

ACTIVITIES DESIGNED TO APPEAL TO DIFFERENT TYPES OF LEARNERS

This workbook uses several different types of activities to help students internalize and apply the information in the textbook. A wide variety of activities is important for appealing to students with different learning styles. Variety also helps to keep students engaged in the assignment. Some of the activity types that you will find in this workbook include:

- **Multiple-choice questions:** Select the single best answer from four choices.
- **Fill-in-the-blanks:** Complete a phrase or sentence.
- **Think About It!** Write a short response to a thought-provoking "what if?" scenario.
- **True or false?** Identify the true statements and correct the false ones.
- **Matching:** Match the terms or pictures to their descriptions.
- **Crossword puzzles:** Decipher the clues to complete the puzzle.
- **Word find puzzles:** Locate key vocabulary words in the grid of letters.
- **Word jumbles:** Use the clues to rearrange scrambled letters and reveal key vocabulary words.
- **Labeling:** Fill in the missing labels on a key piece of artwork.
- **Sequencing:** Put the steps of a procedure or process in the correct order.
- **Identification:** Recognize the phrases or sentences that apply to each situation.

Many workbooks rely heavily on multiple-choice questions. Although multiple-choice questions are important for helping students to prepare for the certification exam, the goal of this workbook is to help prepare students for what comes after the exam. We want students to develop a depth of understanding of this material that will serve them well in their clinical practice, long after the exam is over. Our goal is to help promote good problem-solving abilities and more of a "working" application of the material. Instructors wishing to provide their students with additional practice in answering multiple-choice questions can create worksheets and practice tests using the multiple-choice questions provided on the Instructor's Resource CD and on thePoint, a web-based course and content management system (http://thePoint@lww.com/Carter3e).

OTHER KEY FEATURES

In addition to a variety of activities designed to reinforce the information in Chapters 1 through 45 and Appendix B ("Introduction to the Language of Health Care") of *Lippincott's Textbook for Nursing Assistants*, this workbook contains:

■ **Procedure checklists.** These checklists are very useful during the laboratory portion of the course, when students are practicing the procedures they have just learned.
■ **Pam's pearls:** Scattered throughout the workbook, these words of advice and encouragement from the author serve to reinforce key concepts and remind students of the very important role they will play in providing patient and resident care.

> Preventing the complications of immobility through frequent repositioning and transferring is a major responsibility of the nursing assistant!

Answers to the activities in the *Workbook for Lippincott's Textbook for Nursing Assistants* are provided on the Instructor's Resource CD and on thePoint (http://thePoint@lww.com/Carter3e).

It is our sincere hope that students will find completing assignments from the workbook to be fun as well as educational. As always, we welcome and appreciate feedback from our readers.

Pamela J. Carter
Lippincott Williams & Wilkins

*thePoint is a trademark of WKHealth.

Acknowledgment

I'd like to thank Joellen Shumway, Elizabeth Nieginski, and Eric Van Osten for their assistance during the development of this workbook.

Contents

UNIT VIII

HOME HEALTH CARE

APPENDIX B

CHAPTER 1

The Health Care System

HEALTH CARE DELIVERY, PAST AND PRESENT

Key Learning Points

- The changes that have occurred in how health care is delivered

Activity A *Mark each statement as either "true" (T) or "false" (F). Correct the false statements.*

1. T F   In the 18th, 19th, and early part of the 20th centuries, health care delivery in the United States was focused around care given in health care facilities.

2. T F   A holistic approach focuses on taking care of only the emotional needs of a person.

HEALTH CARE ORGANIZATIONS

Key Learning Points

- Types of health care organizations
- Structure of a health care organization

Activity B *Select the single best answer for each of the following questions.*

1. Which of the following would most likely be the primary mission of a university hospital?

   a. To use the health care industry as a financial investment to turn a profit

   b. To promote health by offering rehabilitation services to people

   c. To train people in the field of health care

   d. To teach people the ways to achieve and maintain physical and mental fitness

2. Who is referred to as a "patient"?

   a. A person who receives the services of a long-term care facility

   b. A person who receives the services of an assisted-living facility

   c. A person who receives the services of a hospital

   d. A person who receives the services of a home health care agency

3. Why are people who are cared for in a long-term care facility referred to as "residents" rather than "patients"?

   a. Because most of the people who are admitted to a long-term care facility are elderly

   b. Because the long-term care facility becomes the person's home, either temporarily or permanently

   c. Because the long-term care facility cares for people of all ages with any number of different medical needs

   d. Because the people in a long-term care facility receive more advanced care than those in a hospital

Activity C *Fill in the blanks using the words given in brackets.*

[inpatient, outpatient]

1. A patient who stays in a hospital for one or more nights receives _____ care.

1

2. A patient with cancer who returns to the hospital every day for a period of time to receive radiation therapy would be receiving _____ care.

Activity D *Observe the figure and answer the following question.*

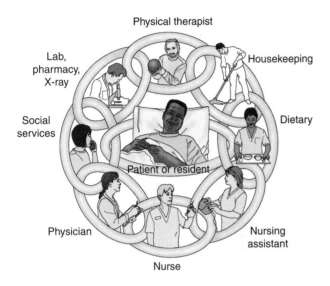

1. In a health care setting, who is always the focus of the health care team's efforts?

    a. The physician

    b. The housekeeping staff

    c. The patient or resident

    d. Social services

> Health care is provided by a team of people, each with different areas of expertise and job responsibilities. As a nursing assistant, you are a critical member of the health care team!

Activity E *Match the health care organization in Column A with its corresponding function in Column B.*

Column A

_____ **1.** Hospice

_____ **2.** Home health care

_____ **3.** Assisted-living facility

_____ **4.** Long-term care facility

_____ **5.** Subacute care unit

Column B

a. Provides rehabilitation and other skilled care and helps the person advance from hospital care to home care

b. Provides limited help with medications, transportation, meals, and housekeeping

c. Provides care for people who are unable to care for themselves at home yet do not need to be hospitalized

d. Provides skilled care in a person's home

e. Relieves pain and provides emotional and spiritual support for both the dying person and the family

Activity F *Look at the organization chart below and match the job title in Column A with its corresponding function in Column B.*

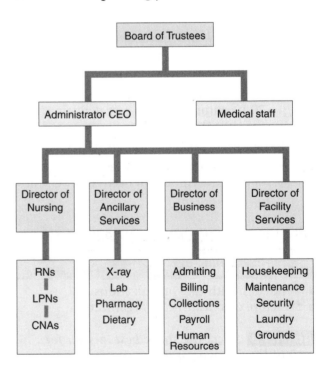

Column A

_____ **1.** Board of trustees

_____ **2.** Director of Nursing

_____ **3.** Administrator or chief executive officer

Column B

a. Manages the organization and is the link between the board and the organization

b. Sets policies to ensure that the care offered by the organization is safe and of good quality

c. Responsible for the quality of the nursing care provided in the facility

OVERSIGHT OF THE HEALTH CARE SYSTEM

Key Learning Points

■ Government and private agencies that provide oversight of the health care system

Activity G *Match the agencies and regulations used to protect health care recipients and providers in Column A with their corresponding function in Column B.*

Column A

_____ **1.** United States Department of Health and Human Services

_____ **2.** Omnibus Budget Reconciliation Act (OBRA), 1987

_____ **3.** Occupational Safety and Health Act, 1970

_____ **4.** The Joint Commission

Column B

a. Established safety and health standards for the workplace

b. Sets national standards for all types of health care organizations

c. Primary government agency responsible for protecting nation's health

d. Improved conditions for people in long-term care facilities

PAYING FOR HEALTH CARE

Key Learning Points

■ How health care is paid for

Activity H *Match the insurance or plan in Column A with its corresponding function in Column B.*

Column A

_____ **1.** Group insurance

_____ **2.** Managed care system

_____ **3.** Medicare

_____ **4.** Medicaid

Column B

a. A federally funded insurance plan by Social Security, under the administration of the Center for Medicare and Medicaid Services (CMMS)

b. A federally funded and state-regulated plan designed to help people with low incomes to pay for health care

c. Insurance that is purchased at group rates by an employer or corporation

d. Assists in delivering health care to people who need it by arranging contacts with various health care providers

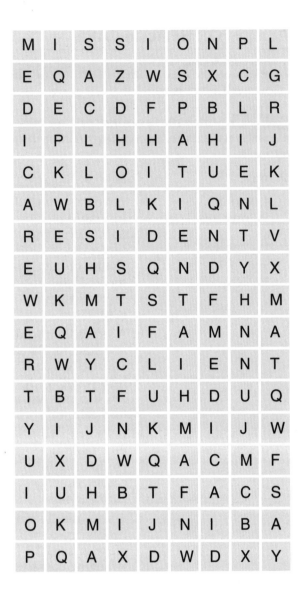

M	I	S	S	I	O	N	P	L
E	Q	A	Z	W	S	X	C	G
D	E	C	D	F	P	B	L	R
I	P	L	H	H	A	H	I	J
C	K	L	O	I	T	U	E	K
A	W	B	L	K	I	Q	N	L
R	E	S	I	D	E	N	T	V
E	U	H	S	Q	N	D	Y	X
W	K	M	T	S	T	F	H	M
E	Q	A	I	F	A	M	N	A
R	W	Y	C	L	I	E	N	T
T	B	T	F	U	H	D	U	Q
Y	I	J	N	K	M	I	J	W
U	X	D	W	Q	A	C	M	F
I	U	H	B	T	F	A	C	S
O	K	M	I	J	N	I	B	A
P	Q	A	X	D	W	D	X	Y

SUMMARY

Activity I *Use the clues to find words that are present in the grid of letters, either horizontally from left to right or vertically from top to bottom.*

Down

1. A type of insurance plan that is federally funded by Social Security and that all people 65 years and older, and some younger disabled people, are eligible to participate in
2. An adjective used to describe care of the whole person, physically and emotionally
3. A federally funded and state-regulated plan designed to help people with low incomes to pay for health care

Across

1. The officially stated purpose of a health care facility or organization
2. A person being cared for in a long-term care facility
3. A person who is receiving the services of a home health care agency

CHAPTER 2

The Nursing Assistant

NURSING, PAST AND PRESENT

Key Learning Points
- The history of nursing

Activity A *Select the single best answer for each of the following questions.*

1. What is Florence Nightingale credited for?
   a. Demonstrating the effect of music on the sick
   b. Establishing nursing as a profession in its own right
   c. Founding the world's first hospital
   d. Discovering the cure for smallpox

2. What were early nursing assistants called?
   a. Helpers
   b. Sub-nurses
   c. Aides
   d. Caretakers

EDUCATION OF THE NURSING ASSISTANT

Key Learning Points
- OBRA requirements for nursing assistant training
- Contents of the registry

Activity B *Select the single best answer for each of the following questions.*

1. What does OBRA stand for?
   a. Overall Budget Reconciliation Act
   b. Omnibus Budget Reconciliation Act
   c. Omnibus Budget Revision Act
   d. Omnibus Budget Reform Act

2. OBRA requires that every state maintain an official database of the people who have successfully completed the nursing assistant training program. What is this record called?
   a. A catalogue
   b. A database
   c. A handbook
   d. A registry

Activity C *Mark each statement as either "true" (T) or "false" (F). Correct the false statements.*

1. T F Many long-term care facilities offer nursing assistant training programs.

2. T F OBRA requires all nursing assistants to undergo a minimum of 50 hours of training.

3. T F A student is given three opportunities to successfully complete the competency evaluation at the end of the training period.

4. T F The principle of reciprocity means that your certificate will not be valid in states other than where you received your training.

5. T F Nursing assistants who have not worked for 2 consecutive years need to undergo retraining and retake the competency evaluation.

Activity D *Place an "X" next to the information that does NOT appear in the registry.*

1. ___ Full name

2. ___ Home address

3. ___ Social Security number

4. ___ Date of birth

5. ___ Date the competency evaluation was passed

6. ___ Educational qualifications

7. ___ Reported incidents of resident abuse or neglect, or theft of resident property

RESPONSIBILITIES OF THE NURSING ASSISTANT

Key Learning Points

■ Responsibilities of the nursing assistant

Activity E *Select the single best answer for each of the following questions.*

1. What important role does the nursing assistant play?
   a. Consultant
   b. Medical advisor
   c. Observer and communicator
   d. Administrator

2. Which one of the following is NOT a basic physical need?
   a. Hygiene
   b. Comfort
   c. Nutrition
   d. Entertainment

3. A nursing assistant's duties do NOT include taking care of the patient's or resident's:
   a. Safety
   b. Exercise
   c. Financial needs
   d. Emotional needs

THE NURSING TEAM

Key Learning Points

■ The members of the nursing team, and the role of each team member

Activity F *Fill in the blanks.*

1. Every nursing team consists of at least a nurse and a nursing assistant. A nurse can either be a _____ _____, or a _____ _____. In some states, an LPN is also referred to as a _____ _____.

   A nursing team could also include a _____ _____, whose duty involves supervising other nurses during a shift, and a _____, who heads a department or section. An RN who directs all the nursing care within a health care organization is called a _____ _____.

Activity G *Think About It! Briefly answer the following question in the space provided.*

Explain the difference between primary nursing, functional (modular) nursing, and team nursing.

_____

_____

_____

DELEGATION

Key Learning Points

■ The delegation process as it relates to the nursing assistant
■ The "five rights" of delegation

Activity H *Mark each statement as either "true" (T) or "false" (F). Correct the false statements.*

1. T F "Scope of practice" refers to the range of tasks that a nursing assistant is morally allowed to perform.

2. T F By delegating a task, a nurse gives a nursing assistant permission to perform the task on his or her behalf.

3. T F Tasks such as assessment, planning, and evaluating can be delegated to nursing assistants.

Activity I *The National Council of State Boards of Nursing (NCSBN) has developed guidelines, called the "five rights" of delegation, to help nurses effectively delegate tasks. Match the rights in Column A with the corresponding guidelines in Column B.*

Column A

_____ 1. The right task

_____ 2. The right circumstance

_____ 3. The right person

_____ 4. The right direction

_____ 5. The right supervision

Column B

a. Will the nurse be available to supervise or answer questions?

b. Will the nurse be able to give the nursing assistant clear directions regarding how to perform the task?

c. What are the needs of the patient or resident at this time?

d. Can this task be delegated?

e. Does the nursing assistant have the right training and experience to safely complete the task?

Activity J *Select the single best answer for each of the following questions.*

1. Which one of the following reasons is NOT an acceptable reason to refuse to perform a delegated task?
   a. The directions given to you by the nurse are not clear.
   b. You do not have the proper equipment to perform the task.
   c. You do not enjoy the task.
   d. The task is illegal or unethical.

2. When a nurse delegates a task to a nursing assistant, the nurse is responsible for any injury that may occur to the patient or resident if:
   a. The nursing assistant is not qualified for the task
   b. The nursing assistant is suitably qualified, but is not supervised by the nurse
   c. The nursing assistant is suitably qualified but makes a mistake while carrying out the task
   d. The nursing assistant is suitably qualified but does not perform the task as requested

> The delegation of tasks cannot be taken lightly by either the nurse or the nursing assistant. Both share responsibility for ensuring that the procedure is carried out without harm to the patient or resident. Know which tasks are within your scope of practice and which are not, and don't be afraid to ask for help or clarification if you need it.

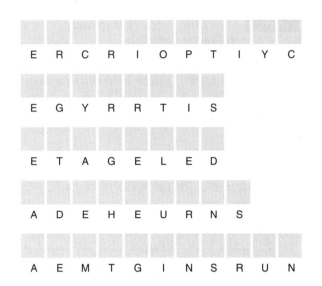

E R C R I O P T I Y C

E G Y R R T I S

E T A G E L E D

A D E H E U R N S

A E M T G I N S R U N

SUMMARY

Activity K *Words shown in the picture have been jumbled. Use the clues to form correct words using the letters given in the picture.*

1. The principle by which one state recognizes the validity of a license or certification granted by another state
2. An official record maintained by the state of the people who have successfully completed the nursing assistant training program
3. To authorize another person to perform a task on your behalf
4. A registered nurse (RN) who is in charge of a department or section
5. A model for organizing the nursing team's efforts in which a team leader (a registered nurse) determines all of the nursing needs for the patients or residents assigned to the team, and assigns tasks according to each team member's skills and level of responsibility

CHAPTER 3

Professionalism and Job-Seeking Skills

WHAT IS A PROFESSIONAL?

Key Learning Points

- The meaning of the terms *professional* and *professionalism*
- Characteristics of a professional health care worker

Activity A *Select the single best answer for the following question.*

1. Which one of the following nursing assistants does NOT show the attitudes characteristic of a professional?

   a. Sara is an experienced nursing assistant who is kind and caring toward the patients and residents in the facility where she works.

   b. Sally is a certified nursing assistant who works only to earn a paycheck.

   c. Sara is a certified nursing assistant who is committed to doing her work to the best of her ability.

   d. Sally is a certified nursing assistant who takes pride in her work at the hospital and is always interested in learning more about her job.

The health care industry relies on all types of professionals to provide quality care to patients and residents. Professionals have certain credentials that are earned through education and training, but being a professional also means having a professional attitude and a good work ethic.

WHAT IS A WORK ETHIC?

Key Learning Points

- The term *work ethic* and how good work habits promote professionalism

Activity B *Select the single best answer for each of the following questions.*

1. A strong "work ethic" is one of the most important qualities that potential employers look for in a nursing assistant. What does this term refer to?

   a. A person's ability to judge whether a nurse has made a correct decision

   b. A person's ability to perform the work assigned to him or her

   c. A person's attitude toward his or her work

   d. A person's awareness of the rules that should be followed in the workplace

2. Which of the following qualities does NOT reflect a strong work ethic?

 a. Punctuality

 b. Competitiveness

 c. Accountability

 d. Reliability

Activity C *Match the words given in Column A with the corresponding meanings in Column B.*

Column A

____ **1.** Punctuality

____ **2.** Reliability

____ **3.** Accountability

____ **4.** Conscientious-ness

____ **5.** Courtesy and respectfulness

____ **6.** Honesty

____ **7.** Cooperative-ness

____ **8.** Empathy

Column B

a. You can be trusted by patients and residents with their private information and valuables.

b. You are polite and do not make negative remarks about your coworkers.

c. Your supervisor can depend on you to finish your assignment properly.

d. You offer a helping hand when you see that a coworker requires help.

e. You take responsibility for your actions and their consequences.

f. You are always on time for work.

g. You are able to show kindness and tolerance by imagining yourself in someone else's situation.

h. You take your work seriously and give your patients or residents the "royal treatment."

> A nursing assistant with a strong work ethic has qualities that make her both pleasant to work with and dependable.

PERSONAL HEALTH AND HYGIENE

Key Learning Points

■ The importance of personal health and hygiene for a health care worker

Activity D *To maintain good physical health, a nursing assistant must take care of himself or herself first. Look at the figures below and fill in the blanks.*

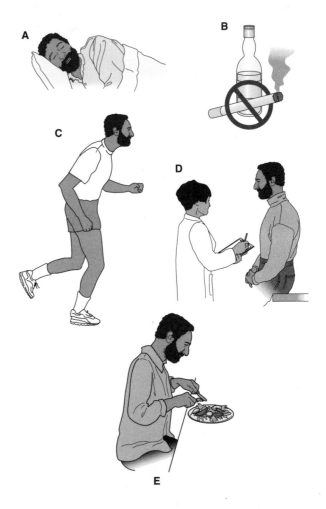

A. You should get enough _____.

B. You should not _____ and you should limit your _____ intake.

C. You should _____ regularly.

D. You should have a routine _____ _____.

E. You should eat _____ meals.

Activity E *Select the single best answer for each of the following questions.*

1. Why is it important for a nursing assistant to maintain good personal hygiene?

   a. Good personal hygiene helps to prevent the spread of infection.

   b. Good personal hygiene sets you apart from other nursing assistants.

   c. Good personal hygiene makes you eligible for a raise in salary.

   d. Good personal hygiene sets an example for your patients and residents.

2. Which of the following activities is NOT a part of maintaining good personal hygiene?

   a. Bathing daily and using a deodorant

   b. Keeping your nails short and clean

   c. Wearing a clean, pressed uniform everyday

   d. Wearing jewelry to improve your appearance

Activity F *Mark each statement as either "true" (T) or "false" (F). Correct the false statements.*

1. T F Physical activity relieves mental and emotional stress.

2. T F Making time for yourself is just not that important when you feel overwhelmed with responsibilities.

3. T F You must never ask to be assigned to different work areas or to different patients or residents.

> To care for your patients or residents to the best of your ability, you must first care for yourself!

JOB-SEEKING SKILLS

Key Learning Points

- Sources of information about employment opportunities in the health care industry
- Factors to consider when seeking employment
- The application process necessary for obtaining employment

Activity G *Match the characteristics of a nursing assistant in Column A with the health care facility that she would be best suited for in Column B.*

Column A	Column B
___ 1. Likes to work with elderly people	a. acute care unit
___ 2. Wants to care for people in their homes	b. long-term care facility
___ 3. Likes a fast-paced work environment	c. home health care agency

Activity H *Sally is searching for a suitable nursing assistant job. Considering her situation, help her make a decision from the given options. Select the single best answer for each of the following situations.*

1. Sally has a child.

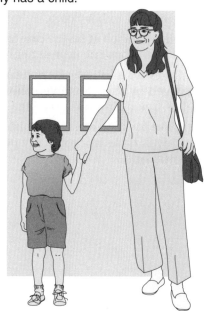

   a. She takes the child to work.

   b. She works whatever shift she is scheduled for, not considering the childcare arrangements.

   c. She tells the employer that she is available to work any shift, even though this is not true.

   d. She tells the employer what shift she is available to work, based on her childcare arrangements.

2. Sally plans to take the bus to get to work.

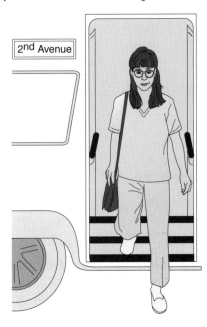

a. She applies for a job at every health care facility, whether or not it is served by the bus line nearest to her home.

b. She applies for a job at health care facilities serviced by the bus line nearest her home.

c. She applies for a job at a health care facility serviced by the train, even though she does not live near a train station.

d. She applies for a job at every health care facility, even those not served by public transportation.

Activity I *Use the clues for sources of employment opportunities to complete the crossword puzzle.*

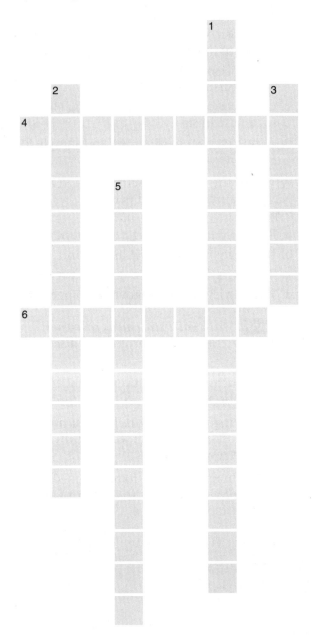

Across

4. Contains classified ads listing employment opportunities
6. Use this to check sites that help people find jobs

Down

1. A department at your school that may have job listings and can often help with writing a résumé

2. Check here for a list of facilities and agencies that hire nursing assistants
3. They may know of possible job openings
5. Many schools and facilities have one of these, where job opportunities may be posted

> Advance planning about the type of employment you want helps to give your job search direction.

Activity J *Match the words given in Column A with their corresponding meanings in Column B.*

Column A

____ 1. Résumé

____ 2. Cover letter

____ 3. Reference list

Column B

a. A letter to introduce yourself to a potential employer

b. List of three or four people willing to talk to a potential employer about your abilities

c. A brief document that gives general information about you, your education, and work experience to a potential employer

Activity K *Place an "X" next to the information that should be included in a résumé.*

1. ____ Full name
2. ____ Employment history
3. ____ Weight
4. ____ Marital status
5. ____ Age
6. ____ Address
7. ____ Education history
8. ____ Sexual preference

Activity L *Think About It! Briefly answer the following question in the space provided.*

Amy Robinson goes on an interview for a position as a nursing assistant at a long-term care facility. The interviewer asks Amy whether or not she is married. How should Amy respond to the interviewer's question?

_____

_____

_____

Activity M *Select the single best answer for the following question.*

1. Why is it a good idea to first ask for a person's permission before including his name and contact information in your reference list?
   a. The person may not want his contact information given out.
   b. The person may not be able to give you a positive reference and therefore might be more comfortable not giving any reference at all.
   c. It is good manners to ask before including someone on a reference list.
   d. All of the above

Activity N *Place an "X" next to the information that should be included in a job application form.*

1. ____ Weight
2. ____ Work history
3. ____ Marital status
4. ____ Education
5. ____ Position applied for
6. ____ Reason you left your previous job
7. ____ Shifts that you can work
8. ____ Contact address and how can you be reached
9. ____ Sexual preference
10. ____ Religion

Activity O *Which one of the nursing assistants pictured below is most likely to make a favorable impression on a potential employer?*

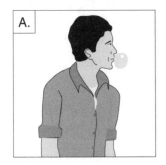

A.

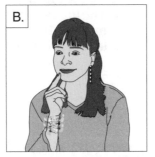

B.

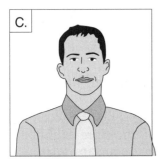

C.

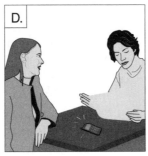

D.

Activity P *Fill in the blanks.*

1. If you haven't heard from your employer in _____ week's time, it is appropriate to call and ask about the status of your application.

2. Write a thank you note within _____ day(s) of interviewing for a position.

SUMMARY

Activity Q *Use the clues to find words that are present in the grid of letters, either horizontally from left to right or vertically from top to bottom.*

Down

1. A meeting between an employer and a potential employee, during which information is exchanged regarding the organization, the job, and the potential employee's qualifications for the job

2. A person who has credentials, obtained through education and training, that enable him or her to become licensed or certified to practice a certain profession; also, a person who demonstrates a professional attitude

3. The side of ourselves that we display to the world, communicating outwardly how we feel about things

4. A brief document that gives a potential employer general information about a job candidate's education and work experience

Across

1. A person's attitude toward his or her work

I	H	R	P	E	R	S	O	N
N	L	I	S	T	S	D	Y	J
T	A	E	N	Y	B	G	P	Q
E	V	S	E	T	L	K	I	D
R	A	Z	W	P	L	I	V	B
V	L	M	R	R	A	E	A	W
I	J	Q	L	O	V	S	T	T
E	T	O	D	F	O	N	T	U
W	O	R	K	E	T	H	I	C
R	S	E	Q	S	V	R	T	I
F	A	S	A	S	A	I	U	T
V	D	U	Z	I	L	E	D	R
Y	Y	M	W	O	J	S	E	U
A	G	E	S	N	T	Z	A	S
S	N	Q	X	A	R	M	E	R
H	F	T	T	L	Y	Q	Y	D

CHAPTER 4

Legal and Ethical Issues

INTRODUCTION TO LEGAL AND ETHICAL ISSUES

Key Learning Points

- Factors influencing behavior in society
- Need for laws and ethics

Activity A *Place an "X" next to the factors that influence a person's behavior in society.*

1. ___ Society's laws

2. ___ Personal ethical code

3. ___ Fear of punishment

4. ___ Spiritual beliefs

5. ___ Values instilled by family

6. ___ Rules established by a governing authority

Activity B *Mark each statement as either "true" (T) or "false" (F). Correct the false statements.*

1. T F   Fear of punishment is what causes a person to act according to an ethical code.

2. T F   Laws and ethics provide guidance to health care providers.

3. T F   Values instilled by a person's family influence the person's ethical code.

PATIENTS' AND RESIDENTS' RIGHTS

Key Learning Points

- Patients' and residents' rights, as set forth by the American Hospital Association (AHA) and the Omnibus Budget Reconciliation Act (OBRA)
- Two major types of advance directives
- Why advance directives play an important role in health care

Activity C *Select the single best answer for each of the following questions.*

1. Which of the following statements is NOT listed in *The Patient Care Partnership*?
   a. The right to information regarding diagnosis, treatment, and prognosis
   b. The right of confidentiality pertaining to all communication
   c. The right to use personal possessions
   d. The right to considerate and respectful care

2. Where is the right to be informed of one's options for care stated?
   a. *The Patient Care Partnership*
   b. *Patients' Bill of Responsibilities*
   c. *Residents' Rights*
   d. *Rights for the Health Care Organizations*

3. Which one of the following is a responsibility of the patient?

   a. The patient is responsible for the consequences of refused treatment or disregarded instructions.

   b. The patient is responsible for withholding information that is confidential.

   c. The patient is responsible for having his medical records explained and interpreted.

   d. The patient is responsible for participating in experimental studies.

4. Which of the following statements is NOT listed in the "Residents' Rights"?

   a. The right to be free from physical or psychological abuse, including the improper use of restraints

   b. The right to organize and participate in groups organized by other residents, or the families of residents

   c. The right to respect the property, comfort, environment, and privacy of other patients

   d. The right to information about advocacy groups

5. Which of the following conditions could result in a loss of the resident's right to remain in the facility?

   a. Planned changes in living arrangements

   b. Harrassing or threatening the safety of other residents

   c. Participation in social or religious activity

   d. Sharing the room with a spouse

Activity D *Fill in the blanks using the words given in brackets.*

[durable power of attorney, advance directive, living, health care agent]

1. An _____ is a document that allows a person to make his wishes regarding health care known to family members and health care workers, in case the time comes when he is no longer able to make those wishes known himself.

2. A _____ is the person who is responsible for making decisions on the person's behalf.

3. A _____ will allows the person to give instructions about what medical treatments he would or would not want to be done in an effort to save his life.

4. A _____ for health care transfers the responsibility for making medical decisions on the person's behalf to a family member, friend, or other trusted individual, in the event that the person is no longer able to make these decisions on her own behalf.

LAWS: A WAY OF PRESERVING PATIENTS' AND RESIDENTS' RIGHTS

Key Learning Points

- The legal aspects of health care delivery
- Common legal violations that are related to the provision of health care
- The awareness that health care workers must have in order to avoid legal dilemmas
- Types of abuse and signs that indicate abuse
- The health care worker's obligations in the reporting of suspected abuse

Activity E *Place an "X" next to the correct answers for the following questions.*

1. Why should laws be enforced?

   ____ Because they preserve citizens' basic human rights

   ____ Because American colonies have gained independence

   ____ Because they protect basic human rights for all people, regardless of race, religion, gender, or income

   ____ Because they help settle disputes in a civilized, orderly way

2. Which of these terms relate to a violation of civil law?

   ____ Litigation

   ____ Defamation

   ____ False imprisonment

   ____ Battery

3. What is the purpose of the Health Insurance Portability and Accountability Act (HIPAA)?

   ____ It regulates who has the right to view a person's medical records, data, or other private information.

_____ It sets standards on how a person's medical information is to be stored and transmitted from one place to another.

_____ It permits a contractual agreement that exists between a nursing assistant and the person he or she cares for.

_____ It requires that health care organizations set policies that allow a patient or resident to have access to his or her medical records.

4. Which of the following may be considered elder abuse?

_____ Larceny

_____ Sexual abuse

_____ Involuntary confinement or seclusion

_____ Failure to provide food, water, care, and medications

5. Which of the following situations may result in abuse?

_____ A desire of one person to overpower and dominate another

_____ A primary caregiver becoming very tired, frustrated, and overwhelmed by the responsibilities of providing care

_____ A relationship that is long term rather than short term

_____ A patient or resident who is "difficult" to manage

_____ A failure to provide medication

Activity F *Mark each statement as either "true" (T) or "false" (F). Correct the false statements.*

1. T F Criminal laws are concerned with the relationship between the individual and society as a whole.

2. T F Libel is an untrue oral statement that hurts another person's reputation.

3. T F Keeping a person in a room alone with the door closed can be considered a form of physical abuse.

Activity G *Think About It! Briefly answer the following question in the space provided.*

Janine works in a long-term care facility located in a small town. One day, Janine runs into Mrs. Jamison at the grocery store. Janine has just learned that Mrs. Jamison's mother-in-law, a resident at the long-term care facility where she works, has been diagnosed with cancer. Assuming that Mrs. Jamison knows about her mother-in-law's condition, Janine tells her how sorry she was to hear the news about her mother-in-law's cancer. . . . and is stunned when Mrs. Jamison says, "What cancer?" Did Janine do anything wrong by expressing her condolences to Mrs. Jamison?

_____

_____

_____

_____

_____

_____

_____

_____

_____

_____

_____

Activity H *Match the terms associated with abuse or legal issues given in Column A with their examples given in Column B.*

Column A

_____ **1.** Assault

_____ **2.** Fraud

_____ **3.** Neglect

_____ **4.** Slander

_____ **5.** Libel

Column B

a. A home health aide fails to change an incontinent client's soiled sheets more than once a week.

b. A nursing assistant tells a potential employer that he passed his certification exam when in fact he has not.

c. A nursing assistant tells Mrs. Smith that if she can't be nice to her roommate, she will slap her.

d. A movie star sues a tabloid newspaper that publishes an untrue report that the movie star had sought and received treatment at a certain well-known mental health clinic.

e. A nurse who feels she has been unfairly treated by a doctor on staff is overheard telling another employee of the hospital that the doctor never actually graduated from medical school.

Always keep in mind the legal responsibilities and obligations that you have as a caregiver. Knowing the tasks that are part of your job description and being aware of your employer's policies are critical to ensure that the care you give is within the legal limits of your job.

ETHICS: GUIDELINES FOR BEHAVIOR

Key Learning Points

- The difference between legal and ethical issues
- The ethical standards that govern the nursing profession in particular and the health care profession in general

Activity I *Fill in the blanks using the words given in brackets.*

[Beneficence, Autonomy, Justice, Nonmaleficence, Fidelity]

1. _____ is when kindness and gentleness are used while administering care.

2. _____ is doing good for patients and residents by preventing harm and promoting the health and welfare of the person above all else.

3. _____ is respecting a person's rights and personal preferences.

4. _____ is acting with integrity to earn others' trust.

5. _____ is treating people fairly and equally, regardless of race, religion, culture, disability, or ability to pay.

Activity J *Place an "X" next to statements that describe the term "ethics."*

1. ___ Ethics are less prescriptive than laws.

2. ___ Ethics are moral principles or standards that govern conduct.

3. ___ Ethics are guidelines pertaining to standards of conduct and practice.

5. ___ Ethics help us to determine the difference between right and wrong in areas where the law fears to tread.

Activity K *Select the single best answer for each of the following questions.*

1. Which act or association provides the guidelines for the code of ethics for nursing?
   a. American Hospital Association (AHA)
   b. Omnibus Budget Reconciliation Act (OBRA)
   c. Health Insurance Portability and Accountability Act (HIPAA)
   d. American Nurses Association (ANA)

2. Which factors influence a person's values?
   a. His culture and heritage
   b. His illness or disability
   c. His income
   d. His gender

SUMMARY

Words shown in the picture have been jumbled. Use the clues to form correct words using the letters given in the picture.

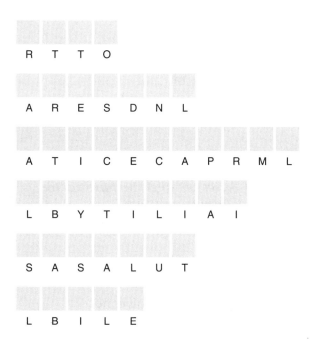

R T T O

A R E S D N L

A T I C E C A P R M L

L B Y T I L I A I

S A S A L U T

L B I L E

1. A violation of civil law
2. Spoken statements that injure someone's reputation; a form of defamation
3. Negligence committed by people who hold licenses to practice their profession, such as doctors, nurses, lawyers, dentists, and pharmacists
4. The responsibility of an individual to act within the confines of the law
5. Threatening or attempting to touch a person without the person's consent
6. Written statement that injures someone's reputation; a form of defamation

CHAPTER 5

Communication Skills

WHAT IS COMMUNICATION?

Key Learning Points

- The definition of the word *communication*
- Two major forms of communication

Activity A *Communication is the exchange of information. Conversation is a form of communication. Look at the following picture and fill in the blanks.*

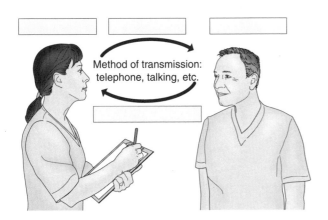

Method of transmission: telephone, talking, etc.

The _____ is the person with information to share, and the _____ is the person for whom the information is intended. The _____ delivers the information in the form of a _____ which the receiver may or may not understand. Through _____, or a return message, the _____ lets the _____ know whether the message was received and understood.

Activity B *Select the single best answer for each of the following questions.*

1. Which of the following activities is a form of communication?
   a. Telling someone something
   b. Giving a gift to someone
   c. Accepting a gift from someone
   d. Driving down to a friend's house to meet him

2. Which of the following is an example of verbal communication?
   a. Unintentional facial expressions
   b. Shaking the hand of a new patient or resident
   c. Sign language or writing out a question to a deaf resident
   d. Body language

3. Which of the following statements indicates that Mrs. Smith is using a form of nonverbal communication?
   a. Mrs. Smith walks over to the room next to hers to talk to another resident.
   b. Mrs. Smith grimaces and groans softly when she gets up from her bed and attempts to stand.
   c. Mrs. Smith talks about a pain in her back to a nursing assistant.
   d. Mrs. Smith listens carefully to the doctor who is informing her about her condition.

Activity C *Place a "V" next to the statements that are examples of verbal communication, and an "N" next to the statements that are examples of nonverbal communication.*

1. ___ Use of language, either spoken or written

2. ___ Gently touching a patient or a resident on the shoulder to reassure her

3. ___ Making a face when you put weight on a painful leg

4. ___ Using sign language to communicate with a person who is deaf

5. ___ Making a telephone call

6. ___ Nodding as someone speaks

7. ___ Tapping your fingers on the table because you are bored

8. ___ Recording vital sign measurements in a patient's or resident's chart

> Nursing assistants are an important link between the patient or resident and other members of the health care team. The nursing assistant is often the first member of the health care team to become aware of a change in a patient's or resident's condition that could be a sign of something serious. This is why it is important for nursing assistants to have good communication skills.

COMMUNICATING EFFECTIVELY

Key Learning Points

- Techniques that promote effective communication
- Blocks to effective communication and methods used to avoid them
- Causes of conflict, and ways of resolving conflicts

Activity D *Select the single best answer for each of the following questions.*

1. How will you create a verbal message as a sender?

   a. Organize relevant facts into a clear statement

   b. Use language that the receiver understands

   c. Speak clearly and in a voice that is loud enough to be heard

   d. All of the above

2. Which one of the following is an example of negative body language?

   a. Nodding encouragingly as someone speaks

   b. Crossing your arms across your chest

   c. Making eye contact when speaking to someone

   d. Gently touching a patient or resident on the shoulder or holding her hand

3. Which one of the following is an open-ended question?

   a. "Mr. John, tell me all about a favorite meal you enjoyed in your younger days."

   b. "Are you Mrs. Smith?"

   c. "Are you feeling okay, Mrs. Broan?"

   d. "Don't you like green beans, Mrs. Jones?"

4. Mr. Zimmer is a new resident at the facility where you work. You have just explained to him how to use the call light control system. What would be the best thing to say to Mr. Zimmer to verify that he understands what you have just explained to him?

   a. "Let me make sure you understand this correctly."

   b. "Let me know if you have any questions."

   c. "Could you just repeat these instructions back to me so I can make sure that I didn't leave anything out?"

   d. "Do you think you've got it now?"

5. Which of the following is a block to effective communication?

   a. Not being an active listener

   b. Being judgmental

   c. Interrupting a person before he finishes speaking

   d. All of the above

6. Conflict between people can occur when one person:

   a. Is unable to understand or accept another's ideas or beliefs

   b. Has expectations that differ from those of the other person

   c. Misunderstands another person's words or intentions

   d. All of the above

Activity E *There are different effective ways to resolve a conflict. Place "T" in front of the sentences that describe effective ways of resolving conflict. Place an "F" next to statements that describe ineffective ways of resolving conflict. Then, correct the statements marked "F."*

1. ____ Arrange to speak privately with the person you have a conflict with.

2. ____ Ask a supervisor to mediate immediately.

3. ____ During the conversation, focus on the area of conflict.

4. ____ Be specific about what you understand the problem to be.

5. ____ Tell the person how you feel about him or her.

6. ____ Say, "You really hurt my feelings by what you said the other day."

7. ____ Agree to disagree.

8. ____ Offer advice to the person.

> Listening is one of the most important communication skills, especially in the health care field.

TELEPHONE COMMUNICATION

Key Learning Points

- Proper telephone communication skills

Activity F *Select the single best answer for the following question.*

1. As a nursing assistant, you are responsible for answering the telephone, either at the nursing station or in a patient's or resident's room. When answering the telephone, what should you NOT do?

    a. Speak in a pleasant and unhurried voice.

    b. Take a message by writing down the caller's name and telephone number and delivering the message to the person it is intended for.

    c. Convey a kind and professional attitude.

    d. Provide information about a patient's or resident's condition to the caller.

COMMUNICATION AMONG MEMBERS OF THE HEALTH CARE TEAM

Key Learning Points

- Methods of reporting and recording information in a health care setting
- How a patient's or resident's medical record makes communication easier among members of the health care team
- Communication technologies that are being used in the health care field today
- Why the nursing assistant is a vital link in the communication chain
- How the nursing assistant communicates information to other members of the health care team
- Steps of the nursing process and how the nursing team uses the nursing process to plan the patient's or resident's care
- Role of effective communication in the provision of quality health care

Activity G *Select the single best answer for the following question.*

1. What usually forms the basis for a subjective observation?

    a. Mrs. Smith, a patient at the hospital, complains of abdominal pain immediately after a meal.

    b. A nursing assistant records Mrs. Smith's temperature.

    c. A nursing assistant measures Mrs. Smith's urine output.

    d. A nursing assistant reports Mrs. Smith's pulse rate to the nurse.

Activity H *As a nursing assistant, you must be a good communicator. What will you use your communication skills for? Place an "X" next to the relevant statements.*

1. ____ To comfort, reassure, and teach your patient or resident

2. ____ To achieve a greater understanding of what your patients or residents are feeling and thinking

3. ____ To diagnose and treat medical problems

4. ____ To relay vital information about a patient's or resident's condition to a nurse

5. ____ To report and record information in a health care unit

Activity I *Match the documents of a medical record given in Column A with their description in Column B.*

Column A

____ **1.** Admission sheet

____ **2.** Medical history

____ **3.** Physician's order sheet

____ **4.** Narrative nurse's notes

____ **5.** Graphic sheet

Column B

a. Document used by the doctor to communicate to other members of the health care team what should be done for the patient or resident

b. Document where information that is gathered routinely, such as vital signs, is recorded

c. Record of previous surgeries and medical conditions, current medications, allergies, and current medical diagnosis

d. Provides standard information about the patient or resident, such as his or her name, address, age, and insurance information

e. Record of a patient's or resident's complaints (symptoms) and the actions taken by the nursing staff to address these complaints

Activity J *Think About It! Briefly answer the following question in the space provided.*

What legal document is used to record information about a person's current condition, the measures that have been taken by the medical and nursing staff to diagnose and treat the condition, and the person's response to the treatment? Write the name of the document in the space provided below.

_____

_____

_____

Activity K *Think About It! Briefly answer the following question in the space provided.*

You are caring for Mrs. Wilson, who has been admitted to a hospital for the treatment of hypertension. One morning, Mrs. Wilson tells you that she feels dizzy when she gets up from the chair. This is your subjective observation. What objective data would you gather to support the subjective data given to you by Mrs. Wilson?

_____

_____

_____

_____

_____

_____

_____

_____

_____

_____

_____

Activity L *Think About It! Mrs. Chang has been admitted to the long-term care facility where you work because her Alzheimer's disease has progressed to the point where she is no longer able to manage many basic activities, such as bathing, dressing, and using the toilet. Susan, the nursing team leader, is responsible for preparing a nursing care plan for Mrs. Chang. Susan will use the nursing process to prepare this plan. The nursing process is organized into a series of steps. Fill in the blanks using the words given in brackets. Then, write down the correct order of the steps in the boxes provided below.*

[Planning, Diagnosis, Implementation, Assessment, Evaluation]

1. _____ The nursing team carries out the interventions detailed in the nursing care plan.

2. _____ The nursing team checks the effectiveness of the plan and revises it as necessary.

3. _____ The nurse describes the problems that Mrs. Chang is having, as well as the cause of the problems.

4. _____ The nurse examines Mrs. Chang and asks questions about her abilities, habits, and needs.

5. _____ The nurse makes a plan for Mrs. Chang's care.

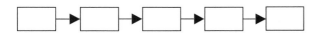

> The nursing assistant plays an important role in the nursing process by carrying out interventions and communicating observations to the nurse.

SUMMARY

Activity M *Use the clues to complete the crossword puzzle.*

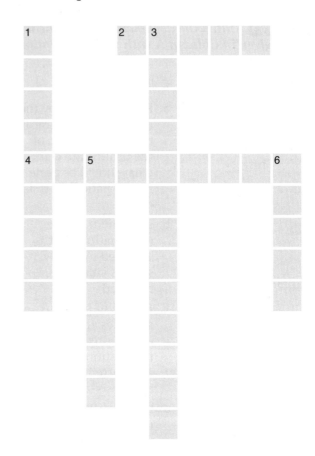

Down

1. The spoken exchange of information between health care team members
3. Actions that are taken by the nursing team to help the patient or resident
5. Discord resulting from differences between people; can occur when one person is unable to understand or accept another's ideas or beliefs
6. Descriptions of what nursing interventions (nursing actions that are taken to help a patient or resident) are meant to achieve

Across

2. Objective observations (that is, observations based on information that is obtained directly, through measurements or by using one of the five senses)
4. Communicating information about a patient or resident to other health care team members in written form; sometimes called charting

Those We Care For

PATIENTS, RESIDENTS, AND CLIENTS

Key Learning Points

- Health care is a people-focused service
- Why people need health care intervention
- Acute, chronic, and terminal conditions
- How the health care industry classifies people
- As a nursing assistant, the types of people that you might have the opportunity to work with

Activity A *As a nursing assistant you care for people who are sick, injured, or unable to care for themselves. Match the types of people you care for, given in Column A, with their descriptions, given in Column B.*

Column A

___ **1.** A client

___ **2.** A patient

___ **3.** A resident

Column B

a. A person who is receiving health care in a hospital, clinic, or extended-care facility.

b. A person who is living in a long-term care facility or an assisted-living facility.

c. A person who is receiving care in his or her own home, from a home health care agency.

> At the most basic level, patients, residents, and clients are "those we care for."

Activity B *There are three general types of illnesses that can cause a person to need health care services. Fill in the blanks using the terms given in brackets.*

[acute, chronic, terminal]

1. A _____ illness is a condition that is ongoing such as diabetes or high blood pressure.

2. A _____ illness is an illness or condition from which recovery is not expected, such as end-stage emphysema.

3. An _____ illness is a condition characterized by a rapid onset and a relatively short recovery time such as pneumonia, appendicitis or a broken bone.

Activity C *Select the single best answer for each of the following questions.*

1. In order to make providing care more efficient, the health care industry groups people according to which of the following criteria?

  a. Their ages

  b. Their illnesses or medical conditions

  c. Their special health care needs

  d. All of the above

2. Which one of the following is an example of a chronic condition?

   a. Pneumonia

   b. Asthma

   c. A broken bone

   d. Appendicitis

Activity D *Use the clues to complete the crossword puzzle.*

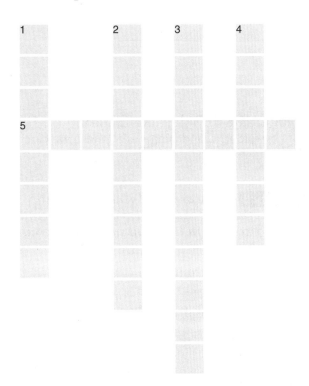

Across

5. People who are elderly

Down

1. People who are in need of surgical treatment
2. People who are children and adolescents
3. People who are pregnant or have just given birth
4. People who need medication, physical therapy or radiation

Activity E *Match the terms that are often used to group people who are in need of health care, given in Column A, with their descriptions given in Column B.*

Column A

____ 1. Psychiatric patient

Column B

a. Person recovering from an acute illness or condition

____ 2. Rehabilitation patient

____ 3. Subacute patient

____ 4. Intensive care patient

b. Person who has undergone a heart or brain surgery or is suffering from a heart attack or stroke.

c. Person with impaired mental health

d. Person undergoing therapy to restore his highest level of physical, emotional or vocational functioning

> People you care for can be classified in many different ways. However, those in need of health care services are not merely defined by their illnesses and disabilities. First and foremost, patients, residents, and clients are human beings.

GROWTH AND DEVELOPMENT

Key Learning Points

■ Stages of human growth and development
■ Developmental changes that are common throughout the life span of a person

Activity F *Select the single best answer for each of the following questions.*

1. Throughout the course of our lives we all pass through a series of changes that are related either to our physical growth or our psychological and social development. Which of the following describes a child who is more advanced in terms of growth than development?

   a. A child begins to walk at 8 months and talk at 12 months.

   b. A child begins to walk at 12 months and talk at 8 months.

   c. A 5-year-old prefers the company of older children but lacks the motor skills that would allow him to ride a bike.

   d. A 5-year-old prefers the company of children similar to his age and often plays with them.

2. From the following examples of changes that can occur in the human body, which one is an example of "growth"?

   a. Changes in the height and weight of a person

   b. Changes in the behavior of a person

   c. Changes in the way a person thinks

   d. Changes in the way a person interacts socially

3. Which one of the following is typical of adolescent behavior?

   a. An adolescent questions the moral teachings of his or her parents.

   b. An adolescent's spirituality and religious beliefs take root.

   c. An adolescent enjoys stable, supporting friendships.

   d. An adolescent assumes the role of caretaker.

Activity G *Think About It! Briefly answer the following question in the space provided.*

1. A 7-year-old does NOT prefer the company of older children, but is certainly as skilled when playing baseball with children older than his age. Write the reasons for such an occurrence in the space provided below.

   _____

   _____

   _____

2. Why is it important for a nursing assistant to become familiar with the various stages of growth and development of a person?

   _____

   _____

   _____

Activity H *The process of growth and development is divided into stages of normal progression. Some of the behaviors that a person exhibits as he or she progresses through the developmental milestones are listed below. Write down the correct order of the milestones as a person ages in the boxes provided below.*

1. Development of the muscular and nervous systems permits greater control of the bladder and bowels, so this is when toilet training begins.

2. Assumes the role of a caretaker and begins to show signs of aging, such as wrinkles or a few gray hairs.

3. Becomes aware of gender differences and roles and curiosity about the differences between boys and girls increases.

4. May suffer the loss of friendship or spouse due to death. Strength diminishes, as do many senses, such as hearing and sight.

5. Begins to recognize parents and siblings, begins to say simple words and laugh.

6. Becomes self conscious about his or her body and aware of his or her own sexuality. Secondary sex characteristics appear and the reproductive organs begin to function with the onset of puberty.

7. Becomes able to write and ability to draw improves, develops logical thinking patterns and learns to incorporate other people's perspectives into his or her own thinking.

8. Enjoys sharing wisdom with younger people.

9. Enjoys stable, supportive friendships and good health. Focuses on completing his or her education, starting a career, and, possibly, finding a partner and marrying.

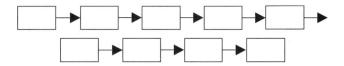

Activity I *Match the stages of growth and development, given in Column A, with their characteristics, given in Column B.*

Column A	Column B
___ 1. Infancy	a. A stage of gender identity
___ 2. Toddlerhood	b. A stage of active imagination
___ 3. Preschool	c. A stage of sharing wisdom but failing health
___ 4. School-age	d. A stage of toilet training
___ 5. Adolescence	e. A stage of assuming a caretaker's role
___ 6. Middle adulthood	f. A stage of rapid physical and psychological growth
___ 7. Older adulthood	g. A stage of questioning the moral teachings of an authority

As a person grows and ages, the physical and psychological changes that occur affect the type of care the person needs, and the way in which we communicate with him or her. Becoming familiar with the various stages of growth and development, and the tasks commonly associated with these stages, will help you to become a more able caregiver.

BASIC HUMAN NEEDS

Key Learning Points

- Maslow's hierarchy of basic human needs
- Ways that a nursing assistant helps patients and residents to meet their needs
- The difference between sex and sexuality
- How a person's sexuality can be affected by illness

Activity J *Maslow's pyramid identifies the hierarchy of human needs. Look at the following picture and write down the correct order of needs as described in Maslow's hierarchy. Also, list an example of a way that a nursing assistant may be able to help a patient or resident meet each level of these needs.*

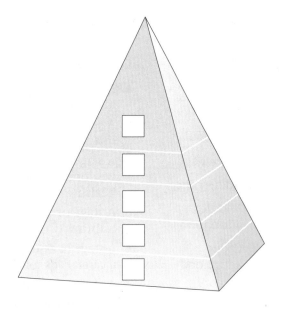

A. Self esteem needs _____

B. Physiological needs _____

C. Safety and security needs _____

D. Self actualization needs _____

E. Love and belonging needs _____

Activity K *Fill in the blanks by using the words given in brackets.*

[Bisexuals, Transsexuals, Heterosexuals, Transvestites, Homosexuals]

1. _____ are people attracted to members of the opposite sex.

2. _____ are people attracted to members of the same sex.

3. _____ are people attracted to members of both sexes.

4. _____ are people who believe that they should be members of the opposite sex.

5. _____ are people who get excited by dressing as a member of the opposite sex.

Activity L *Select the single best answer for each of the following questions.*

1. When a nursing assistant assists a patient or resident with toileting, which one of Maslow's needs does the nursing assistant help the person to meet?

   a. Love and belonging need

   b. Self esteem need

   c. Self actualization need

   d. Physiological need

2. Which one of the following actions helps to fulfill a patient's or resident's need for love and belonging?

   a. A gentle touch

   b. Tucking the patient or resident into bed at night

   c. Helping the patient or resident set realistic goals

   d. Assisting the patient or resident with basic grooming

3. Which of the following is not a physical need?

   a. Shelter

   b. Food

   c. Acceptance

   d. Air

4. Which one of the following is NOT a basic human need?

   a. Safety and security

   b. Self-esteem

   c. Self-actualization

   d. Fear

5. A resident in a long-term care facility shows the desire to have a sexual relationship with you. What would you do?

   a. Ignore the resident

   b. Complain to the nurse

   c. Giggle and tease the resident in a flirtatious manner

   d. Tell the resident kindly, yet firmly, that you are not going to do what he or she is asking you to do

6. Which of the following medical conditions could affect a person's sexuality?

   a. Mrs. Robinson has to undergo surgery for the removal of a cancerous breast.

   b. Mr. Smith's gangrenous right leg has to be amputated.

   c. Mrs. Ching is burnt from the face down to her chest.

   d. All of the above.

Activity M *Think About It! Briefly answer the following questions in the space provided.*

1. Mrs. Amico broke her hip when she fell while taking a load of laundry to the washing machine in her basement. She is returning home today. By achieving her goal of making a full recovery and coming home following her injury, Mrs. Amico has met her need for self-actualization. List the difficulties that Mrs. Amico has had to overcome in order to be able to return home and how each of those goals was met.

   _____

   _____

   _____

2. What would you do if you see that a person is masturbating in a public room?

   _____

   _____

   _____

Clearly, all patients and residents are not alike. The people you will care for will be in different growth and development stages, and as such, they will have different needs. The primary mission of a health care professional is to administer to the physical and emotional needs of those you care for.

CULTURE AND RELIGION

Key Learning Points

- The concept of diversity
- Why it is important for health care workers to recognize their patients' and residents' diversity

Activity N *Place a "C" next to the statements that are related to a person's culture, an "RE" next to the statements that are related to a person's religion, and an "RA" next to the statements that are related to a person's race.*

1. ____ A person of African descent has dark skin and curly, black hair.

2. ____ A Jewish person does not want to have his long beard shaved.

3. ____ An Asian person has great respect for his elders.

4. ____ A Middle Eastern woman is not allowed to be questioned or examined by a male health care provider unless her husband is present.

5. ____ An Asian person has almond-shaped eyes and straight black hair.

6. ____ A person from Panama believes that wearing strings on the wrist will relieve pain.

7. ____ A Catholic person does not want to eat meat on Fridays during Lent.

Activity O *Think About It! Briefly answer the following question in the space provided.*

Write a brief essay about the beliefs and values that you have because of your culture or religion.

_____

_____

_____

_____

_____

> Throughout your career, you may be lucky enough to care for people from many different cultural and religious backgrounds. You will most likely encounter situations, practices, and beliefs that no book could have prepared you for! Take time to listen to your patients or residents, and to learn from them. Exposure to cultures other than your own is enriching, both professionally and personally.

QUALITY OF LIFE

Key Learning Points

- The concept of quality of life
- How it would feel to be a patient or resident

Activity P *Think About It! Briefly answer the following question in the space provided.*

1. Mr. Pyne was treated for heart problems a few months ago. He continues to smoke heavily, despite his heart problems. He also won't eat anything but steak, and he rarely exercises. The first time that he was hospitalized for his heart problems, the health care team advised Mr. Pyne to stop smoking and to begin eating a heart-healthy diet and exercising, but he seems not to have taken that advice. Now Mr. Pyne is back in the hospital again. If you were a member of the health care team who cared for Mr. Pyne the first time, how would you feel toward him now?

_____

_____

_____

Activity Q *Think About It! Briefly answer the following question in the space provided.*

1. Mr. Simon is a resident at the health care facility where you work. He has severe arthritis, and his children live far away and rarely come to visit. He is very critical, and rarely has anything pleasant to say to you or to anyone else. Why might Mr. Simon be acting this way?

_____

_____

_____

_____

_____

> Each of your patients and residents must be allowed to make decisions concerning his or her quality of life. In order to provide holistic care for your patients or residents, you must respect their decisions related to maintaining their quality of life.

A PERSON'S FAMILY

Key Learning Points

- How family members may be affected by a person's illness or disability

Activity R *Think About It! Briefly answer the following questions in the space provided.*

1. Modern families can be made up of many different members. Describe the different types of members that make up three families that you know personally.

_____

_____

2. Illness, injury, or disability can have a significant impact on a person's family. List three particular areas that may affect a person's family.

_____

_____

_____

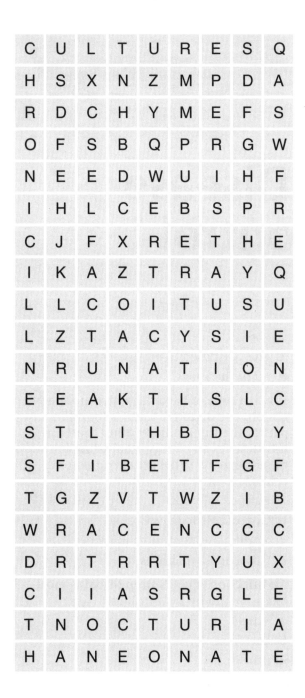

C	U	L	T	U	R	E	S	Q
H	S	X	N	Z	M	P	D	A
R	D	C	H	Y	M	E	F	S
O	F	S	B	Q	P	R	G	W
N	E	E	D	W	U	I	H	F
I	H	L	C	E	B	S	P	R
C	J	F	X	R	E	T	H	E
I	K	A	Z	T	R	A	Y	Q
L	L	C	O	I	T	U	S	U
L	Z	T	A	C	Y	S	I	E
N	R	U	N	A	T	I	O	N
E	E	A	K	T	L	S	L	C
S	T	L	I	H	B	D	O	Y
S	F	I	B	E	T	F	G	F
T	G	Z	V	T	W	Z	I	B
W	R	A	C	E	N	C	C	C
D	R	T	R	R	T	Y	U	X
C	I	I	A	S	R	G	L	E
T	N	O	C	T	U	R	I	A
H	A	N	E	O	N	A	T	E

SUMMARY

Activity S *Use the clues to find words that are present in the grid of letters, either horizontally from left to right or vertically from top to bottom.*

Down

1. An illness that is ongoing and often needs to be controlled through continuous medication or treatment
2. The highest level in Maslow's hierarchy of needs
3. The period during which the secondary sex characteristics appear and the reproductive organs begin to function
4. The most basic level in Maslow's hierarchy of needs such as oxygen, water, food, shelter, elimination, rest and sleep, physical activity, and sexuality and is essential for survival

Across

1. The beliefs (including religious or spiritual beliefs), values, and traditions that are customary to a group of people; a view of the world that is handed down from generation to generation
2. Something that is essential for a person's physical and mental health
3. Sexual intercourse
4. A general characterization that describes skin color, body stature, facial features, and hair texture
5. A newborn infant, 28 days or younger

Communicable Disease and Infection Control

COMMUNICABLE DISEASE

Key Learning Points

■ Definition of *communicable disease*

Activity A *Select the single best answer for the following question.*

1. What is a communicable disease?
   a. A disease that cannot be transmitted from one person to another
   b. A disease that can be transmitted from one person to another
   c. A physical injury like a burn or a cut
   d. A disease that results in an inability to communicate effectively

WHAT IS A MICROBE?

Key Learning Points

■ Types of "germs" (microbes) that cause diseases
■ The conditions that are essential for the survival and growth of microbes
■ Meaning of the terms *normal flora* and *pathogen*

Activity B *Select the single best answer for each of the following questions.*

1. Which one of the following is a microbe?
   a. The virus that causes chicken pox
   b. The bacterium that causes "strep throat"
   c. The yeast used to make beer
   d. All of the above

2. When a type of bacteria, which normally lives in the digestive tract, is found in any part of the human body other than the intestine it can change from being harmless to pathogenic. What are such microbes called?
   a. Escaped microbes
   b. Opportunistic microbes
   c. Normal (resident) flora microbes
   d. Nosocomial microbes

3. An infection such as strep throat is most likely caused by a:
   a. Virus
   b. Bacteria
   c. Parasite
   d. Fungus

4. What are the characteristics of the microbe known as *Staphylococcus aureus*?
   a. A rod-shaped bacterium that arranges itself in clusters
   b. A round bacterium that arranges itself in chains
   c. A round bacterium that arranges itself in clusters
   d. A rod-shaped bacterium that arranges itself in pairs

5. Which one of the following diseases is caused by a virus?

   a. Strep throat

   b. Rocky mountain spotted fever

   c. Common cold

   d. Malaria

Activity C *The diagram below shows the four major types of microbes (bacteria, viruses, fungi, and parasites). Fill in the blanks using the words given in brackets, according to what type of microbe causes the disease.*

[malaria, urinary tract infection, AIDS, Rocky Mountain spotted fever, strep throat, common cold, athlete's foot, lice, ringworm, hepatitis]

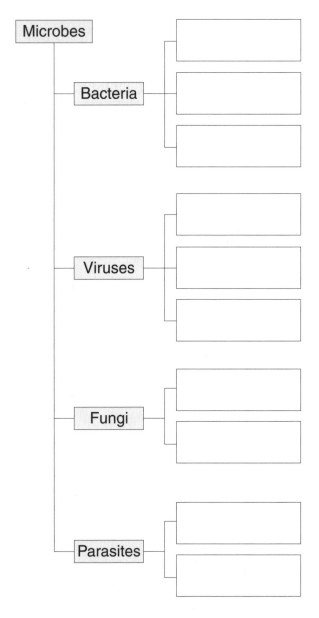

Activity D *Place an "F" next to the diseases that are caused by a fungi and a "P" next to the diseases that are caused by parasites.*

1. ___ Pinworms

2. ___ Thrush (a yeast infection in the mouth)

3. ___ Amebic dysentery

4. ___ Athlete's foot (tinea pedis)

5. ___ Pediculosis (lice)

6. ___ Candidiasis (a vaginal yeast infection)

7. ___ Ringworm (tinea corporis)

8. ___ Tape worms

Activity E *Match the terms related to microbes, given in Column A, with their descriptions given in Column B.*

Column A

___ 1. Normal flora

___ 2. Pathogen

___ 3. Opportunistic microbe

___ 4. Endospore

___ 5. Aerobic bacteria

___ 6. Anaerobic bacteria

Column B

a. Microbe that can change from harmless to pathogenic

b. Hard shell that makes it difficult to kill some types of bacteria using standard infection control methods

c. Bacteria that die if oxygen is present

d. Microbe that can cause illness

e. Harmless microbes that live on our skin and in our bodies

f. Bacteria that need oxygen to live

DEFENSES AGAINST COMMUNICABLE DISEASE

Key Learning Points

- Defense mechanisms used by the body to fight infection

Activity F *Select the single best answer for each of the following questions.*

1. What does the non-specific defense system do?

   a. It protects us only from viruses.

   b. It protects us only from certain pathogens.

   c. It protects us from all pathogens.

   d. It protects us only from bacterial infections.

2. Which one of the following is an example of a non-specific defense mechanism?

   a. Receiving a vaccination

   b. Taking an antibiotic

   c. Sneezing or coughing

   d. Producing antibodies

Activity G *Match the terms related to bodily defense mechanisms, given in Column A, with their descriptions, given in Column B.*

Column A

_____ 1. Immune system

_____ 2. Non-specific defense mechanism

_____ 3. Antibiotic

_____ 4. Antibodies

_____ 5. Methicillin-resistant *Staphylococcus aureus* (MRSA)

_____ 6. C.diff

Column B

a. A drug that is able to kill bacteria or make it difficult for them to reproduce and grow

b. Specialized proteins that help our bodies to fight off specific microbes

c. A defense system that protects us from infection

d. A type of Multi-drug-resistant organism

e. Skin that is without cuts, scrapes, or wounds

f. A major cause of healthcare-associated diarrhea

Activity H *Think About It! Briefly answer the following question in the space provided.*

1. If a pathogen manages to get past the first lines of defense of the human body, such as the skin and the mucous membranes, and an infection results, the body activates a general immune response that helps to fight off the infection. List and briefly describe signs that you may observe in a person who has an infection.

   _____

   _____

2. Why do most of us get the "childhood diseases" such as measles and chicken pox only once?

   _____

   _____

COMMUNICABLE DISEASE AND THE CHAIN OF INFECTION

Key Learning Points

■ The term *infection*

■ The chain of events required for infection to occur

Activity I *Select the single best answer for each of the following questions.*

1. Which one of the following could be a fomite?

   a. A patient's wound

   b. Linens that have just come back from the laundry

   c. A dirty spoon

   d. A mosquito

2. All of the following can be portals of entry for a pathogen EXCEPT:

   a. The mouth

   b. Non-intact skin

   c. The nose

   d. Intact skin

Activity J *There are six key elements in the chain of infection that are essential for an infection to spread. Complete the following diagram with the six key elements that must be present for an infection to spread. We have filled in one to get you started.*

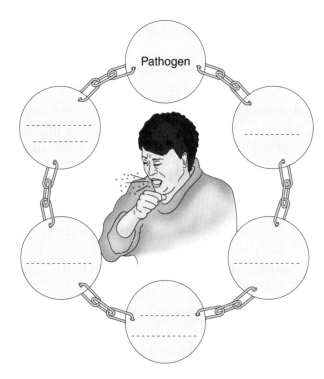

Pathogen

Activity K *The chain of infection can be broken by removing just one of the six elements that must be present for an infection to occur. Match each link in column A with the action in Column B that will remove it, breaking the chain of infection.*

Column A

____ **1.** Reservoir

____ **2.** Portal of exit

____ **3.** Method of transmission

____ **4.** Portal of entry

____

Column B

a. Covering an infected wound with a dressing

b. Washing your hands and making sure that linens, utensils, glassware, and other possible fomites are properly cleansed

c. Wearing gloves and keeping your skin healthy and intact

5. Susceptible host

d. Receiving required immunizations and maintaining general good health

e. Taking the right antibiotic for a bacterial infection

Activity L *Match the terms related to infection, given in Column A, with their definitions, given in Column B.*

Column A

____ **1.** Infection

____ **2.** Chain of infection

____ **3.** Fomite

____ **4.** Vector

____ **5.** Contagious disease

____ **6.** Indwelling medical devices

Column B

a. A living creature that transmits pathogens

b. A communicable disease that is easily transmitted from one person to the next through casual contact

c. Medical equipment that is inserted into a person's body; catheters, intravenous lines, and feeding tubes are examples

d. A non-living object that has been soiled by pathogens

e. The elements that must be present for a person to get an infection

f. Illness caused by a pathogen

Activity M *Think About It! Briefly answer the following question in the space provided.*

1. What factors make people more susceptible to getting infections in the health care setting?

_____

_____

Some of the people you will care for will be receiving health care because they have a serious communicable disease. Others may have a serious communicable disease and not even know it. In addition, many of the people you will care for will be more at risk for catching a communicable disease because they are not entirely healthy to begin with. Therefore, infection control is very important in the health care setting.

INFECTION CONTROL IN THE HEALTH CARE SETTING

Key Learning Points

- The term healthcare-associated infection (HAI)
- Ways a person could get an infection within the health care system
- Techniques of medical asepsis and infection control
- Methods used in the health care setting to destroy microbes
- How personal protective equipment (PPE) is used in infection control
- The standard precautions that are taken with every patient or resident
- How isolation (transmission-based) precautions are used to help prevent the spread of infection
- Proper hand washing, gloving, masking, gowning, and double-bagging techniques

Activity N *Place an "X" in front of those situations where it would be necessary to wear gloves:*

1. ____ When you are providing perineal care (cleaning the area between the legs)

2. ____ Before and after inserting contact lenses

3. ____ When picking an object up off the floor

4. ____ When you have a cut or abrasion on your hands

5. ____ When you are shaving a patient or resident

6. ____ Before obtaining clean linen from a linen cart

7. ____ When you are performing care on a patient or resident who has an open wound or a break in the skin

8. ____ When there is a possibility that you will come in contact with body fluids or substances

Activity O *Select the single best answer for each of the following questions.*

1. What is an infection that is gotten while in a hospital or other health care setting called?
   a. A viral infection
   b. A healthcare–associated infection (HAI)
   c. A bacterial infection
   d. A fungal infection

2. What type of chemical is safe to use on the skin to kill pathogens or keep them from growing?
   a. Disinfectant
   b. Antiseptic
   c. Sterilant
   d. Bleach

3. Which of the following procedures best destroys all bacteria?
   a. Sterilization
   b. Washing with bleach
   c. Soaking in alcohol
   d. All of the above

Activity P *Mark each statement as either "true" (T) or "false" (F). Correct the false statements.*

1. T F There are four major methods of infection control—medical asepsis, surgical asepsis, barrier methods, and isolation (transmission-based) precautions.

2. T F Medical asepsis involves removing or killing pathogens through the use of antibiotics.

3. T F Sanitization by using soap and water cleans your hands after you use the bathroom.

4. T F There are two main types of microbes found on a person's hands. They are normal flora and transient flora.

5. T F When caring for patients or residents, a nursing assistant should keep her fingernails short and unpolished.

6. T F Alcohol-based hand rubs can be used instead of soap and water to cleanse the hands.

7. T F Resident flora are easily removed from the hands by routine handwashing.

Activity Q *Think About It! Briefly answer the following question in the space provided.*

List the three new elements that have been added to existing standard precaution guidelines and give an example of steps the nursing assistant would take to follow them.

_____

_____

_____

Activity R *Place an "A" next to the situations where you would take airborne precautions, a "D" next to the situations where you would take droplet precautions, and a "C" next to the ones where you would take contact precautions. Also mention the precautionary measure you will take in each situation.*

1. ____ You are caring for a person who is suffering from whooping cough.

2. ____ You have to change the soiled linens of a person with a draining wound.

3. ____ You are caring for a person infected with measles.

4. ____ You are helping an incontinent person to change her clothes.

Activity S *Some of the steps in the procedure for removing more than one article of personal protective equipment (PPE) are listed below. Write down the correct order of the steps in the boxes provided below.*

1. Remove and dispose of your gloves.
2. Remove and dispose of your mask.
3. Remove your protective eyewear.
4. Untie the gown's waist ties.
5. Wash your hands.
6. Remove and dispose of your gown.

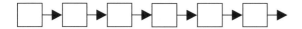

Activity T *Mark each statement as either "true" (T) or "false" (F). Correct the false statements.*

1. T F Medical asepsis involves chemically removing or killing pathogens.

2. T F Surgical asepsis is required when inserting an intravenous catheter.

3. T F Personal protective equipment (PPE) includes disposable gloves, masks, gowns and protective eyewear.

4. T F The single most important method of preventing the spread of infection is by using personal protective equipment (PPE).

5. T F When your hands are visibly soiled with dirt, blood, or other bodily fluids you should use an alcohol-based hand rub to disinfect your hands.

Activity U *Think About It! Briefly answer the following question in the space provided.*

You have just received your shift report and will be caring for Mrs. Wilson, who is recovering from a stroke. Her roommate, Miss Blair, is receiving intravenous antibiotic therapy for a foot infection caused by methicillin-resistant Staphylococcus aureus (MRSA). What types of precautions are necessary to prevent spreading the MRSA to Miss Blair or the other patients in the hospital? Briefly describe the infection control methods you would use in this situation.

_____

_____

_____

_____

_____

_____

_____

_____

_____

Activity V *The following picture shows four techniques that make up the practice of medical asepsis. Identify the four techniques used in the figures and label them. Also write down their definitions.*

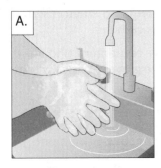
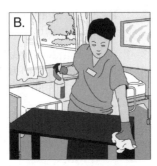
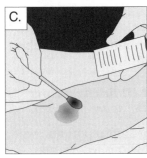
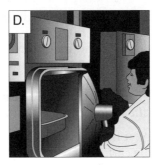

A. _____

B. _____

C. _____

D. _____

Activity W *Think About It! Briefly answer the following question in the space provided.*

1. Handwashing is the most important safeguard against spread of infection and is one of the OSHA standard precautions. List below four other standard precautions.

_____

_____

_____

_____

SUMMARY

Activity X *Words shown in the picture have been jumbled. Use the clues to form correct words using the letters given in the picture.*

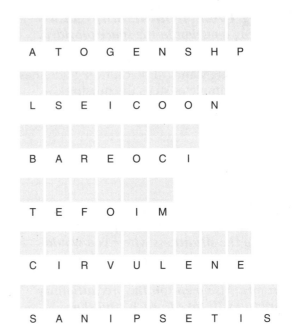

A T O G E N S H P

L S E I C O O N

B A R E O C I

T E F O I M

C I R V U L E N E

S A N I P S E T I S

1. Microbes that can cause illness
2. Groups of bacteria
3. An adjective used to describe bacteria that need oxygen in order to live
4. A non-living object that has been contaminated (soiled) by pathogens
5. The strength or disease-producing potential of a pathogen
6. Practices that kill microbes or stop them from growing; one of the techniques of medical asepsis

CHAPTER 8

Bloodborne and Airborne Pathogens

BLOODBORNE DISEASES

Key Learning Points

■ Types of bloodborne pathogens and the risks they pose to a health care worker
■ The OSHA standards for bloodborne pathogens
■ Body fluids that can contain bloodborne pathogens
■ Requirements for an exposure control plan

Activity A *Select the best answer for each of the following questions.*

1. All of the following fluids are considered to be body fluids EXCEPT:
   a. Blood
   b. Breast milk
   c. Sweat
   d. Water

2. A vaccination for all of the following types of hepatitis is available EXCEPT:
   a. Hepatitis A
   b. Hepatitis E
   c. Hepatitis D
   d. Hepatitis B

3. Which one of the following diseases is the health care worker at highest risk to catch on the job?
   a. HIV
   b. Tuberculosis
   c. Hepatitis B
   d. Hepatitis E

Activity B *Consider the ways by which bloodborne pathogens can be transmitted and list four of those ways in the space provided below.*

_____

_____

_____

Activity C *Place an "X" next to each of the following pathogens that are bloodborne.*

1. ____ Hepatitis A
2. ____ Hepatitis B
3. ____ Hepatitis C
4. ____ Hepatitis D
5. ____ Hepatitis E
6. ____ Tuberculosis
7. ____ HIV

Activity D *Place an "X" next to each of the following methods by which hepatitis B virus (HBV) can be transmitted.*

1. ____ Transfusion of infected blood
2. ____ Transfusion of infected blood products
3. ____ Across the placenta
4. ____ Through unprotected heterosexual intercourse
5. ____ Wound drainage

6. ___ Breast milk

7. ___ Needlestick injuries

8. ___ Oral–fecal route

Activity E *Match each term related to pathogens, given in Column A, with its description given in Column B.*

Column A

___ **1.** Bloodborne pathogen

___ **2.** Hepatitis

___ **3.** Oral–fecal route

___ **4.** HIV

Column B

a. The method by which hepatitis A is transmitted

b. The virus that causes AIDS

c. Inflammation of the liver

d. A disease-producing microbe that is transmitted through blood or body fluid

Activity F *Fill in the blanks using the words given in brackets.*

[1 thousand, T cell, goggles, 1 billion, gloves, an approved viricidal cleaning agent]

1. The main target of HIV is a type of cell called the _____.

2. The amount of hepatitis B virus particles per cc/mL of blood is _____.

3. The amount of HIV particles per cc/mL of blood is _____.

4. If the possibility exists that the hands could come in contact with blood or other body fluids, the type of PPE you should wear would be _____.

5. If the possibility exists that blood or other body fluids could splash or spray, the type of PPE you should wear would include _____.

6. Spills of blood or other body fluids should be cleaned up promptly with _____.

Activity G *The following figure shows the digestive system. Place an "X" next to the organ affected by the hepatitis B virus (HBV).*

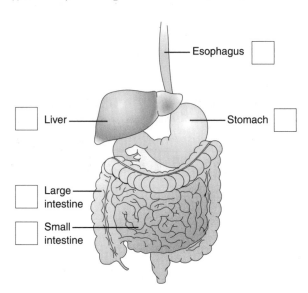

Esophagus

Liver

Stomach

Large intestine

Small intestine

Activity H *Place an "A" next to the pathogens that can be classified as airborne, and a "B" next to the pathogens that can be classified as bloodborne.*

1. ___ Hepatitis B virus

2. ___ Measles

3. ___ Hepatitis C virus

4. ___ Hepatitis D virus

5. ___ Chicken pox

6. ___ HIV

7. ___ Tuberculosis (TB)

Activity I *Think About It! What is wrong in the following series of pictures?*

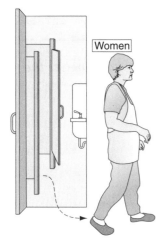

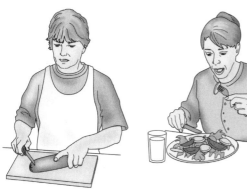

_____

_____

Activity J *Think About It! Briefly answer the following questions in the space provided.*

1. You are caring for Mr. Watson, who is HIV-positive. Mr. Watson has been hospitalized for a respiratory tract disorder. This morning, while you are helping Mr. Watson to brush his teeth, he coughs and soils your uniform and arms with bloody mucus. You are wearing gloves but not a gown or mask.

   a. Is it possible that you may have been exposed to an infectious disease?_____

   _____

   b. What is the first step you would take as dictated by the OSHA Bloodborne Pathogens Standard?_____

   _____

   c. What is the duty of your employer toward you in the current circumstance as dictated by the OSHA Bloodborne Pathogens Standard?_____

   _____

2. OSHA has created certain standards that all employers must follow, called the OSHA Bloodborne Pathogens Standard. These standards include: training on risks and methods to safeguard against the risks; vaccination against hepatitis B; provision of personal protective equipment; environmental control methods; and an exposure control plan. Choose one of these precautions and in the space below, explain what it is and why it is important.

   _____

   _____

   _____

   _____

> You will face exposure to many infections, some life-threatening, while caring for others. Learning about these infections and how they are transmitted, as well as staying well-informed about new developments and treatments for these diseases, will allow you to provide quality care to those you are responsible for.

AIRBORNE DISEASES

Key Learning Points

- The various methods used to protect against tuberculosis (TB) exposure
- Types of airborne pathogens and the risks they pose to the health care worker
- Engineering and work practice controls that help protect the nursing assistant (and others) from exposure to bloodborne and airborne diseases

Activity K *Think About It! Briefly answer the following question in the space provided.*

1. Describe how airborne pathogens are spread.

_____

_____

2. Over the past 20 years, the number of new cases of tuberculosis has increased. List three reasons that caused the increase.

_____

_____

3. A simple skin test is used to screen for exposure to tuberculosis. Describe the TB skin test.

_____

_____

4. Describe two precautions that you need to use for a resident or patient who is known or suspected to be infected with an airborne pathogen.

_____

_____

SUMMARY

Activity L *Look at the following series of pictures. Explain how a pathogen or a disease can be transmitted through each of them.*

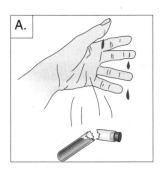

A.

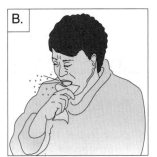

B.

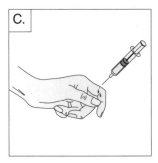

C.

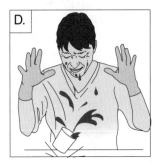

D.

A. _____

B. _____

C. _____

D. _____

Activity M *Use the clues to complete the crossword puzzle.*

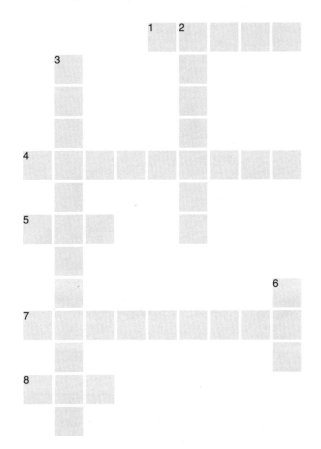

ACROSS

1. A leukocyte that is targeted by HIV
4. Inflammation of the liver
5. A bloodborne virus that can eventually lead to cirrhosis, liver failure, or liver cancer
7. Liquid or semi liquid substance produced by the body
8. The virus that causes AIDS

DOWN

2. A person who is infected with a virus but never develops symptoms of the disease
3. An airborne infection caused by a bacterium that usually infects the lungs
6. A bloodborne virus found in people who are also infected with hepatitis B virus

CHAPTER 9

Workplace Safety

PROTECTING YOUR BODY

Key Learning Points

- The definition of the term "ergonomics"
- Why people who work in a healthcare setting are at an increased risk for developing musculoskeletal disorders
- The definition of the term *body mechanics*
- Actions that make the body more effective when working
- Use of good body mechanics when lifting
- Ways to prevent back injury

Activity A *Select the single best answer for each of the following questions.*

1. As a nursing assistant, which of the following activities places physical stress on your body?
   a. Assisting a person out of bed
   b. Recording a person's temperature
   c. Showing a person how to use the call light control
   d. Arriving late at work

2. Which one of the following is one of the basic components of good body mechanics?
   a. Using the powerful muscles in your back to lift
   b. Using coordinated body movement
   c. Standing with your shoulders hunched
   d. Standing with your feet close together

3. When you are standing, which part of your body is the center of gravity?
   a. The torso
   b. The head
   c. The feet
   d. The thigh muscles

4. When lifting, remember to use the large muscles of your:
   a. Back
   b. Hips and thighs
   c. Shoulders
   d. Chest

5. What work-related injury are nursing assistants most at risk for?
   a. Communicable infection
   b. Back injury
   c. Electrical shock
   d. Falls

6. The most common causes of musculoskeletal disorders include all of the following except:
   a. Pinched nerves
   b. Emotional burn-out
   c. Ligament sprains
   d. Herniated spinal discs

7. The practice of designing equipment and work tasks to conform to the capability of the worker is known as:
   a. Standard precautions
   b. Body alignment
   c. Economics
   d. Ergonomics

Activity B *The figure shows a person who is holding her body in proper alignment. Draw an imaginary line that indicates the person is in good alignment.*

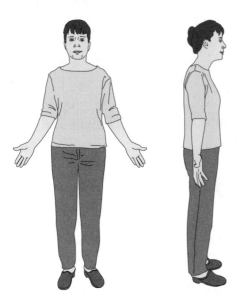

Activity C *Think About It! Briefly answer the following question in the space provided.*

You need to help Mr. Tompkins out of his wheelchair and into bed. List two ways you can stabilize your body and maximize your ability to remain balanced.

_____

_____

_____

Activity D *Look at the figure given below. Is this the correct way of moving a person up in bed? Which component of good body mechanics is involved here?*

_____

_____

_____

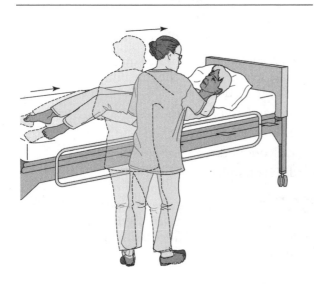

Activity E *Think About It! Briefly answer the following questions in the space provided.*

1. A weightlifter's lifting technique is an excellent example of good body mechanics being used. Describe briefly the maneuvers that the weightlifter uses to lift weights in excess of 500 pounds that allows the large, strong muscles of the body to do the work of lifting and also protect his back from injury.

_____

_____

_____

2. The figures below show examples of good lifting techniques. Write down what each figure represents.

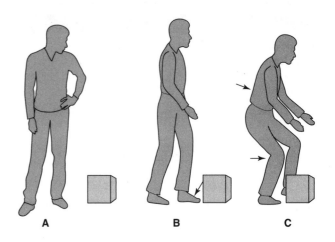

A   B   C

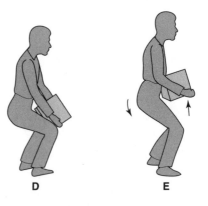

D   E

A. _____

B. _____

C. _____

D. _____

E. _____

Back injuries are painful and costly (in terms of medical care and missed work), and can be serious enough to end your career and prevent you from participating in other activities you enjoy. Practice good body mechanics and use proper lifting techniques to minimize your risk for physical injury.

FOLLOWING PROCEDURES

Key Learning Points

- The steps that are taken before and after every patient or resident care procedure

Activity F *Procedures, such as those that are followed when applying a restraint, are lists of routine steps or actions that are followed to ensure that the care you provide is safe and correct. Some actions, called "Pre-Procedure" or "Getting Ready" actions, are taken before performing any procedure on a patient or resident. Other actions, called "Post-Procedure" or "Finishing Up" actions, are taken after every patient or resident care procedure. Fill in the blanks using the words given in brackets, then place the "Getting Ready" and "Finishing Up" steps in the proper order by filling in the boxes below.*

1. **Getting Ready Actions**
   [gloves, wrist bands, photographs, drape, body mechanics, equipment use, infection control, lower, raise]

   a. Gather needed supplies.

   b. Provide privacy by closing the door and the curtain. _____ the person for modesty as appropriate.

   c. Knock on the door and identify yourself by name and title to the person.

   d. Identify the person, and greet him or her by name. Methods of identifying patients and residents will vary depending on where you work. Common methods of identifying people in health care facilities include _____ _____ and _____ .

   e. See to safety. Take safety precautions by following standards of _____ _____ , _____ , and _____ . In

procedures that involve getting a person out of bed, you will be instructed to _____ the bed to its lowest position. This is to decrease the distance between the bed and the floor, should the person fall. In procedures that involve providing care while the person remains in bed, you will be instructed to _____ the bed to a comfortable working height. This is to protect your back.

   f. Wash your hands. Apply _____ and follow standard precautions if contact with blood or body fluids is possible.

   g. Explain the procedure and encourage the person to participate as appropriate. Show any visitors where they may wait, if necessary, until you have completed the procedure.

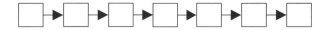

2. **Finishing Up Actions**
   [alignment, call light control, lowest, raise, wash, record]

   a. Confirm that the person is comfortable and in good body _____ .

   b. Wash your hands. If gloved, remove and discard the gloves following facility policy, and then _____ your hands.

   c. Open the curtain and door if desired by the patient or resident, and inform visitors that they may return to the room.

   d. Leave the _____ , telephone, and fresh water within easy reach of the person.

   e. Report and _____ actions as required by your facility.

   f. See to safety. Return the bed to the _____ position, lock the wheels, and _____ the side rails (if side rails are in use).

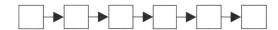

PREVENTING FALLS

Key Learning Points

- Hazards that increase the risk of falls in the health care setting
- How to assist a person who is falling

Activity G *Several factors in the workplace put the nursing assistant at risk for falling. Fill in the blanks using the words given in brackets.*

[help, surroundings, fluids]

1. Be aware of your _____ and move only as fast as you are safely able.

2. If you see _____ or other substances on the floor, immediately stop what you are doing and dry the area.

3. When helping a very weak, unsteady, or uncooperative person to walk or transfer from one place to another, ask for _____ from another nursing assistant or the nurse.

Activity H *Think About It! Briefly answer the following question in the space provided.*

You are helping Mrs. Bowman to walk down the hall. Mrs. Bowman is recovering from pneumonia, and she is very weak and unsteady on her feet. All of a sudden, Mrs. Bowman starts to fall! Describe the steps you should take to help minimize your risk of injury, as well as Mrs. Bowman's.

_____

_____

_____

PREVENTING CHEMICAL INJURIES

Key Learning Points

- Chemical hazards found in the health care setting

Activity I *One way of communicating information about chemicals present in the workplace to employees is through a Materials Safety Data Sheet (MSDS). Place an "X" next to the information provided by the MSDS.*

1. ____ What the chemical is made from

2. ____ What the chemical is used for

3. ____ Which exposures may be dangerous

4. ____ Which disease the chemical is used to treat

5. ____ Which type of bottle should be used to carry the chemical from one place to another

6. ____ What to do if an exposure occurs

7. ____ How to clean up spills

PREVENTING ELECTRICAL SHOCKS

Key Learning Points

- Electrical hazards found in the health care setting and ways to avoid them

Activity J *Knowing how to safely operate and maintain electrical equipment is necessary to prevent electrical shocks. Fill in the blanks using the words given in brackets.*

[frayed, grounded, power strip, loose, water]

1. Use _____ appliances, which have special three-prong plugs.

2. If more than two items must be plugged into an outlet, use a facility-approved _____.

3. If you notice anything unsafe about an appliance that is being used, such as _____ wires or _____ plugs, remove the appliance from use immediately.

4. Never operate electrical equipment around _____.

FIRE SAFETY

Key Learning Points

- The elements necessary for a fire to start and continue to burn
- The RACE fire response plan
- How to use a fire extinguisher

Activity K *The figure shows three elements that must be present for a fire to occur. Write the names of the three elements and list at least two sources of each alongside.*

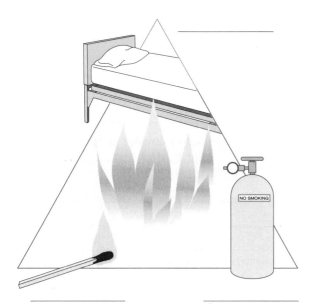

Activity L *Match the type of extinguisher, given in Column A, with the type of fire that it is used to extinguish, given in Column B.*

Column A

____ **1.** Type A

____ **2.** Type B

____ **3.** Type C

Column B

a. Fire that is fueled by a petroleum product (e.g., gasoline, automotive oil), cooking oil, or grease

b. An electrical fire

c. Fire that is fueled by ordinary material such as wood, paper, cloth, leaves, and grass

Activity M *Water is a readily available source. Write a "YES" against the type of fire that can be extinguished with water, and a "NO" next to the type of fire that should not be extinguished with water. If "NO," give the reason why not.*

1. ____ Fire that is fueled by ordinary material such as wood, paper, cloth, leaves, and grass _____

2. ____ Fire that is fueled by a petroleum product (e.g., gasoline, automotive oil), cooking oil, or grease _____

3. ____ An electrical fire _____

Activity N *Think About It! Briefly answer the following question in the space provided.*

Miss Wray has an "oxygen in use" sign posted outside of her room. Why is it especially important to follow safety precautions designed to prevent fires when you are in Miss Wray's room?

_____

_____

_____

Activity O *Look at the following pictures. Fill in the labels and write down the correct order of events, using the RACE sequence.*

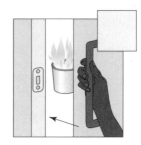

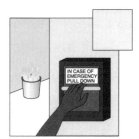

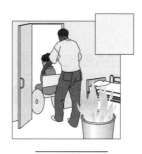

_____

_____ _____

_____

_____

_____

Activity P *A fire has started in a wastebasket at the nurses' station. Look at the following picture and write down the correct order of steps for using a fire extinguisher.*

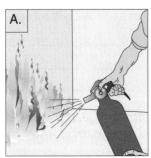

A.

Spray the contents at the base of the fire, using a sweeping motion.

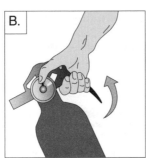

B.

Squeeze the handle.

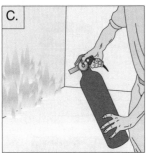

C.

Aim the hose toward the base of the fire.

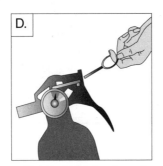

D.

Pull the safety pin out.

A. ☐ ☐ ☐ ☐
B. ☐ ☐ ☐ ☐
C. ☐ ☐ ☐ ☐
D. ☐ ☐ ☐ ☐

DISASTER PREPAREDNESS

Key Learning Points

- Disaster situations that may affect a health care facility
- The focus of a disaster preparedness plan in a hospital, versus in a long-term care facility

Activity Q *Think About It! Briefly answer the following question in the space provided.*

1. List five reasons a health care facility might have to enact a disaster preparedness plan.

   _____

   _____

   _____

   _____

   _____

2. Briefly describe how a disaster preparedness plan in a hospital might differ from one in a long-term care facility.

   _____

   _____

   _____

WORKPLACE VIOLENCE

Key Learning Points

- Factors that may lead to workplace violence in the health care setting

Activity R *Think About It! Briefly answer the following questions in the space provided.*

1. List two different sources that may cause a health care worker to become a victim of a violent act.

   _____

   _____

   _____

2. Describe a situation of workplace violence in a health care setting that you have heard of recently and discuss possible reasons why this situation occurred.

   _____

   _____

   _____

SUMMARY

Activity S *Words shown in the picture have been jumbled. Use the clues to form correct words using the letters given in the picture.*

1. The "A" in the ABCs of good body mechanics

2. Necessary for good body mechanics

3. Adjective used to describe electrical equipment that helps lower the risk of electrical shock by returning stray current to the outlet

4. An unexpected event that causes injury, major damage to property, or both

5. The practice of designing equipment and work tasks to conform to the capability of the worker.

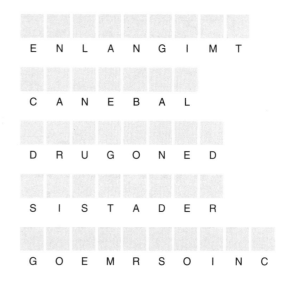

E N L A N G I M T

C A N E B A L

D R U G O N E D

S I S T A D E R

G O E M R S O I N C

CHAPTER 10

Patient Safety and Restraint Alternatives

ACCIDENTS

Key Learning Points

- The terms "accident" and "incident," and how each can threaten the safety of a person in a health care setting
- OBRA requirements related to accidents and incidents
- Risk factors that may put people in a health care facility at higher risk for accidents and injury
- Basic safety methods designed to prevent accidents and incidents in a health care facility
- The importance of reporting and recording accidents and incidents

Activity A *Each of the people described in Column A is at risk for an accident. Match each person in Column A with one of the risk factors given in Column B.*

Column A

____ **1.** Mr. Levine is being treated for extreme pain.

____ **2.** Miss Janey is 93 years old and is becoming more forgetful with every passing day.

____ **3.** Both of Mrs. Markus' knees are affected by very bad arthritis, which makes it painful for her to walk.

____ **4.** Joshua had an accident at work and is in a coma.

____ **5.** Mr. Thompson uses glasses, which he often forgets to wear.

____ **6.** Mrs. Orwell had a stroke and now has lost all sensation on the left side of her body.

Column B

a. Limited awareness of surroundings

b. Limited mobility

c. Medication

d. Sensory impairment

e. Paralysis

f. Age

Activity B *Think About It! Briefly answer the following question in the space provided.*

A major responsibility of a nursing assistant is to protect patients and residents from falling and injuring themselves seriously. List five situations that could cause a patient or resident to fall.

_____

_____

_____

Activity C *Select the single best answer for each of the following questions.*

1. Which of the following can cause confusion and disorientation?

a. Dementia

b. Head injury

c. Pain medication

d. All of the above

2. You regularly assist Mrs. Martin to the facility garden in her wheelchair. One evening, she has an accident because her wheelchair brakes would not lock. Which of the following actions would you take?

a. Avoid reporting the accident to the nurse because Mrs. Martin's injuries are minor and you can take care of them.

b. Report the accident immediately to the nurse and then fill out an incident (occurrence) report.

c. Report the accident to the doctor but not to the nurse.

d. Complete an incident (occurrence) report since the cause of the accident was equipment malfunction.

3. Which of the following precautions would you take to avoid accidental burns to a person while bathing him or her?

a. Always encourage a cold water bath

b. Measure the water temperature with a bath thermometer before bathing the patient or a resident

c. Allow the patient or resident to choose the temperature of the water to be used

d. There is no need to take any precautions because the water heaters in the facility pre-set the water temperature for bathing

Activity D *Think About It! Briefly answer the following question in the space provided.*

What is the difference between an "accident" and an "incident"? Give an example of each.

_____

_____

_____

Activity E *Mark each statement as either "true" (T) or "false" (F). Correct the false statements.*

1. T F   Only children are at risk for accidental food poisoning.

2. T F   Burns are the leading cause of accidental deaths amongst elderly people.

3. T F   Before assisting a person with a reduced sense of touch with bathing, always check the temperature of the water by placing your hand in it.

4. T F   An incident (occurrence) report is completed whenever an accident or incident occurs in a health care facility.

5. T F   Entrapment can occur if the mattress is too small for the bed frame.

Activity F *Match the terms representing different types of paralysis, given in Column A, with their descriptions given in Column B.*

Column A

____ 1. Paraplegia

____ 2. Quadriplegia

____ 3. Hemiplegia

Column B

a. Paralysis from the neck down

b. Paralysis on one side of the body

c. Paralysis from the waist down

Activity G *Sensory impairment can lead to serious accidents. Match the type of sensory impairment, given in Column A, with the accident it could cause in Column B.*

Column A

____ 1. Reduced sense of touch

____ 2. Poor vision

____ 3. Reduced sense of smell and taste

____ 4. Reduced sense of hearing

Column B

a. Mrs. Vincent took her medication more often than was written on the bottle

b. Mr. Watson did not hear his smoke alarm in time to escape from a fire in his home

c. Mrs. Vas, a resident with diabetes, suffered hot water burns

d. Mr. Simon had food poisoning from drinking spoiled milk

Activity H *Think About It! Briefly answer the following question in the space provided.*

Falls are the leading cause of accidental deaths in a health care setting. As a nursing assistant, you will take many measures to prevent your patients or residents from falling and injuring themselves. Briefly explain the rationale behind each of the following fall prevention guidelines.

a. Check the patient's or resident's clothing and shoes. _____

b. Check equipment used by the patient or resident, such as wheelchairs, canes, and walkers. _____

c. Keep the patient's or resident's bed as low as possible. _____

d. Remove clutter from pathways used for walking. _____

e. Report your observations to the nurse immediately. _____

f. Keep a disoriented patient or resident who could be at a high risk of falling close to the nurses' station. _____

> Safety is a basic human need. If we feel safe, we can relax and rest because we feel secure and comfortable. You will play a very important role in helping those you care for to feel safe.

RESTRAINTS

Key Learning Points

- Different types of restraints
- Methods used to reduce the need for restraints
- Safety concerns of restraint use
- The proper application of a vest restraint, a wrist or ankle restraint, and a lap or waist (belt) restraint

Activity 1 Select the single best answer for each of the following questions.

1. Which one of the following statements suggests the correct use of restraints?
   a. The restraint should be removed every 2 hours, for a total of 10 minutes.
   b. The restraint should be changed every day.
   c. If the patient or resident complains about the restraint, disregard the complaint because it is beyond the nursing assistant's scope of practice to remove a restraint.
   d. If the patient or resident complains about the restraint, disregard the complaint because the purpose of the restraint is to reduce the patient's or resident's risk for accidents.

2. Restraints are used for all of the following reasons EXCEPT:
   a. To provide postural support
   b. To protect the patient or a resident from harm
   c. To protect the staff from a combative patient or a resident
   d. For staff convenience

3. Which one of the following is your responsibility with regard to the use of restraints?
   a. To order a restraint for a patient or resident
   b. To provide care for the patient or a resident while he or she is in a restraint
   c. To administer a sedative to an agitated or combative patient or resident
   d. To order the removal of a restraint for a patient or resident, on the person's request

4. You are caring for Mrs. Miller, a resident at the long-term care facility where you work. Mrs. Miller suffers from dementia and is receiving intravenous antibiotic therapy. Because she cannot understand the purpose of the IV line, Mrs. Miller keeps trying to pull it out. You report your observations to the nurse. What might the doctor order to prevent Mrs. Miller from pulling out her IV line?
   a. A sensor alarm
   b. A mitt restraint
   c. A vest restraint
   d. A wanderer monitoring system

5. Each time you attend to a patient or a resident who is wearing a restraint, you should be alert to signs and symptoms related to the use of the restraint. Which of the following observations should you report to the nurse immediately?
   a. The restrained person is resting quietly
   b. The restrained person's arm is cool to the touch and pale or blue
   c. The restrained person asks for a drink of water
   d. The restrained person has visitors

Activity J *Write the name of the knot shown below and explain why this type of knot is used to secure a restraint.*

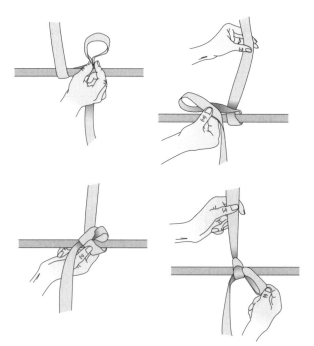

This knot is called a _____ knot. It is used to secure a restraint because _____

_____

_____

Activity K *Write the name of the restraint shown in each figure below.*

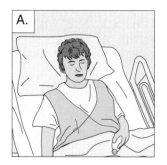

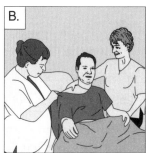

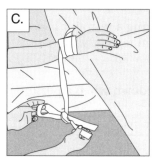

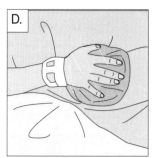

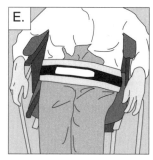

A. _____

B. _____

C. _____

D. _____

E. _____

Activity L *Think About It! Briefly answer the following questions in the space provided.*

What could happen if:

a. A vest restraint is put on backwards, with the back of the vest on the person's chest and the flaps crossed across her back?

_____

b. A restraint is put on too tight? _____

_____

c. A person is left in a restraint for a long time? _____

d. A person who is wearing a restraint is not taken to the bathroom regularly?

_____

e. The side rails are left down when a person is restrained in bed?

_____

Activity M *Think About It! Briefly answer the following question in the space provided.*

Restraints should only be used as a last resort. Briefly describe four things a nursing assistant can do to eliminate or reduce the need for restraints.

_____

_____

_____

_____

_____

Physically and emotionally, restraints have a very negative impact on a person's quality of life. The use of restraints requires extra care on the part of the nursing assistant to protect the patient's or resident's safety and dignity.

Positioning, Lifting, and Transferring Patients and Residents

POSITIONING PATIENTS AND RESIDENTS

Key Learning Points

- Complications of immobility
- Concept of proper body alignment
- Different body positions and the purpose of regular, frequent repositioning

Activity A *Place an "X" next to the reasons why a person might need to be repositioned.*

1. ____ The person may be recovering from a particular procedure.

2. ____ The person may be weak due to an illness or disease.

3. ____ The person may be completely or partially paralyzed.

4. ____ The person may be unconscious or in a coma

Activity B *A patient who is unable to reposition himself is at risk for developing serious complications involving several body systems. Name three of these body systems, and a complication likely to occur in each.*

BODY SYSTEM	COMPLICATION
A _____	A _____
B _____	B _____
C _____	C _____

Activity C *Select the single best answer for the following question.*

1. Mrs. Jones suffers from partial paralysis. You need to position her on the bed in proper body alignment. Which figure below shows the proper way to position Mrs. Jones? _____

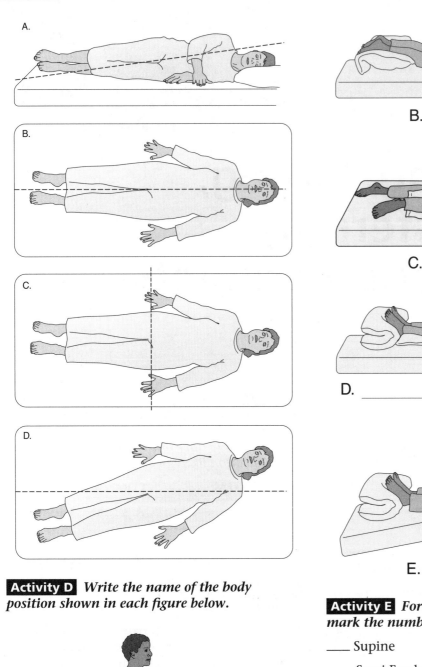

A.

B.

C.

D.

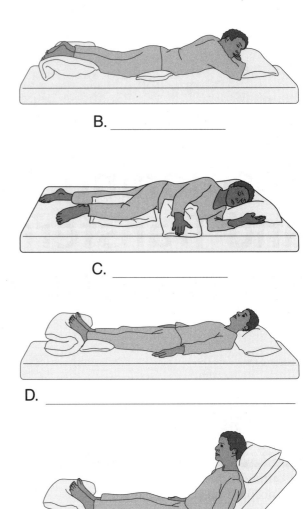

B. _____

C. _____

D. _____

E. _____

Activity D *Write the name of the body position shown in each figure below.*

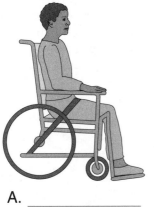

A. _____

Activity E *For each body position listed below, mark the number of its correct use next to it.*

___ Supine

___ Semi Fowler's

___ Sims'

___ Lateral

___ High Fowler's

1. Tube feeding

2. Sleeping

3. Relief from back pain

4. Grooming

5. Receiving enema

Activity F *List at least three items that can be used as a supporting device to ensure proper body alignment.*

a. _____

b. _____

c. _____

Activity G *Mark each statement as either "true" (T) or "false" (F). Correct the false statements.*

1. T F   Good body alignment is dependent upon proper body position.

2. T F   In proper body alignment, an imaginary line runs through the person's nose, breastbone, pubic bone, and between the person's knees and ankles.

3. T F   When a person's legs are spread apart, proper body alignment is attained if each leg is equidistant from the imaginary line.

4. T F   The imaginary line of proper body alignment could run diagonally through the body when a person lies on his side.

> ● Preventing the complications of immobility through frequent repositioning and transferring is a major responsibility of the nursing assistant!

TRANSFERRING PATIENTS AND RESIDENTS

Key Learning Points

- Safety measures related to lifting and transferring people
- Techniques of safe lifting and transfer

Activity H *Think About It! Briefly answer the following question in the space provided.*

A nursing assistant needs to help Mr. Burns transfer from his bed to a wheelchair. Write down four safety measures the nursing assistant should keep in mind when helping Mr. Burns to transfer.

_____

_____

_____

Activity I *Select the single best answer for the following question.*

1. Which of the following devices will you use to help transfer a person to or from a wheelchair safely?

   a. A transfer belt

   b. A walker

   c. Crutches

   d. A cane

Activity J *Some of the steps in the procedure for transferring a person from a bed to a wheelchair are listed below. Place the steps in the proper order by filling in the boxes below.*

1. Position the person's feet on the footrest of the wheelchair and buckle the wheelchair safety belt. Cover the person's lap with a lap blanket.
2. Help the person put on shoes and a robe, and then apply a transfer belt.
3. Lower the person into the wheelchair by bending your hips and knees.
4. Help the person to move toward the side of the bed, where the wheelchair is located.
5. Lock the wheelchair wheels and swing the footrest to the side.

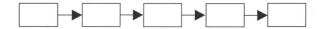

Activity K *Some of the steps in the procedure for transferring a person from a bed to a stretcher are listed below. Place the steps in the proper order by filling in the boxes below.*

1. Raise the level of the bed and lower the head of the bed.
2. Grasp the edge of the lift sheet and roll it over as close to the person's body as possible.
3. Position the lift sheet under the person's shoulders and hips.
4. Position the stretcher alongside the bed and lock the stretcher wheels.

5. Position the person on the stretcher, making sure that his or her body is in proper body alignment. Buckle the stretcher safety belts across the person and raise the side rails on the stretcher.

6. Ask your three co-workers to lift the person using the lift sheet in unison at the count of three.

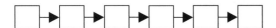

Activity L *Think About It! Briefly answer the following question in the space provided.*

A patient or resident sitting on the side of the bed is described as "dangling." This is the first step for someone who is getting up from bed to walk. Explain the importance of dangling.

_____

_____

_____

> Encouraging and assisting patients and residents to walk enhances their quality of life by providing both physical and emotional benefits.

SUMMARY

Activity M *Use the clues to complete the crossword puzzle.*

Across

2. One of the basic positions in which the person lies on his abdomen with his head turned to one side
5. A term used to describe the force created when two surfaces rub against each other

Down

1. A condition that occurs when a joint is held in the same position for too long
3. This can lead to skin breakdown
4. To move a person from one place to another

CHAPTER 12

Basic First Aid and Emergency Care

RESPONDING TO AN EMERGENCY

- The role of the nursing assistant in an emergency situation
- Terms used to describe a person's condition in an emergency situation

Activity A *Select the single best answer for the following question.*

1. Nursing assistants are encouraged to seek training in which of the following areas?

   a. Basic life support (BLS) techniques

   b. Cardiopulmonary resuscitation (CPR)

   c. First aid techniques

   d. All of the above

Activity B *Returning from work one day, you notice that your neighbor is lying in his yard next to a ladder and he's not moving! You rush over to assist him. Place the steps that you would take to help your neighbor in this emergency situation in the correct order by filling in the boxes below.*

1. You activate the emergency medical services (EMS) system

2. You gently touch your neighbor's shoulder and say, "Mr. Veracruz, are you OK?"

3. You recognize that an emergency exists

4. You provide appropriate care until the EMS personnel arrive

5. You decide to act

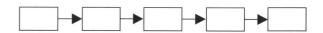

Activity C *Mark each statement as either "true" (T) or "false" (F). Correct the false statements.*

1. T F General training programs in basic emergency care are available and cover principles of first aid and basic life support (BLS).

2. T F Your familiarity with your patients or residents makes you less likely to notice signs and symptoms that could alert the health care team to the fact that an emergency situation is lurking.

3. T F When an emergency situation occurs, you should stay calm, organize your thoughts, and then act.

4. T F In case of an emergency, you should not speak to the patient or resident.

⬤ Your knowledge of your patient's or resident's usual condition, combined with keen observation skills, may allow you to recognize a potential emergency situation. By communicating what you have observed to the nurse, you may be able to prevent the emergency from occurring, or to minimize the effects if it does occur.

BASIC LIFE SUPPORT (BLS) MEASURES

Key Learning Points

- The steps of basic life support (BLS)
- Some of the organizations that offer approved training in first aid and basic life support (BLS) measures

Activity D *Select the single best answer for the following question.*

1. What is the goal of basic life support (BLS)?

   a. To prevent respiratory arrest

   b. To prevent cardiac arrest

   c. To keep a person who is in respiratory or cardiac arrest alive until help arrives

   d. All of the above

Activity E *Think About It! Briefly answer the following question in the space provided.*

The medical chart of a terminally ill patient contains a do not resuscitate (DNR) order. One morning, the patient goes into cardiac arrest. What should you do under these circumstances?

_____

_____

_____

_____

Activity F *Mark each statement as either "true" (T) or "false" (F). Correct the false statements.*

1. T F   An emergency is a condition that requires immediate medical or surgical evaluation or treatment in order to prevent the person from dying or having a permanent disability.

2. T F   A person who has no pulse or is not breathing is said to be clinically dead, a condition that is irreversible.

3. T F   Human beings can live for days without oxygen.

4. T F   Biological death is not reversible.

Activity G *Think About It! Which situation is most important to correct first—cardiac arrest or respiratory arrest? Explain your answer below.*

_____

_____

_____

_____

_____

_____

_____

_____

Activity H *One day, you are driving down the highway when you see the car in front of you swerve suddenly. The car crashes through the guard rail and rolls down a small hill on the side of the road, landing upside down. You immediately pull over to assist the driver. By the time you get to the scene, another motorist has pulled the unconscious driver out of the car and away from the wreckage. You use your training to provide basic life support to the driver. Look at the following images depicting the steps of BLS and place them in the correct order.*

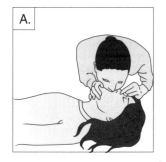

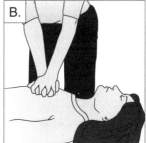

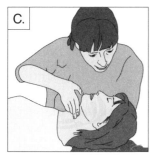

A. _____

B. _____

C. _____

EMERGENCY SITUATIONS

Key Learning Points

- The signs and symptoms of a "heart attack"
- The actions that you would take to assist a person with signs and symptoms of a "heart attack"
- The signs and symptoms of a stroke
- The actions that you would take to assist a person who complains of feeling faint or who has fainted
- The actions that you would take to assist a person who is having a seizure
- The actions that you would take to assist a person who is bleeding uncontrollably (hemorrhaging)
- Some of the types and causes of shock, and how you would assist a person who is in shock
- The actions that you would take to clear the airway of a choking adult or child older than 1 year by using abdominal or chest thrusts
- The method used to clear the airway of a choking infant

Activity I *Match the terms, given in Column A, with their descriptions, given in Column B.*

Column A

___ **1.** May be an early sign of a serious medical condition

___ **2.** Blood flow to the myocardium is blocked

___ **3.** Results when the organs and tissues of the body do not receive enough oxygen-rich blood

___ **4.** Caused by blocked blood flow to the brain

___ **5.** Occurs when electrical brain activity is interrupted

___ **6.** Can be caused by trauma to a blood vessel or by certain illnesses, such as gastric ulcers

Column B

a. Heart attack

b. Stroke

c. Fainting (syncope)

d. Seizures

e. Hemorrhage

f. Shock

Activity J *Place an "H" next to signs and symptoms of a heart attack and an "S" next to signs and symptoms of stroke.*

1. ___ Pain or tightness in the chest that might extend to the neck, back, or arm

2. ___ Muscle weakness or paralysis

3. ___ Disorientation or loss of consciousness

4. ___ Pale, gray or blue skin

5. ___ Excessive sweating

6. ___ Drooping of an eyelid or mouth

7. ___ Trouble breathing

8. ___ Nausea or heartburn-like pain

9. ___ Severe headache

Activity K *Think About It! Briefly answer the following questions in the spaces provided.*

You are a home health care aide. One day, you are at Mrs. Gillepsie's house and while you are cleaning the bathroom, she decides to go downstairs to her basement. You hear a loud crash and a scream and when you go to investigate, you find that Mrs. Gillepsie has fallen down the stairs and has a very deep wound on her leg, which is gushing blood.

1. How could you tell whether the client is bleeding from an artery or a vein?_____

_____

2. What should you do first to help the client? _____

_____

3. What should you do to control the blood loss until help arrives? _____

_____

Activity L *Mark each statement as either "true" (T) or "false" (F). Correct the false statements.*

1. T F During a heart attack, the muscular heart is not able to contract normally, which means that oxygen-rich blood is not circulated throughout the body efficiently.

2. T F If you observe that a person is having signs or symptoms of a heart attack, have the person lie down and elevate his legs 12 inches.

3. T F A stroke may cause only a mild physical change in a person.

4. T F If you believe that a person is about to faint, have the person lie down or sit down and bend forward.

5. T F A person who is having a grand mal seizure may show no signs other than appearing to be momentarily absent from the present situation.

6. T F Grand mal seizures cause a loss of consciousness and, because of the violent jerking of the muscles, place the person who is having the seizure at risk of injuring herself.

7. T F Anaphylactic shock is caused by severe bacterial infections that involve the entire body.

8. T F People who are not conscious are not at risk for aspiration.

Activity M *Use the clues to complete the crossword puzzle.*

Across

1. This condition occurs when the blood supply to the brain suddenly decreases
6. Caused by severe bacterial infections that involve the entire body

Down

2. A condition that requires immediate medical or surgical evaluation
3. A condition that is caused by trauma to a blood vessel or by certain illnesses, such as gastric ulcers
4. Points where the large arteries run close enough to the surface of the skin to be felt as a pulse
5. Caused by a severe allergic reaction (for example, to medications, bee stings, or certain foods, such as nuts)

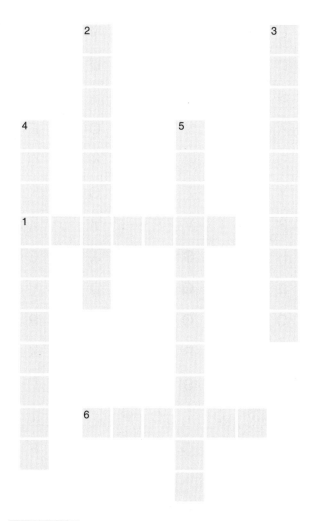

Activity N *Identify what is wrong with the following picture.*

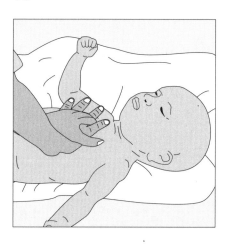

_____

_____

_____

Activity O *Think About It! Briefly answer the following question in the space provided.*

It is lunch time at Longwood Meadows, the long-term care facility where you work. The residents are eating and talking, when suddenly, Mrs. Lowell, one of the residents, starts to choke and can't seem to get her breath. In the space provided, describe how you would perform abdominal thrusts to clear Mrs. Lowell's airway.

_____

_____

_____

Activity P *Place an "X" next to the scenarios that place people at increased risk for choking and aspiration.*

1. ___ Poorly fitting dentures

2. ___ Missing teeth

3. ___ Young age

4. ___ Unconscious state or weak coughing or swallowing reflexes

5. ___ Impaired gag reflex

THE CHAIN OF SURVIVAL

Key Learning Points

■ The steps of the chain of survival

Activity Q *Some of the steps in the chain of survival are listed below. Place the steps in the correct order by filling in the boxes below.*

1. Medical intervention, such as that provided by a paramedic, a nurse, or a doctor, must be provided as soon as possible.

2. First responder care (basic first aid, including BLS if applicable) must be given by able people at the scene of the emergency.

3. Someone must recognize that an emergency situation exists, and activate the emergency medical services (EMS) system.

4. Rehabilitation, a step that focuses on improving the general health status of the person, must occur.

5. After the immediate crisis passes, hospital care might be required to help the person survive.

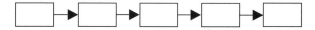

SUMMARY

Activity R *Use the clues to find words that are present in the grid of letters, either horizontally from left to right or vertically from top to bottom.*

Down

1. A person who is unconscious and cannot be aroused, or conscious but not responsive when spoken to or touched
2. A state of confusion
3. The accidental inhalation of foreign material into the airway

Across

1. A condition that requires immediate treatment to prevent the person from dying or having a permanent disability
2. Fainting
3. The condition that results when the organs and tissues of the body do not receive enough oxygen-rich blood

E	M	E	R	G	E	N	C	Y
D	E	D	O	G	I	D	I	O
S	U	I	K	J	F	S	R	O
A	N	S	Y	N	C	O	P	E
D	R	O	J	A	H	K	P	G
Y	E	R	F	S	H	O	C	K
S	S	I	V	P	U	W	D	X
H	P	E	S	I	H	J	T	C
E	O	N	Q	R	M	D	X	V
O	N	T	O	A	P	C	M	P
Y	S	E	R	T	F	U	S	K
W	I	D	S	I	B	T	N	L
G	V	O	T	O	R	J	S	T
C	E	S	O	N	X	J	E	P

CHAPTER 13

The Patient or Resident Environment

THE PATIENT OR RESIDENT UNIT

Key Learning Points

- The types of rooms and areas that are commonly found in different health care settings

Activity A *Select the single best answer for each of the following questions.*

1. Which of the following factors might determine the setup of a patient's or a resident's unit?

    a. Mr. Wilson has tuberculosis

    b. Mrs. Wilhelm is in labor

    c. Mrs. Pierson, who had a stroke, is not well enough to go home but not quite sick enough to be in a hospital

    d. All of the above

2. Which one of the following rooms in a hospital has special equipment to monitor and care for a patient who is critically ill?

    a. A single occupancy room

    b. A double occupancy room

    c. An intensive care unit

    d. A sub-acute care unit

3. Which of the following work areas commonly found in a healthcare facility often has a hopper where bed pans can be emptied and cleaned?

    a. The clean utility room

    b. The nurses' station

    c. The staff restroom

    d. The soiled utility room

Activity B *Think About It! Briefly answer the following question in the space provided.*

The pictures below show units of two different facilities. Identify the type of unit shown in each picture, and write a few sentences about how rooms in these two types of facilities are similar, and how they are different.

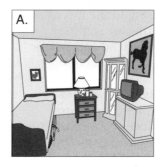 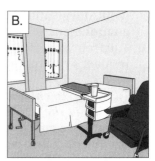

_____ _____

_____

_____

_____

Activity C *Match the health care facilities, given in Column A, with the patient or resident need, given in Column B.*

Column A

___ **1.** Long-term care facility

___ **2.** Assisted living facility

___ **3.** Sub-acute care unit

___ **4.** Home health care

Column B

a. Mr. Watson is somewhat independent but needs help taking his medications and getting groceries.

b. Mary is not quite well enough to go home, but not quite sick enough to be in a typical hospital room.

c. Mr. Johnson receives health care services in his apartment.

d. Mrs. Tang is not able to care for herself independently.

ENSURING COMFORT

Key Learning Points

- The Omnibus Budget Reconciliation Act (OBRA) regulations relating to the physical environment in long-term care facilities
- Your role in helping to keep the patient's or resident's environment clean and comfortable

Activity D *To enhance the comfort and well-being of the residents, long-term care facilities have policies designed to regulate the environment. These policies are set by Omnibus Budget Reconciliation Act (OBRA) regulations. Look at the pictures below and identify which of the following aspects of the resident's environment are specified by the OBRA regulations, by placing an "X" in the boxes.*

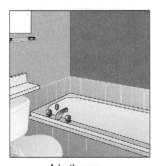

A bathroom without a handrail

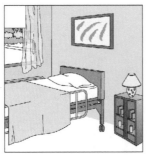

A room that is clean and comfortable

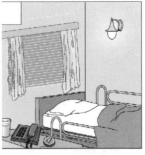

A room with very bright lighting

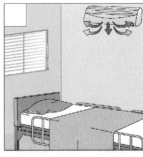

A room with a well-functioning ventilation system

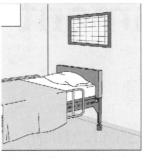

A room with noise-absorbing tiles and carpeting

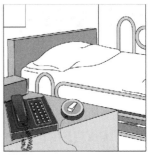

A room with a call light system

Activity E *Nursing assistants perform many tasks to help ensure cleanliness and a good quality of life for the people they care for. Mark each statement as either "true" (T) or "false" (F). Correct the false statements.*

1. T F Each member of the health care team is responsible for keeping the facility clean.

2. T F A nursing assistant does major, routine cleaning of the facility.

3. T F The housekeeping or custodial staff is responsible for changing the bed linens according to facility policy.

4. T F A nursing assistant helps to keep the personal belongings of the patient or resident neat and clean.

5. T F If you notice something spilled on the floor or a countertop, you should call for the housekeeping staff immediately.

6. T F If you see a stray piece of trash, you should pick it up and dispose of it properly.

7. T F If you notice that there is an ongoing problem, such as wastebaskets not being emptied or bathrooms not being cleaned properly, you should report this observation to the housekeeping department, so that they can follow up with the appropriate people.

Activity F *Think About It! Briefly answer the following questions in the space provided.*

1. You are caring for Mrs. Mariwell, who has asthma. After smoking a cigarette on your break, you enter Mrs. Mariwell's room to assist her with lunch. The odor from smoking clings to your hands and your breath smells like smoke. Not only does Mrs. Mariwell find the odor offensive, she is also having difficulty breathing and she asks you to find someone else to help her. What should you have done before entering the room?

   _____

   _____

   _____

2. As a nursing assistant, what would you do to control odor and maintain a pleasant environment in the given situations?

   a. A resident is sick with the stomach "flu" and vomits frequently

   _____

   b. A resident is incontinent of urine

   _____

   c. A resident has used the bedpan to have a bowel movement and is embarrassed by the odor

   _____

   d. A resident who is incontinent of feces must wear disposable briefs

   _____

Activity G *Look at the pictures and fill in the blanks.*

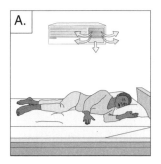 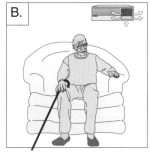

1. These patients may be feeling _____. They may require an extra blanket or a _____.

2. The bed and the chair are positioned poorly because they are in a _____ area.

3. Avoid placing furniture and wheelchairs right underneath a circulation _____.

Activity H *Select the single best answer for each of the following questions.*

1. You are working in a long-term health care facility. While moving around, you feel warm but your patient or resident is quite comfortable. What would you do under these circumstances?

   a. Switch on a fan

   b. Increase the air flow by turning up the air conditioning

   c. Open a window

   d. Plan for the warmer temperatures and dress accordingly

2. Which one of the following will help decrease unnecessary noise in a hospital or a health care facility?

   a. Answering the phones promptly

   b. Reporting noisy equipment that needs to be oiled

   c. Being aware of the volume of your own voice

   d. All of the above

3. Which one of the following types of lighting helps to prevent eye strain while reading?

   a. Task lighting

   b. General lighting

   c. Sunlight

   d. A night light

> Many people judge a facility according to its level of cleanliness. In addition, a clean environment is essential for odor and infection control.

FURNITURE AND EQUIPMENT

Key Learning Points

■ The standard equipment and furniture found in a person's room in a health care facility

Activity I *On the line next to its description, write the name of each piece of furniture or object shown below that is typically found in a patient or resident unit.*

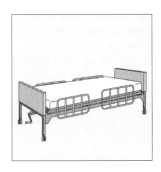
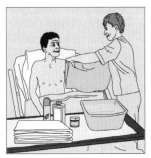

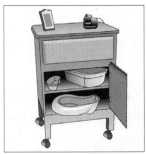
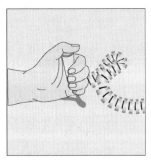

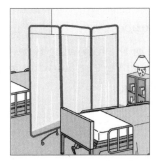

1. _____ Has unique features such as wheels, side rails, and controls for adjusting bed height and the position of the mattress

2. _____ Fits over a bed or chair and is used as a work surface

3. _____ Storage unit for personal care items and equipment

4. _____ Used to communicate with the health care staff

5. _____ Used to protect the patient's or resident's modesty when providing care

Activity J *Think About It! Briefly answer the following question in the space provided.*

Adjustable beds have several features that regular beds do not have: controls for adjusting the height of the bed and the position of the mattress, wheels, and side rails. Explain the purpose of each of these special features. Also explain when to lock the wheels on the bed, and why it is important to remember to do this.

_____

_____

_____

Activity K *Think About It! Look at the picture below and find the items that are inappropriately placed according to OBRA regulations. Briefly record your observations in the space provided.*

_____

_____

_____

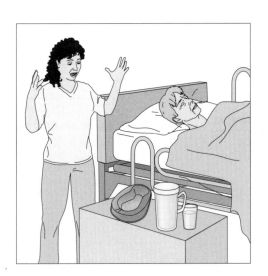

Activity L *Fill in the blanks using the words given in brackets.*

[Fowler's position, Trendelenburg's position, reverse Trendelenburg's position]

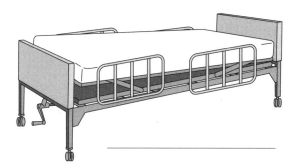

_____

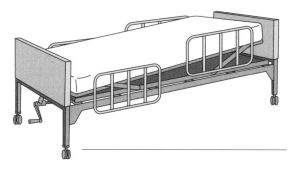

_____

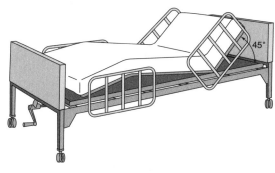

_____

Activity M *Many of the beds used in health care settings have controls for adjusting the bed height and the position of the mattress. These controls can be electric or manual. Look at the pictures below and identify what each control does.*

A. Electric controls

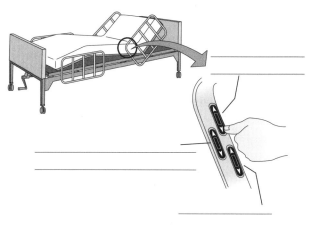

_____

_____

_____

_____

B. Manual controls

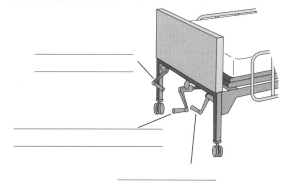

_____

_____

_____

_____

PERSONAL ITEMS

Key Learning Points

■ The importance of allowing a person to have and display personal items

Activity N *Think About It! Briefly answer the following question in the space provided.*

Mr. Albright is a brand-new resident at the long-term care facility where you work. He has brought along with him a few personal belongings, two reclining chairs, and an accompanying table. Mr. James, who shares the room with Mr. Albright, complains that Mr. Albright's items are cluttering up the room. Briefly write what you would do in this situation.

_____

_____

_____

_____

_____

_____

_____

_____

SUMMARY

Activity O *Use the clues to complete the crossword puzzle.*

Across

2. A patient's or resident's room
3. Lighting that supplies overall illumination
4. Bright light directed toward a specific area

Down

1. Necessary to provide fresh air and keep the air in the room circulating
3. Joints that allow the mattress to "break" so that the person's head can be elevated or his knees bent

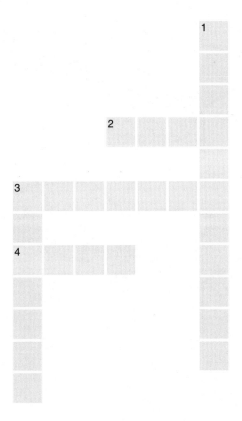

CHAPTER 14

Admissions, Transfers, and Discharges

ADMISSIONS

Key Learning Points

- Why admission to a health care facility may be emotionally difficult for a person and his or her family members
- How the nursing assistant can help to make a person's admission into a health care facility a more pleasant experience
- The duties of the nursing assistant during the admission process

Activity A *Think About It! Briefly answer the following question in the space provided.*

Explain some of the reasons why admission to a health care facility might be traumatic for a patient or resident.

_____

_____

_____

Activity B *Place an "X" next to the measures that will help ease the patient's or resident's emotional difficulties during the admission process.*

1. ___ Include the person's family members in the admissions process

2. ___ Ask the person about his or her personal preferences

3. ___ Rush the person through the admissions process

4. ___ Refer to the person by room number and medical problem

5. ___ Introduce yourself to the person

6. ___ Do not interact with the person

7. ___ Treat the person as if he were a guest in the facility

Activity C *A nursing assistant plays an important role in ensuring that the admissions process is as pleasant and orderly as possible. Mark each statement as either "true" (T) or "false" (F). Correct the false statements.*

1. T F A nursing assistant should prepare the patient's or resident's room only after his or her arrival.

2. T F It is important to give the patient or resident a "tour" of the room.

3. T F Helping the patient or resident unpack is considered to be inappropriate.

4. T F The resident inventory sheet must be completed by the resident.

5. T F While helping the patient or resident settle into the facility, you must not strike up a conversation with him or her.

Activity D *Place an "X" next to the items that a typical admissions pack would contain.*

1. ___ A basin

2. ___ A water pitcher

3. ___ Magazines

4. ___ A drinking cup

5. ___ A walkman

6. ___ Cookies

7. ___ A whistle

8. ___ A package of tissues

9. ___ An alarm clock

10. ___ Assorted personal care items (such as toothpaste, soap, and shampoo)

Activity E *Select the single best answer for the following question.*

1. What is the resident inventory sheet used for?

   a. To record standard information about the person, such as her name, address, date of birth and age, Social Security number, and gender

   b. To list and briefly describe the person's personal belongings

   c. To identify the person

   d. To gather information about the person's preferences, abilities, disabilities, and habits

> Becoming a patient or resident can be very traumatic for a person. Therefore, the person's physical and emotional needs must always remain the focus of the admissions process.

TRANSFERS

Key Learning Points

- Some of the reasons a person in a health care facility might need to be moved to another room or to another facility
- A nursing assistant's duties when assisting with the transfer of a patient or resident

Activity F *Fill in the blanks using the words given in brackets.*

[room, unit, health care facility]

1. A transfer occurs when a patient or resident is moved from one _____ to another, from one _____ to another, or from one _____ to another.

Activity G *Think About It!* *Briefly answer the following question in the space provided.*

List three reasons why a patient or resident may be transferred.

_____

_____

_____

Activity H *Place an "X" next to the duties of a nursing assistant during a patient's or a resident's transfer.*

1. ___ Gathering and packing the person's belongings

2. ___ Arranging for an ambulance, car, or taxi

3. ___ Assisting the nurse in transporting the person to the new room or unit, or to the ambulance, car, or taxi

4. ___ Informing the receiving nurse about the person's medical condition, medications, and other treatments

5. ___ Offering to transfer along with the person to the new facility

6. ___ Reporting information about the person's preferences and habits to the receiving nursing assistant

DISCHARGES

Key Learning Points

- The purpose of discharge planning
- A nursing assistant's duties during the discharge process

Activity I *Select the single best answer for the following question.*

1. What does AMA stand for?
   a. Against Medical Assistance
   b. Against Medical Advice
   c. After Medical Approval
   d. After Medical Allocation

Activity J *Mark each statement as either "true" (T) or "false" (F). Correct the false statements.*

1. T F Preparations for a patient's or resident's discharge begin as soon as he or she is admitted to the health care facility.

2. T F Discharge planning makes sure that a patient or resident continues to receive quality care after leaving the health care facility.

3. T F The purpose of discharge planning is to evaluate the amount of money that the person will owe after he or she is discharged.

Activity K *Place an "X" next to the duties of a nursing assistant regarding a patient's or resident's discharge from a health care facility.*

1. ____ Making sure that the person and his family members have been taught how to monitor and care for the person's condition

2. ____ Helping the person gather and pack his belongings

3. ____ Helping the person say goodbye to friends and caretakers

4. ____ Finding out the estimated time of discharge so that you can help the person get ready to leave on time

5. ____ Asking the person to evaluate the quality of your services during his or her stay in the health care facility

6. ____ Assisting the person out of the facility

SUMMARY

Activity L *Use the clues to complete the crossword puzzle.*

Across

3. Official entry of a person into a health care setting
4. When a person leaves a health care facility without a doctor's order

Down

1. To move a patient or resident within or between health care settings
2. The official release of a patient or a resident from a health care facility to his or her home

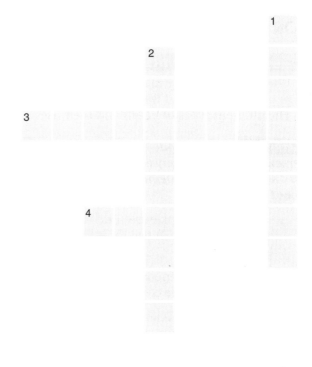

Bedmaking

LINENS AND OTHER SUPPLIES FOR BEDMAKING

Key Learning Points

- Ways that a properly made bed can increase a person's comfort and well being
- The different types of linens and their uses

Activity A *A well-made bed is essential to a person's mental and physical well-being. Place an "X" next to the statements that are true about bedmaking.*

1. ____ Clean, dry, wrinkle-free linens help make a person who is ill feel cared for and more comfortable.

2. ____ Clean woolen linens help to make a person feel more comfortable and homey.

3. ____ Clean, dry, wrinkle-free linens help to prevent complications, such as pressure ulcers, for people who are bedridden or seldom get out of bed.

4. ____ Clean linens made of silk help to make a person feel wanted and give a "rich" feeling.

5. ____ Damp linens help to keep a person's skin moist, preventing skin breakdown, especially during the summer.

6. ____ Clean, dry linens are important for odor and infection control.

Activity B *Fill in the blanks.*

1. A _____ is a thick layer of padding that is placed on the mattress to help make the bed more comfortable for the patient or resident, and to protect the mattress from moisture and soiling.

2. A bed is made with two sheets, a _____ sheet and a _____ sheet.

3. A _____ sheet is a small, flat sheet that is placed over the middle of the bottom sheet, covering the area of the bed from above the person's shoulders to below his or her buttocks.

4. A _____ sheet is simply a draw sheet that is used to help lift or reposition a person who needs assistance with moving in bed.

5. A _____ is a square of quilted absorbent fabric backed with waterproof material that measures approximately 3 feet by 3 feet, to be used for people who are incontinent.

6. _____ provided by a facility are usually woven cotton and should be available as requested by a person for his or her comfort.

7. A _____ adds the finishing touch to a well-made bed and can add a decorative touch to a person's room.

8. _____ are used for comfort and to aid in positioning. They are available in many sizes and made from a variety of materials. They are always covered with clean _____.

9. A _____ _____ is a lightweight cotton blanket or flannel sheet that is used to provide modesty and warmth during a bed bath or a linen change.

Activity C *Select the single best answer for each of the following questions.*

1. Why is it necessary to place a mattress pad between the bottom sheet and a rubberized mattress?
   a. To help provide warmth
   b. To help the person get out of bed without difficulty
   c. To help pull moisture away from the person's skin
   d. To help in positioning a person with a draining wound

2. The top sheet used to make a patient's or resident's bed should be:
   a. Fixed
   b. Flat
   c. Fitted
   d. Folded in half

3. An incontinent resident's bed is to be prepared. The nursing assistant uses a rubberized draw sheet in place of a rubberized mattress. What should she place over the plastic draw sheet to protect the person's skin from contact with the rubber?
   a. A bottom sheet
   b. A moisture-absorbent mattress pad
   c. A cotton draw sheet
   d. A flat sheet

4. How can you provide more efficient and economical care to a patient with a draining wound?
   a. By placing a rubberized sheet next to the person's skin
   b. By using a bed protector
   c. By avoiding the use of rubberized or plastic mattresses, which are expensive
   d. By adding extra blankets

5. Which linen might a resident bring from home and use?
   a. A top sheet
   b. A mattress pad
   c. A fitted sheet
   d. A bedspread

6. Which of the following linens is not made into the bed?
   a. A bed blanket
   b. A draw sheet
   c. A bath blanket
   d. A fitted mattress pad with elasticized sides

7. What is a pressure-relieving mattress used for?
   a. To help people maintain normal blood pressure
   b. To stabilize people with low blood pressure
   c. To help prevent skin breakdown in people who must stay in bed for long periods of time
   d. To help incontinent people by absorbing body fluids

8. What is a bed board?
   a. The wooden board that is used to make the bed frame in most health care settings
   b. A fixture that helps a person to climb in or out of the bed
   c. A clipboard that is kept next to a person's bed displaying his medical record
   d. A piece of wood placed under the mattress that keeps the mattress from sagging, helping to keep the body properly aligned

Activity D *Identify the equipment shown in the pictures that may be used depending on the specific needs of the patient or resident.*

1. This is often used for people who are recovering from burns or for people who are at risk for developing pressure ulcers on their feet. It has a metal frame.

_____

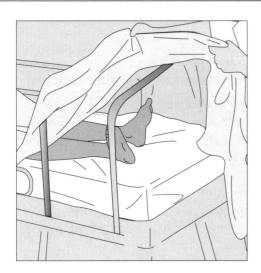

2. This is a padded board that is placed upright at the foot of the bed. The person's feet rest flat against the footboard, helping to keep the feet in proper alignment.

_____

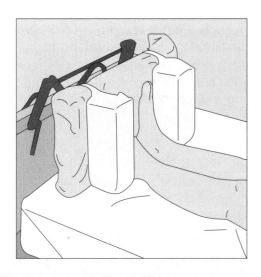

> A well-made bed is essential to a person's mental and physical well-being. In addition, a neat, well-made bed is a sign to visitors that the facility provides capable, competent care to its patients or residents.

HANDLING OF LINENS

Key Learning Points

- The proper way to handle and care for linens
- The infection control measures that are used during bedmaking

Activity E *Randall is on his way to make up Mr. Walker's bed. What is wrong with this picture?* _____

_____

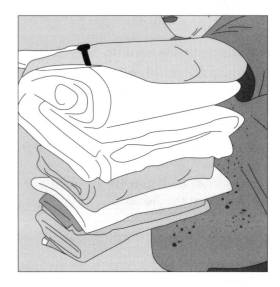

Activity F *Match the guidelines for bedmaking given in Column A with the reasons for their use given in Column B.*

Column A

____ 1. Washing your hands before collecting clean linens

____ 2. Collecting only those linens that you will need for that person's bed

____ 3. Collecting linens in the order that they will be used

Column B

a. Saves money and manpower

b. Helps you to remember which linens you need to collect and allows you to make the bed more efficiently

c. Prevents microbes from being transferred to the clean linens

_____ **4.** Wearing gloves when removing used linens from a bed

    d. Helps to control the spread of infection from dirty linens

_____ **5.** Placing dirty linens in the linen hamper immediately after removing them from the bed

    e. Helps to minimize your exposure if the linens are soiled with blood or other body fluids

> Because linens soiled with body fluids and substances can act as fomites, it is important to use good infection control practices when handling soiled linens.

STANDARD BEDMAKING TECHNIQUES

Key Learning Points

■ Techniques of proper bedmaking, including making a closed bed, opening a bed, preparing a surgical bed, and making an occupied bed

Activity G *Mitering is a way of folding and tucking the sheet so that it lies flat and neat against the mattress. The figure shows the steps to make a mitered corner. Look at the figure and write down the correct order of the steps.*

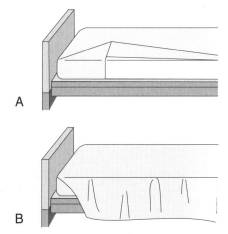

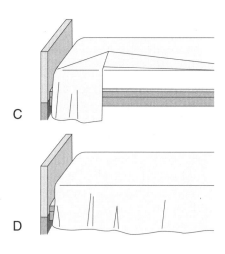

A. _____

B. _____

C. _____

D. _____

Activity H *Fill in the blanks.*

1. Mr. James has gone to visit his family for the day. While he's gone, his bed should be a _____ bed.

2. When the top sheet, blanket, and bedspread of a closed bed are turned back, or _____, the closed bed becomes an _____ bed.

3. Mr. Ming will be returning to his hospital room on a stretcher following his surgery. His bed is prepared as a _____ bed.

Activity I *Mark each statement as either "true" (T) or "false" (F). Correct the false statements.*

1. T F When preparing a surgical bed, the top sheet, blanket, and bedspread are folded toward the foot of the bed, clearing the way for the patient.

2. T F A surgical bed that is readied to receive a patient should be positioned at a height slightly lower than that of the stretcher on which the patient arrives.

3. T F A bed that is unoccupied because the patient or resident is simply not in it at the moment (and is not expected back any time soon) is considered an open bed.

4. T F A bed that is reserved for a patient or resident is called an occupied bed. Preparing the bed to receive the person is called making an occupied bed.

5. T F Always wear gloves when making an occupied bed and when it is possible you will be handling linens soiled with body fluids or other substances.

SUMMARY

Activity J *Use the clues to find words that are present in the grid of letters, either horizontally from left to right or vertically from top to bottom.*

Down

1. A corner that is made by folding and tucking the sheet so that it lies flat and neat against the mattress
2. A metal frame that is placed between the bottom and top sheets to keep the top sheet, the blanket, and the bedspread away from the person's feet; used when pressure on the person's feet could result in pain or skin breakdown
3. An empty, made bed
4. A lightweight cotton blanket used to cover a person during a bed bath or linen change to help provide modesty and warmth

Across

1. Loosening of the top linens over a person's feet to relieve pressure and promote comfort

F	G	H	T	E	K	B	D	S
M	H	S	P	A	B	T	Q	J
I	G	B	R	C	G	B	D	F
T	O	E	P	L	E	A	T	C
E	T	D	U	O	T	T	P	F
R	H	C	T	S	G	H	O	G
E	N	R	W	E	H	B	I	H
D	J	A	I	D	J	L	D	J
C	J	D	N	B	U	A	J	J
O	K	L	C	E	T	N	H	I
R	E	E	R	D	E	K	H	K
N	Q	I	G	W	E	G	S
E	N	Y	J	I	Q	T	R	E
R	K	T	F	I	S	S	R	D
Z	O	G	A	K	C	Q	F	F

CHAPTER 16

Vital Signs, Height, and Weight

WHAT DO VITAL SIGNS TELL US?

Key Learning Points

- The definition of the term *vital signs* and how vital signs reflect changes in a person's medical condition

Activity A *Place an "X" next to the key measurements that make up the vital signs.*

1. ___ Body temperature

2. ___ Weight

3. ___ Blood pressure

4. ___ Height

5. ___ Respiration

6. ___ Heart beat

Activity B *Mark each statement as either "true" (T) or "false" (F). Correct the false statements.*

1. T F   Health care professionals refer to certain key measurements that provide essential information about a person's health as vital signs because they are necessary to life.

2. T F   It is the duty of a nursing assistant to routinely measure and record a person's vital signs and report promptly to the doctor if abnormal changes are detected.

3. T F   Although height and weight are not technically vital signs, the nursing assistant is responsible for obtaining and recording these measurements as frequently as vital signs.

4. T F   A change in a person's normal vital sign measurements can be a sign of illness.

> Vital signs provide insight into a person's overall health status. Measuring and recording vital signs will be a routine part of your daily duties. Many people are counting on you to provide this information accurately, and to report any abnormalities quickly. Your knowledge of your patient or resident will allow you to know whether the vital sign measurements you have obtained are normal readings for the person you are caring for.

Activity C *Select the single best answer for each of the following questions.*

1. Which functions are regulated automatically by the body?

    a. Height

    b. Food intake

    c. Weight

    d. Heart rate, internal temperature of the body, respiratory rate

2. Why should you know the normal ranges for each vital sign?

    a. Because a person's vital sign measurements may vary over the course of a day

    b. Because a patient or resident might ask you for this information

    c. Because knowing normal ranges will allow you to quickly recognize measurements that are not within the range of normal and may indicate a response to illness or injury

    d. Because blood pressure has to be measured frequently

3. What does a change in a vital sign indicate?

    a. Of all the activities going on inside the body, one of them has ceased

    b. Something has put the body out of balance, and the body is attempting to get back that balance

    c. Regulation of body functions such as temperature and breathing

    d. A state of complete physical balance

> Your ability to quickly recognize and report changes in vital signs may prevent a medical emergency from occurring.

MEASURING AND RECORDING VITAL SIGNS

Key Learning Points

■ The importance of accurately measuring and recording vital signs, and of reporting any changes to the nurse

Activity D *Place an "X" next to the circumstances under which a person's vital signs should be measured and compared.*

1. ____ While visiting the doctor

2. ____ Every shift or every few hours, if admitted to a hospital

3. ____ After every meal

4. ____ Once daily or weekly, if admitted to a long-term care facility

5. ____ Before and after certain medications are given

6. ____ Before, during, and after a surgical or diagnostic procedure

7. ____ At odd hours

8. ____ To compare with normal values

9. ____ In an emergency situation

10. ____ Continuously if the person is critically ill

11. ____ If the person complains of dizziness, nausea, or pain

12. ____ If the person is not looking or acting like he or she normally does

13. ____ If the person is participating in an activity that may affect her vital signs

Activity E *Mark each statement as either "true" (T) or "false" (F). Correct the false statements.*

1. T F A patient who is critically ill may be attached to machines that measure his vital signs continuously and display the results on a monitor.

2. T F If a person has been participating in activities that may affect her vital signs, it is not necessary to wait before measuring them.

3. T F Facilities and agencies will have different policies regarding how vital signs are recorded.

4. T F The flow sheet where a person's vital signs are recorded may be kept in the person's medical record or at the bedside.

5. T F Asking for help when one is unsure is a sign of failure or an inability to do one's job.

Activity F *Select the single best answer for the following question.*

1. Where might a nursing assistant look to learn how often a particular person's vital signs are to be measured and recorded?

   a. In the facility's policy manual

   b. The nursing care plan, the doctor's order sheet, or both

   c. The medication record

   d. The state registry

Activity G *Think About It! Briefly answer the following question in the space provided.*

You have recently become employed at a long-term care facility and are still not comfortable with measuring vital signs. While measuring one of your resident's vital signs, you find it to be significantly higher than the normal range indicated by the flow sheet. What should you do?

_____

_____

_____

BODY TEMPERATURE

Key Learning Points

- The factors affecting a person's body temperature
- The various terms used to describe an abnormal body temperature
- Common sites used for measuring a person's body temperature, and the advantages and disadvantages associated with each site
- The proper use of a glass thermometer, an electronic or digital thermometer, and a tympanic thermometer

Activity H *Select the single best answer for each of the following questions.*

1. What is meant by the term *body temperature*?

   a. The physical and chemical changes that occur when the cells of the body change the food that we eat into energy

   b. How rapidly the heart beats

   c. How hot the body is; or the difference between the heat produced by the person's body and the heat lost by the person's body

   d. Muscle movement

2. What is metabolism?

   a. The heat loss that occurs normally through the skin

   b. Process of readying the body to respond to the source of a given stress

   c. The state of being more sensitive to environmental temperature changes

   d. The physical and chemical changes that occur when the cells of the body convert the food that we eat into energy

3. Which of the following steps must you NOT do while using a glass thermometer?

   a. Wash the thermometer with warm water and soap

   b. Rinse the thermometer with cold water

   c. Place the thermometer in hot water

   d. Soak the thermometer in a disinfectant solution

4. What is one way that heat is lost from the body?

   a. Shivering

   b. Muscle movement

   c. Sweating

   d. Increased metabolism

Activity I *Fill in the blanks using the words given in brackets.*

[sheath, thermoregulatory, fever, hypothalamus, metabolism, vagal nerve]

1. The human body produces heat as a result of the process of _____.

2. The thermoregulatory control center is located in the _____ (part of the brain).

3. Infants often have immature _____ centers, which mean that their bodies are slow to adjust to changes in external temperature.

4. A clear plastic disposable cover called a _____ is used to cover the thermometer.

5. When taking the temperature rectally, the thermometer could stimulate the _____.

6. The state of having a body temperature that is much higher than normal is called _____.

Activity J *Mark each statement as either "true" (T) or "false" (F). Correct the false statements.*

1. T F Stress causes the release of hormones, which increase the rate of metabolism and the heart rate. This increased metabolism may raise the body temperature.

2. T F Heat loss occurs normally through the skin by sweating and by the passing of urine and feces.

3. T F A man's body temperature tends to change more frequently than that of a woman.

4. T F A person who is recovering from rectal surgery may still have a rectal temperature taken.

Activity K *Body temperature can be measured using different thermometers. Place a "G" next to the statements that relate to glass thermometers, an "E" next to statements that relate to electronic or digital thermometers, a "TY" next to statements that relate to tympanic thermometers, and a "TA" next to statements that relate to temporal artery thermometers.*

1. ____ This is inserted into the ear canal where it rests near the eardrum and measures the temperature.

2. ____ In this thermometer, the Fahrenheit thermometer is scaled from 94°F to 108°F, while the Celsius thermometer is scaled from 34°C to 43°C.

3. ____ It is considered to be the least invasive of all of the thermometers available because it does not have to be inserted into any body cavity.

4. ____ The thermometer is powered by batteries and a probe is used to measure the temperature.

5. ____ This device, when passed over a person's forehead, detects the body temperature at numerous points, and then performs a series of calculations on the readings to arrive at the person's peak body temperature.

6. ____ This is more often used for children because it allows temperature to be measured in a safe, quick, and relatively painless manner.

7. ____ Most facilities have stopped using this type of thermometer because of the dangers associated with breakage and spilled mercury.

Activity L *Match the temperature types, given in Column A, with their characteristics, given in Column B.*

Column A	Column B
____ 1. Oral temperature	a. The least reliable measurement
____ 2. Rectal temperature	b. Obtained from the person's forehead
____ 3. Axillary temperature	c. Simple and causes minimal discomfort

____ **4.** Tympanic temperature

____ **5.** Temporal temperature

d. Quite accurate but can be most risky

e. Taken with a tympanic thermometer

Activity M *Think About It! Briefly answer the following question in the space provided.*

You have been asked to measure the rectal temperature of a person using an electronic thermometer. The nurse has stressed that you should remain with the person during the entire procedure. Why is this?

_____

_____

_____

PULSE

Key Learning Points

- The definition of the term *pulse* and factors that may affect a person's pulse
- The different qualities of the pulse that a nursing assistant should be aware of when taking a person's pulse
- The parts of a stethoscope and how it is used
- The proper way to measure and record a radial pulse and an apical pulse

Activity N *Place an "X" next to the correct answers for each of the following questions.*

1. Which of the following statements is true about the pulse?

a. ____ With each heart beat, a wave, or pulse, of blood passes through the arteries.

b. ____ The pulse, a throbbing sensation just underneath the skin, can be felt by placing fingers gently over an artery that runs close to the surface of the skin.

c. ____ You can measure the pulse rate, detect the pulse rhythm, or evaluate the pulse amplitude.

d. ____ Only arteries that run closest to the surface of the skin have a pulse.

2. What can be evaluated when taking a person's pulse?

a. ____ How fast the heart is beating

b. ____ The pattern of the pulsations and the pauses between them

c. ____ How much oxygen is in the blood

d. ____ The force or quality of the pulse known as the pulse amplitude or the pulse character

3. Which factors affect a person's pulse rate?

a. ____ Functioning of the central nervous system

b. ____ Requirements of nutrients and oxygen by tissues

c. ____ Feelings such as anger, anxiety, illness, pain, fever, and excitement

d. ____ Medications

4. Which of the following statements is true about taking a person's radial pulse?

a. ____ The thumb should be placed over the radial artery to count the number of pulses.

b. ____ The middle two or three fingers should be placed over the radial artery to count the number of pulses that occur in either 30 seconds or 1 minute.

c. ____ Although the pulse may be taken at other pulse points, taking the pulse at the radial artery is easiest for the patient or resident.

d. ____ The radial pulse is a common way of measuring the pulse rate.

5. Under which circumstances is the apical pulse checked?

a. ____ When a person has a weak or irregular pulse that may be difficult to feel in the radial artery

b. ____ When an infant's heart rate is to be measured

c. ____ When a person has a known heart disease

d. ____ In an emergency situation

Activity O *Mark each statement as either "true" (T) or "false" (F). Correct the false statements.*

1. **T F** An irregular pulse rhythm is called a pulse amplitude, which means that the pulse rhythm is not smooth and regular, with the same amount of time in between each pulsation.

2. **T F** The rate at which the heart beats is controlled automatically by the body's central nervous system.

3. **T F** A weak or thready pulse usually means that the heart is having trouble circulating blood throughout the body.

4. **T F** The radial pulse is measured by listening over the apex of the heart with a stethoscope.

5. **T F** The apical pulse rate will be equal to or higher than the radial pulse rate, because it is easier to hear a heartbeat at the source than to feel it.

Activity P *Fill in the blanks using the words given in brackets.*

[pulse deficit, stethoscope, bradycardia, bell, cardiopulmonary resuscitation, tachycardia, diaphragm]

1. The carotid or femoral arteries may be used to check the pulse during an emergency situation when _____ is being administered.

2. A _____ is a device that makes sound louder and transfers it to the listener's ears.

3. The _____ is the large flat surface that is used to hear loud, harsh sounds like an apical pulse, blood rushing through the arteries, or respiratory sounds.

4. The _____ is a small rounded surface that is designed to pick up faint sounds like heart murmurs or difficult-to-hear blood pressures.

5. The difference between the apical pulse rate and the radial pulse rate is known as the _____.

6. _____ is a rapid heart rate, or a pulse rate of more than 100 beats per minute for an adult.

7. A heart rate that is slower than normal, that is, a pulse rate of less than 60 beats per minute, is called _____.

Activity Q *You have been asked to measure a person's apical pulse using a stethoscope. Look at the following pictures and write down the correct order of the steps.*

A.
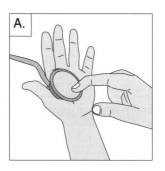

B.
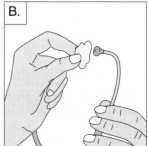

C.
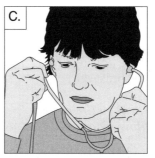

D.
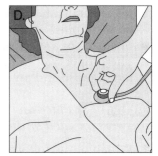

A. _____

B. _____

C. _____

D. _____

RESPIRATION

Key Learning Points

- The definition of the term *respiration* and the factors that may affect a person's respirations
- The terms used to describe a person's respirations
- The proper way to measure and record a person's respirations

Activity R *Some of the steps in the respiration process are listed below. Write down the correct order of the steps in the boxes provided below.*

a. As the body's cells use the oxygen and nutrients delivered to them by the blood, they give off carbon dioxide, which the blood takes back to the lungs.

b. The oxygen in the air passes across a thin membrane into the bloodstream, where it is carried by the red blood cells to all of the cells in the body by the action of the heart, which pumps the oxygen-rich blood throughout the body.

c. During exhalation, carbon dioxide from the lungs is breathed out.

d. In the lungs, the carbon dioxide crosses the same thin membrane, moving from the blood into the air still remaining in the lungs.

e. During inhalation or inspiration, oxygen-containing air is taken into the body.

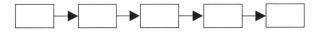

Activity S *Mark each statement as either "true" (T) or "false" (F). Correct the false statements.*

1. T F Ventilation is the exchange of gases between the body and the environment.

2. T F Waste products such as carbon dioxide are created as a result of normal cellular function, namely metabolism.

3. T F During the inhalation phase, the chest deflates as air moves out of the lungs while during the exhalation phase, the chest expands as air is brought into the lungs.

4. T F Control centers, called chemoreceptors, are located in the hypothalamus and in some of the major arteries.

Activity T *Select the single best answer for each of the following questions.*

1. What points should you record when you check for respiration in a person?
   a. The quality of each breath
   b. The number of times the person breathes each minute
   c. The regularity with which a person breathes
   d. All of the above

2. If a person's breathing is irregular, what is the best way to obtain an accurate respiratory rate?
   a. By asking the person to consciously control his respirations
   b. By watching the rise and fall of a person's chest and counting the number of breaths that occur in 1 minute
   c. By placing your hand either near the collarbone or on the person's side to feel the breathing
   d. By watching the rise and fall of a person's chest, counting the number of breaths that occur in 30 seconds, and multiplying that number by two

3. Which vital sign is acceptable to measure without the consent of the patient?
   a. Respiratory rate
   b. Pulse rate
   c. Body temperature
   d. Height and weight

4. A person having difficult or labored breathing is said to be experiencing:
   a. Eupnea
   b. Tachycardia
   c. Dyspnea
   d. Bradypnea

BLOOD PRESSURE

Key Learning Points

- The definition of the term *blood pressure* and factors that may affect a person's blood pressure
- Terms used to describe an abnormal blood pressure
- The various methods used to measure a person's blood pressure
- How a sphygmomanometer works, and how it is used to assess a person's blood pressure
- The Korotkoff sounds

Activity U *Select the single best answer for each of the following questions.*

1. What is measured when taking a person's blood pressure?
   a. Pulse pressure
   b. The force that the blood exerts against the arterial walls
   c. Blood volume
   d. Cardiac output

2. What term is used to describe blood pressure that is lower than normal?
   a. Hypertension
   b. Bradycardia
   c. Orthopnea
   d. Hypotension

3. Mr. John is undergoing a surgical procedure. Which one of the following instruments will most likely be used to monitor his blood pressure during the procedure?
   a. An automated sphygmomanometer
   b. A manually operated sphygmomanometer
   c. A manometer
   d. A stethoscope

4. Mr. Harmon suffers from orthostatic hypotension. He has been lying in bed, but needs to get up for his regular evening walk. What precaution should you take with Mr. Harmon?
   a. Allow him to sit for a moment before standing up, to allow time for his body to adjust
   b. Have him ride in a wheelchair instead; he doesn't really need the exercise
   c. First determine his pulse deficit
   d. Have him stand up quickly from his bed

Activity V *Fill in the blanks using the words given in brackets.*

[hypertension, blood pressure, arteriosclerosis, pulse pressure, sphygmomanometer]

1. The force that the blood exerts against the arterial walls is known as the _____.

2. The difference between the systolic and diastolic pressures is known as the _____.

3. Resistance to blood flow could be due to _____.

4. The most common method to measure blood pressure is by using a manually operated _____ and a stethoscope.

5. If a person has a blood pressure that is consistently higher than 140 mm Hg (systolic) and/or 90 mm Hg (diastolic), then that person is said to have _____.

Activity W *Some of the steps in the procedure for taking a person's blood pressure are listed below. Write down the correct order of the steps in the boxes below.*

   a. Inflate the cuff slowly until the pulse can be heard through the stethoscope.
   b. Continue to inflate the cuff until the pulse cannot be heard.
   c. Pump the bulb, which will result in air entering the pouch in the cuff.
   d. Wrap the cuff around the person's upper arm where the brachial artery is located.
   e. Turn the valve on the bulb slightly counterclockwise to allow air to escape from the cuff slowly.
   f. Continue to inflate the cuff 30 mm Hg more.
   g. Note the reading on the manometer when the first Korotkoff sound is heard.

h. Place the diaphragm of the stethoscope directly over brachial artery and close the valve on the pumping bulb by turning it clockwise.

i. Continue to deflate the cuff and note the reading on the manometer when the last Korotkoff sound is heard.

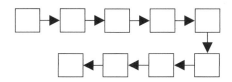

Activity X *Observe the pictures given below. The readings on the manometer for all "A" figures are systolic pressures and for all "B" figures are diastolic pressures. Write the pressure readings for each pair and specify whether the reading falls within the range of normal.*

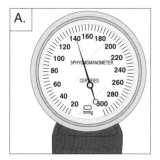 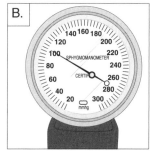

1. _____

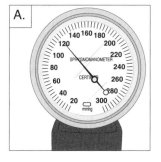 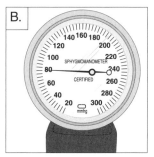

2. _____

HEIGHT AND WEIGHT

Key Learning Points

- Factors that can lead to a change in a person's weight
- The proper way to measure a person's height and weight using an upright scale
- The proper way to measure a person's weight using a chair scale
- The proper way to measure a person's height when the person is in bed

Activity Y *Place an "X" next to the correct answers for each of the following questions.*

1. Why is it useful to obtain a "baseline" height and weight?

   a. ____ Because these measurements provide an insight into the person's overall health and nutritional status

   b. ____ Because weight is often used to calculate medication dosages

   c. ____ Because a change in height or weight could provide insight into a change in a patient's or resident's condition

   d. ____ Because facility policy usually requires it

2. What unit of measurement is used to record a person's height?

   a. ____ Inches (″)

   b. ____ Millimeters of mercury (mm Hg)

   c. ____ Kilograms (kg)

   d. ____ Pounds (lb)

3. Which of the following are found on an upright scale?

   a. ____ A wheelchair

   b. ____ A scale platform

   c. ____ A balance bar

   d. ____ A height rod

Activity Z *Look at the figures below and write down the weight measurement shown on each.*

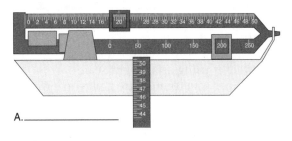

A._____

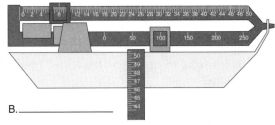

B._____

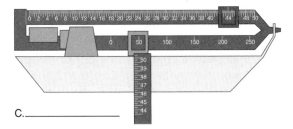

C._____

Activity AA *Think About It! Briefly answer the following question in the space provided.*

1. The nurse has asked you to obtain the height and weight of several residents. How will you do it?

   a. Ms. Quinlan is in a coma.

   _____

   b. Mrs. Lorenz cannot stand for a very long period of time. _____

   c. Mr. Pepper, who weighs more than 250 pounds, is able to get out of bed and walk with help. _____

MEASURING VITAL SIGNS IN CHILDREN

Key Learning Points

■ How vital signs in children differ from those in adults

Activity BB *Select the single best answer for each of the following questions.*

1. How long should you measure the pulse rate and respiratory rate in a child younger than 12 years?

   a. For 1 minute

   b. For 30 seconds

   c. For 2 minutes

   d. For 5 minutes

2. When measuring a child's blood pressure, what determines which cuff size to use?

   a. The child's developmental stage

   b. The child's age and weight

   c. The child's ability to cooperate

   d. The same cuff is used in adults and children

SUMMARY

Activity CC *Use the clues to complete the crossword puzzle.*

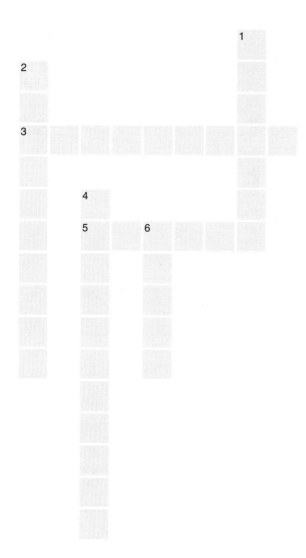

Across

3. A respiratory rate that is higher than normal
5. A normal respiratory rate

Down

1. The state of having a body temperature that is much higher than normal
2. Describes the physical and chemical changes that occur when the cells of the body convert the food that we eat into energy
4. The mechanical process of moving air in and out of the lungs
6. The wave of blood sent through the arteries each time the heart beats

CHAPTER 17

Comfort and Rest

PHYSICAL AND EMOTIONAL BENEFITS OF REST AND SLEEP

Key Learning Points

- The importance of rest and sleep for a person's overall well-being
- The normal sleep cycle
- The factors that can affect a person's ability to obtain a good night's sleep
- The actions that a nursing assistant can take to help patients and residents get the rest and sleep they need

Activity A *Select the single best answer for the following question.*

1. Mrs. Sanders has a new roommate who snores. She is having difficulty sleeping. You notice that she is having difficulty concentrating on the activity this afternoon. You notify the nurse that:

   a. you think she may have had a stroke

   b. her lack of sleep may have caused decreased cognition

   c. her lack of sleep may have caused disinterest in activities

   d. you think she should have a nap instead of going to activities

2. Mrs. Quince has a lot on her mind. She is selling her house and her son is packing up her things. This is the third night that you have noticed that she hasn't slept. You should notify the nurse because Mrs. Quince is at risk for:

   a. illness

   b. pain

   c. fear

   d. anger

3. Mrs. Quince falls the next day and her son becomes angry and states she is punishing him for selling the house you understand that lack of sleep can cause:

   a. anger and the son is right

   b. jealousy and the son is right

   c. fatigue and decreased physical ability

   d. fatigue and Mrs. Quince wants her son to feel guilty

4. The two different types of sleep are:

   a. REM and NREM

   b. MRE and NMRE

   c. SEM and NSEM

   d. SRM and NSRM

5. The average adult requires 7 to 8 hours of sleep in a 24-hour period. How may the average older person achieve this goal?

   a. they do not require as much sleep

   b. they sleep throughout the night

   c. they nap

   d. they take sleeping medication

Activity B *Mark each statement as either "true" (T) or "false" (F). Correct the false statements.*

1. T F Each stage of NREM sleep lasts from 5 to 15 minutes.

2. T F During sleep, the eyes are closed and the muscles are energized.

3. T F On average, a person completes seven or eight sleep cycles during a night's sleep.

Activity C *Match the factors that affect the person's ability to sleep in Column A with the patient or resident in Column B.*

Column A

_____ **1.** Environment

_____ **2.** Insomnia

_____ **3.** Pain and chronic condition

_____ **4.** Sleep apnea

Column B

a. Mr. Watson complains that no matter how hard he tries he cannot sleep. He has not slept in 5 days.

b. Mr. Yang snores and has periods where he stops breathing altogether.

c. Mr. Smith complains that he can't sleep because he can hear the call lights all night long.

d. Mrs. Angier complains that she can't sleep because of her arthritis.

Activity D *Fill in the blanks.*

Remember that a _____, _____ environment promotes rest and sleep. Sometimes the routines in health care facilities make it difficult for patients and residents to _____. When working during the evening and night hours, be especially mindful of things that you do that could affect a person's ability to _____. Take care to keep _____ at a minimum, particularly at the change of shift when there is a lot of staff _____. Keep your voice _____ and encourage others to do the same. Avoid _____ out to co-workers unless you need help in an _____. Finally, be thoughtful about the use of _____. If you need to enter a person's room to provide care, try to avoid turning on _____ _____ _____. Use night-lights or other soft lighting if possible. _____ awaken the person who needs care, and be sure to _____ to the person who you are and what you are there to do. If more light is needed to safely complete the task, turn on only the lights you need. When you have finished providing care, make sure the person is _____ comfortably, and _____ _____ the lights as soon as you can.

PAIN

Key Learning Points

■ The definition of pain and the difference between acute pain and chronic pain

Activity E *Select the single best answer for each of the following questions.*

1. Mrs. Singleton fell at home and fractured her ulna. She states that the pain she experiences is sharp and sudden whenever she moves "just the wrong way." This is an example of:

a. chronic pain

b. escalating pain

c. the pain scale

d. acute pain

2. You are working the 11-7 shift and find Mrs. Hilton awake at 2 AM. She states that her arthritis is acting up again and she needs "a little something" to get the pain under control. This is an example of:

a. chronic pain

b. escalating pain

c. the pain scale

d. acute pain

HOW PEOPLE RESPOND TO PAIN

Key Learning Points

■ The factors that affect a person's response to pain

Activity F *Select the single best answer for each of the following questions.*

1. Mr. Todd is in your sub-acute unit, recovering from a total knee replacement. He has not asked for pain medication since his admission. When asked, he tells you that his pain is at a 2, and very tolerable. You would define his ability to experience pain as a:

a. low pain threshold

b. high pain threshold

c. drug addiction

d. drug tolerance

2. Mr. Gains told the nurse that he waited as long as he could before he asked for pain medication. This is an example of:

 a. pain tolerance

 b. pain threshold

 c. drug addiction

 d. drug tolerance

RECOGNIZING AND REPORTING PAIN

Key Learning Points

- The non-verbal signs of pain that a person may show
- The methods that a nursing assistant can use to gather more information about the person's pain
- The importance of promptly and accurately reporting a patient's or resident's pain

Activity G *As a nursing assistant, you may be the first to notice that one of your patients or residents is in pain. One of the methods that you will use to assess pain is your observational skills. Mark each statement as either "true" (T) if it is a non-verbal sign of pain or "false" (F) if it is not. Correct the false statements.*

1. T F   Facial expressions (such as grimacing or gritting the teeth)

2. T F   Moaning and crying "I can't take the pain anymore."

3. T F   Guarding (avoiding use of) the area of the body that is in pain

4. T F   Redness or swelling in an area, and the resident tells you not to touch the area

5. T F   Profuse sweating

Activity H *Place an "X" next to the information that is important to report to the nurse regarding your patient's or resident's pain.*

1. ___ Location of pain

2. ___ Person's name

3. ___ Characteristics of the pain

4. ___ Intensity of the pain

5. ___ Pain tolerance

6. ___ Circumstances surrounding the pain

7. ___ Pain threshold

Activity I *Select the single best answer for each of the following questions.*

1. Mrs. Case states that her arm hurts her; she fell yesterday and didn't want to bother anyone. It is important to notify the nurse immediately because:

 a. the nurse will have to notify the family that there has been a fall.

 b. the nurse will need to take steps to find out what is causing the pain.

 c. the nurse will have to notify the doctor that there has been a fall.

 d. the nurse will have to re-educate Mrs. Case regarding reporting falls.

2. Mrs. Yates tells you that she can't go to activities today because her arthritis is bothering her. She tells you that it is something that she just has to live with. You should report this pain to the nurse because:

 a. there may still be something the nurse can do to help make Mrs. Yates more comfortable.

 b. activities is an integral part of Mrs. Yates's care plan.

 c. Mrs. Yates may be depressed and require a referral to psychiatric services.

 d. Mrs. Yates may have developed a pain tolerance to her arthritis medication.

3. Mr. Smith, is a hospice resident in your facility, he states that he just can't take the pain anymore and just wants to "get it over with." You should notify the nurse because:

 a. the nurse may wish to call the doctor for medication to make him unconscious

 b. the nurse may wish to give him an extra dose of pain medication

 c. there may still be a pain medication that will also treat his depression

 d. there may still be a medication that may help with Mr. Smith's pain management

TREATMENTS FOR PAIN

Key Learning Points

- The use of medications, physical therapy, and heat and cold applications to relieve pain and promote comfort
- How to safely use heat and cold applications in the health care setting

Activity J — Fill in the blanks.

1. Some people may experience _____ _____ (pain that occurs before the next regularly scheduled dose of pain medication). It is important to recognize and report _____ so that the person does not have to be unnecessarily _____ while waiting for the next scheduled dose of _____. You can help the doctor and nurse plan the person's medication _____ by reporting your _____ about the person's _____ to the nurse _____.

Activity K — Think About It! Briefly answer the following question in the space provided.

Discuss two methods used by physical therapy for the management of pain.

_____

_____

_____

Activity L — Older people and very young children are at very high risk for injury from the application of heat or cold, because their skin is very fragile and sensitive. Other factors that can increase the persons risk for injury from the application of heat or cold are listed below. Mark each statement as either "true" (T) or "false" (F). Correct the false statements.

1. T F People with impaired sensation, such as those who are paralyzed or who have diabetes, are not at risk for injury because they are able to detect whether an application is too hot or too cold.

2. T F People who are disoriented or taking pain medications may be unaware that an application is too hot or too cold, or unable to communicate discomfort caused by the application to others.

3. T F Fair skin tends to be less sensitive to temperature changes than darker skin.

Activity M — Heat and cold applications can be used to provide comfort to a person in pain. Match the applications listed in Column A with the corresponding use in Column B.

Column A	Column B
___ 1. Heat	a. used for people who have musculoskeletal injuries resulting from trauma, such as sprains and fractures
___ 2. Burns	b. a special type of electric heating pad that heats water to a preset temperature
___ 3. Aquamatic Pad	c. reduces pain and swelling, causes blood vessels to constrict, and causes a reduction in bleeding
___ 4. Cold	d. most common complication of heat applications
___ 5. Cold applications	e. relaxes the muscles, relieves pain, and promotes blood flow to the area

THE NURSING ASSISTANT'S ROLE IN MANAGING PAIN

Key Learning Points

- The actions that a nursing assistant can take to help a person who is experiencing pain

Activity N — Select the single best answer for each of the following questions.

1. Mrs. Janis just received her pain medication. She is anxious and is fearful that the medication won't work. What can you do to help her to relieve her pain?
   a. Tell her the medication will work in about 20 minutes.
   b. Provide a quiet environment and stay with her until she relaxes.
   c. Tell her you will check in on her in 10 minutes to make sure that the medication worked.
   d. Give her supper and tell her the medication will work better if she has food in her stomach.

2. Mr. Gainsborough states that his left leg is bothering him. Since his stroke, he just can't get comfortable. To relieve his pain and discomfort you will:

a. place his leg in proper body alignment

b. get him out of bed and into the dining room

c. ask the nurse for pain medication

d. tell the resident that the pain is now a fact of life for him

SUMMARY

Activity O *Fill in the Blanks.*

1. Pain can be acute or _____.

2. Common treatments for pain include _____, physical therapy, and heat and cold applications.

3. Factors that can negatively affect a person's ability to sleep include environmental conditions, pain and other symptoms of _____, and sleep disorders.

4. Nursing assistants can help patients and residents to get the rest and sleep they need by ensuring a restful _____.

5. Adequate rest and sleep are very important for a person's overall health and _____.

CHAPTER 18

Cleanliness and Hygiene

THE BENEFITS OF PERSONAL HYGIENE

Key Learning Points

- The activities that make up personal hygiene
- The importance of good hygiene in relation to a person's physical and emotional well-being

Activity A *Think About It! Briefly answer the following question in the space provided.*

Helping your patients or residents with personal hygiene provides both physical and emotional benefits. List two ways that caring for the skin and mouth helps to promote physical health by preventing infection. Then, list two ways that caring for the skin and mouth helps to promote emotional health.

PHYSICAL HEALTH

1. _____

2. _____

EMOTIONAL HEALTH

1. _____

2. _____

SCHEDULING OF ROUTINE CARE

Key Learning Points

- Specific times for routine activities
- Reasons for schedule
- PRN (as-needed) care

- How personal and cultural preferences influence a person's hygiene practices

Activity B *Following are routine activities associated with personal hygiene that are performed at different times during the day. Place an "EM" next to activities that are a part of early morning care, an "M" next to activities that are a part of morning care, an "A" next to activities that are part of afternoon care, and an "E" next to activities that are part of evening (hs, hour of sleep) care.*

1. ____ General housekeeping duties, such as tidying the person's room and changing the bed linens

2. ____ Straightening the bed linens and fluffing the pillows

3. ____ A general "freshening up" involving assistance with using the toilet, washing of the hands and face, and oral care

4. ____ Preparing the person for breakfast or early diagnostic testing or treatment

5. ____ Helping the person to change into pajamas

6. ____ Assisting with insertion of dentures prior to eating breakfast

7. ____ Providing "extras," such as a bath, soft music and a back massage, or reading in bed

8. ____ Assisting with using the toilet, bathing, oral care, shaving, hair care, dressing, and putting on make-up

Activity C *Think About It! Briefly answer the following question in the space provided.*

Sometimes a patient or a resident may need PRN (as-needed) care. Next to each of the following conditions, write down why the person will need PRN care and how you will meet this need.

a. Mr. Ludwig has been in a coma for 3 weeks

_____

_____

b. Mrs. O'Brien has advanced dementia and is incontinent of urine and feces

_____

_____

c. Mr. Johnson has a very high fever and is sweating a great deal

_____

_____

Activity D *Select the single best answer for each of the following questions.*

1. Why should you try to accommodate a patient's or resident's personal preferences with regard to personal hygiene practices?

   a. As a nursing assistant you are bound to do so

   b. To abide by the policies of the hospital or long-term care facility

   c. To protect the person's physical health

   d. To help the person feel appreciated and respected

2. Mr. Symington, one of your residents with dementia, is frightened when you tell him it is time for his bath. Worse, he is also creating a big ruckus. What step will you take to resolve this situation?

   a. Tell Mr. Symington firmly that he must bathe or he will get sick

   b. Adopt a calm, efficient attitude and seek extra help from a coworker if necessary

   c. Restrain Mr. Symington and give him a bed bath

   d. Tell Mr. Symington that you do not have time to argue with him so you will let him skip his bath today

Make an effort to accommodate your patients' or residents' individual requests with regard to when personal hygiene activities are carried out whenever possible. Also, remember: people with wet or soiled skin, linens, or clothing require immediate attention!

ASSISTING WITH ORAL CARE

Key Learning Points

- Practices that are considered to be a part of oral hygiene
- Situations that may require a person to need more frequent oral hygiene
- Actions that promote the safe handling of a person's dentures
- Proper technique for providing oral care for a person's natural teeth, for a person with dentures, and for an unconscious person

Activity E *Select the single best answer for each of the following questions.*

1. What is the preferred method of cleaning natural teeth in a conscious person?

   a. Placing a padded tongue blade between the upper and lower back teeth to keep the mouth open

   b. Cleaning the teeth using saline water

   c. Brushing the teeth with a soft toothbrush and fluoride toothpaste

   d. Cleaning the gums using a sponge-tipped swab

2. Mrs. Jones wears dentures. What should you do when assisting Mrs. Jones with oral care?

   a. Dry the dentures before placing them in her mouth

   b. Rinse her mouth with water or mouthwash and a soft toothbrush or a sponge-tipped swab to clean her gums, tongue, and the insides of the cheeks

c. Place the dentures in a denture cup and cover them with hot water

d. Write Mrs. Jones' name and age on the denture cup

3. Where do you place dentures when cleaning them?

a. In a sink lined with a washcloth

b. In the palm of your hand

c. In the patient's or resident's mouth

d. On the counter or over-bed table

Activity F *Mark each statement as either "true" (T) or "false" (F). Correct the false statements.*

1. T F It is important to practice standard precautions when assisting patients with brushing and flossing the teeth or cleaning dentures because you will come in contact with saliva.

2. T F A denture brush (or a toothbrush) and a denture cleaner (or toothpaste) are used to clean all surfaces of the denture, and then the dentures are rinsed with lukewarm water.

3. T F When brushing a person's teeth, the toothbrush is positioned at a 90-degree angle to the gums, and moved briskly in a straight up-and-down motion.

4. T F Oral care is usually provided on awakening, after meals, and before bed.

Activity G *Think About It! Briefly answer the following question in the space provided.*

One of your residents, Mr. Brentwood, is in a coma. When providing oral care for Mr. Brentwood, why do you turn his head to the side? What is the purpose of using a padded tongue blade when providing oral care to Mr. Brentwood?

_____

_____

_____

Activity H *Some of the steps based on brushing the teeth are listed below. Write down the correct order of the steps in the boxes provided below.*

a. Wet the toothbrush. Put a small amount of toothpaste on the toothbrush.

b. Get ready by gathering oral care supplies and covering the over-bed table with paper towels.

c. Offer the person the cup of water and ask her to rinse her mouth completely.

d. Brush the tongue.

e. Raise the head of the bed as tolerated. Place a towel under the person's chin.

f. Hold the emesis basin underneath the person's chin so that she can spit the water into the basin.

g. Position the toothbrush at a 45-degree angle to the gums, and move gently in a circular motion.

h. Dry the person's mouth and chin thoroughly using a towel.

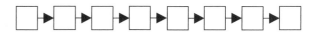

> A clean, healthy mouth makes food taste better and provides a line of defense against infection.

ASSISTING WITH PERINEAL CARE

Key Learning Points

- Why perineal care is an essential aspect of daily hygiene
- Sensitivity issues that a nursing assistant should be aware of when assisting with perineal care
- Proper technique for providing perineal care for males and for females

Activity I *Following are pictures of the male and female perineum and associated structures. Label the figures.*

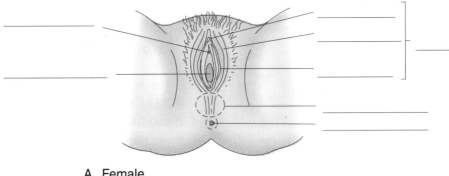

A. Female

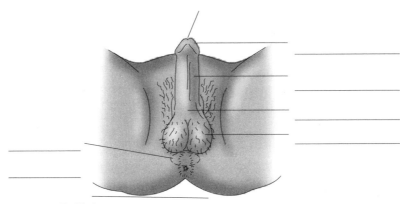

B. Male

Activity J *Think About It! Briefly answer the following question in the space provided.*

Explain how poor hygiene in the perineal area can put a person at risk for infection and skin breakdown.

_____

_____

_____

Activity K *Select the single best answer for each of the following questions.*

1. What is perineal care?

    a. Cleaning the anus

    b. Cleaning the perineum and anus, as well as the vulva (in women) and the penis (in men)

    c. Cleaning the area between the bottom of the vagina and the anus (in women) and the root of the penis and the anus in men

    d. Cleaning only the penis in men and the vulva in women

2. What can cause skin breakdown and odor in the perineal area?

    a. Irritants on the skin, such as feces, urine, and menstrual blood

    b. Frequent perineal care with a soapless cleanser

    c. An unwillingness to shave the private area

    d. Not being circumcised

3. What can happen if you forget to pull the foreskin back up over the head of the penis of a male patient or resident who has NOT been circumcised?

    a. The penis cannot be cleaned thoroughly the next time

    b. The patient or resident may face a cultural or religious dilemma

    c. The foreskin can create a band around the penis, causing pain and swelling

    d. The patient's or resident's sexual drive may be affected

4. Which of the following should be done when providing perineal care?

    a. Rinse away all soap and dry the skin thoroughly

    b. Ask the person's consent for the procedure before beginning

    c. Take standard precautions

    d. All of the above

Activity L *Mark each statement as either "true" (T) or "false" (F). Correct the false statements.*

1. T F   When providing female perineal care, make sure to wipe from the anal area upwards toward the vulva.

2. T F   Perineal care is the first part of the person's bathing routine.

3. T F   Circumcision is a procedure involving the removal of the foreskin, the fold of loose skin that covers the head of the vulva.

Activity M *Think About It! Briefly answer the following question in the space provided.*

Assisting a patient or resident with perineal care can be embarrassing for both the patient or resident and the nursing assistant. Write down how you would handle each of the following potentially embarrassing situations.

a. You have to provide perineal care for a member of the opposite sex

_____

_____

_____

b. A male patient or resident becomes sexually aroused while you are providing perineal care

_____

_____

_____

ASSISTING WITH SKIN CARE

Key Learning Points

- How bathing and skin care benefit a person's health
- The methods of bathing a nursing assistant may be asked to assist with
- Observations that a nursing assistant should make while assisting a person with bathing and skin care
- The benefits of massage
- The proper technique for bathing a person (in bed or in a shower or bathtub) and giving a back massage

Activity N *Place an "X" next to each correct answer for the following questions.*

1. Which of the following are benefits of a bath?

    a. ____ Helps the person feel relaxed and refreshed

    b. ____ Eliminates bad breath

    c. ____ Exercises muscles that might otherwise not be used

    d. ____ Stimulates blood flow to the skin

    e. ____ Helps a person meet cultural and religious needs

    f. ____ Gives the nursing assistant an opportunity to observe skin problems

    g. ____ Reduces the risk of infection

2. What points must you keep in mind while giving a massage to a person?

   a. ____ A massage takes about 4 to 6 minutes to complete

   b. ____ You should not provide a massage to a person with fractured ribs, a back injury, or a recent back surgery

   c. ____ You should not provide massage to an elderly person with dementia because doing so is likely to irritate the person

   d. ____ You can provide massage with the person in either the prone or the lateral position.

Activity O *Select the single best answer for each of the following questions.*

1. Mrs. Ray developed an itching sensation and redness after using a bath product given to her by her daughter. What action should you take?

   a. Throw away the bath product

   b. Apply a hydrocortisone cream to reduce the itching and redness

   c. Allow only limited use of the product and only in your presence

   d. Stop the use of the product until the source of the skin irritation has been determined

2. When giving a bed bath, when is the water in the basin changed?

   a. After washing each body part

   b. Whenever it becomes cool or soapy

   c. When the resident requests fresh water

   d. Before bathing the next resident

3. Which one of the following is an acceptable temperature for a tub bath?

   a. 110°F

   b. 98.6°F

   c. 125°F

   d. 212°F

4. When giving a person a bed bath, where is the bath blanket placed?

   a. Under the person

   b. Over the person

   c. Over the top linens

   d. Under the wash basin

5. When assisting a person with a tub bath or shower, which of the following should you do?

   a. Place a nonskid mat on the floor of the tub or shower

   b. Take standard precautions

   c. Leave the door unlocked

   d. All of the above

Activity P *Mark each statement as either "true" (T) or "false" (F). Correct the false statements.*

1. T F   Touching and massaging of the skin leads to skin breakdown.

2. T F   It may be better for elderly people to use a soapless cleanser because it is drying to the skin.

3. T F   After each use, the tub or shower stall and the shower chair is disinfected.

4. T F   Bath oil and body powder are an especially important part of skin care for elderly people.

Activity Q *In the picture given below, draw in the sequence of strokes for each phase of the back massage.*

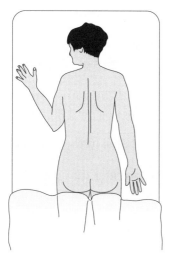

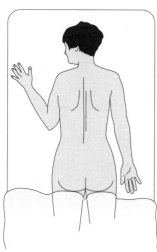

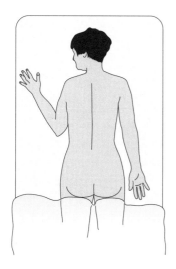

Activity R *Match the skin care products, given in Column A, with their descriptions, given in Column B.*

Column A

___ **1.** Soapless cleanser

___ **2.** Bath oil

___ **3.** Lotion or cream

___ **4.** Body powder

___ **5.** Deodorant

___ **6.** Antiperspirant

Column B

a. Covers or masks odor

b. Prevents drying and chapping

c. Perfumes bath water and moistens skin

d. May not need to be rinsed away; often used to clean the perineal area

e. Stops or slows the secretion of sweat

f. Absorbs sweat and reduces friction between skin

Activity S *You are getting ready to assist Mr. Granger with a tub bath. Write down the correct order of the steps in the boxes below.*

a. Assist Mr. Granger with undressing.

b. Ask Mr. Granger if he needs to use the toilet.

c. Assist Mr. Granger out of the bath and onto a towel-covered chair.

d. Fill the tub with warm water at the proper temperature.

e. Assist Mr. Granger with washing his face.

f. Assist Mr. Granger with perineal care.

g. Assist Mr. Granger to the tub room.

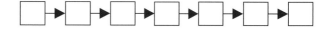

Activity T *Think About It! Briefly answer the following question in the space provided.*

You are assigned to assist one of your residents, Mrs. Scott, with her daily personal hygiene. But today, Mrs. Scott, who is usually very cooperative, tells you that she just doesn't feel like bathing and asks you if she can skip her bath. How would you handle this situation?

_____

_____

_____

SUMMARY

Activity U *Words shown in the picture have been jumbled. Use the clues to form correct words using the letters given in the picture.*

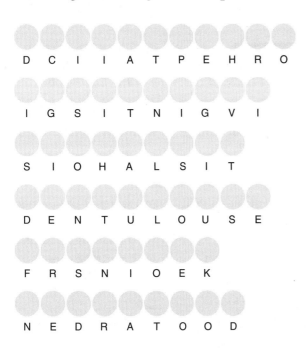

D C I I A T P E H R O

I G S I T N I G V I

S I O H A L S I T

D E N T U L O U S E

F R S N I O E K

N E D R A T O O D

Allowing people to participate in their own self-care helps to maintain independence, but assisting as necessary helps to ensure that hygiene is performed thoroughly.

1. Adjective used to describe a person who has a medical condition that causes him to sweat a great deal
2. Inflammation of the gums
3. Bad breath that does not go away
4. Without teeth
5. The fold of loose skin that covers the head of the penis
6. A grooming product that covers or masks odor

CHAPTER 19

Grooming

INTRODUCTION TO GROOMING

Key Learning Points

- How grooming differs from hygiene
- Factors that influence a person's grooming habits
- The effect that illness or disability may have on a person's grooming habits

Activity A *Place an "X" next to the activities that are considered "grooming" activities.*

1. ___ Shampooing and styling the hair

2. ___ Bathing

3. ___ Applying make-up

4. ___ Providing nail care

5. ___ Assisting with exercise

6. ___ Shaving

Activity B *Think About It! Briefly answer the following question in the space provided.*

List five factors that can influence a person's grooming practices.

_____

_____

_____

Grooming, or activities related to maintaining a neat and attractive appearance, goes beyond basic personal hygiene. Helping a person to complete his or her routine grooming practices meets many of the person's emotional needs, as well as some physical ones.

ASSISTING WITH HAND AND FOOT CARE

Key Learning Points

- Changes that occur in a person's feet as a result of aging or illness
- The importance of proper hand and foot care
- The proper technique for assisting with hand and foot care

Activity C *Select the single best answer for each of the following questions.*

1. Which statement regarding nail care is true for a disoriented or comatose person?

   a. A disoriented or comatose person is not aware of his fingernails' length or appearance, so it is not important to provide nail care for him.

   b. A disoriented or comatose person is more likely to have hangnails, a fungal infection of the nails.

   c. A disoriented or comatose person's fingernails should be kept smooth and short.

   d. It is best to provide nail care for a person who is disoriented or comatose when the nails are hard and dry.

2. The condition of a person's nails can provide clues to the person's overall health. Which of the following are signs of good health that might be observed when providing nail care?

 a. The nail beds are pink.

 b. There is no gap between the nail and the nail bed.

 c. The cuticles are smooth and unbroken.

 d. All of the above

3. When is the best time to perform nail care?

 a. At least 2 hours before a meal.

 b. At least 2 hours following a bath.

 c. During or immediately following a bath.

 d. There is no ideal time for this activity.

4. In a long-term care facility, who is usually NOT permitted to trim a patient's or resident's toenails?

 a. The nurse

 b. The nursing assistant

 c. The doctor

 d. The podiatrist

5. When caring for a person's feet, what should you NOT do?

 a. Soften the nails by soaking them for a short time in warm water

 b. Trim or file corns or calluses

 c. File the nails so that the edges are smooth

 d. Apply foot powder or lotion to the feet after they are dry

Activity D *Use the clues to complete the crossword puzzle.*

Across

1. A tool used to trim nails
5. A doctor who specializes in the care of the feet

Down

2. A condition where the nail curves down and back into the skin, causing injury and pain
3. A fungal infection of the skin and nails of the feet
4. Broken pieces of cuticle that cause injury and pain

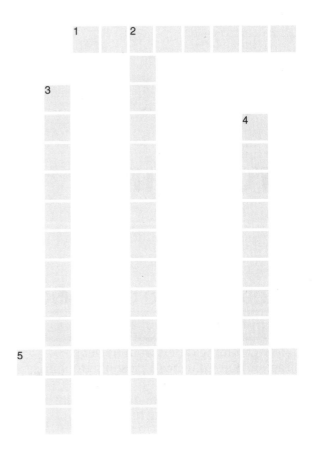

Activity E *Think About It! Briefly answer the following question in the space provided.*

Mrs. McAndrews has diabetes. What sorts of changes would you inspect her feet for while you are assisting her with foot care? Why is being observant for changes in the feet of a person with diabetes especially important?

_____

_____

_____

> Assisting with hand and foot care gives you the chance to observe for potential health problems, including poor blood flow and infections.

ASSISTING WITH DRESSING AND UNDRESSING

Key Learning Points

■ The various dressing needs that a patient or resident may have

■ Different methods of helping a person to dress and undress

Activity F *Place an "X" next to the statements that are true about helping a person to dress.*

1. ____ All patients and residents wear the same clothing, per facility policy.

2. ____ Allowing a person to choose the clothing he or she wishes to wear is a top priority when assisting with dressing.

3. ____ Patients and residents are used to dressing and undressing in the presence of others.

4. ____ The type of clothing a person wears will differ according to the person's abilities.

Activity G *A person who has an intravenous (IV) line in place needs your help to dress. Look at the following picture and write down the correct order of the steps.*

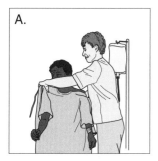

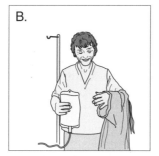

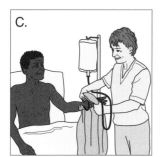

1. _____

2. _____

3. _____

Activity H *Mark each statement as either "true" (T) or "false" (F). Correct the false statements.*

1. T F If you are unsure about how to manage an intravenous (IV) line when assisting a person to dress or undress, you should first disconnect the IV line to avoid any accident during the process.

2. T F When helping a person with a paralyzed extremity (arm or leg) to dress, you should place the garment's sleeve or leg onto the affected extremity first.

Activity I *Think About It! Briefly answer the following question in the space provided.*

Mr. David, one of your residents, is going on a facility-sponsored outing to a baseball game this afternoon. He insists on wearing a short-sleeved cotton shirt with the team's logo on it and no jacket, but you think it will be chilly at the game because it is early May and there is rain in the forecast. What should you do?

_____

_____

_____

> Dressing is usually a routine part of morning and evening care. As with other personal care routines, the amount of help that each person needs for dressing will vary. Some conditions may make helping the person to dress or undress a bit more challenging, but good planning on your part can simplify the situation.

ASSISTING WITH HAIR CARE

Key Learning Points

■ Disorders a nursing assistant may observe when assisting with hair care

■ Methods used to assist a person with shampooing his or her hair

■ Methods used to style a person's hair

■ Proper technique for shampooing a bedridden person's hair and combing a person's hair

Activity J *Fill in the blanks.*

1. _____ is itching and flaking of the scalp.

2. _____ causes severe scaling of the scalp.

3. _____ is a fungal infection of the scalp.

4. _____ is baldness.

5. _____, or head lice, is commonly transferred through person-to-person contact.

Activity K *Think About It! Briefly answer the following question in the space provided.*

The doctor has ordered complete bed rest for Ms. Loyd, who is 7 months pregnant with triplets and is in the hospital due to complications with her pregnancy. Ms. Loyd leaves bed only to use the bathroom, but not long enough for a shower. The nurse has asked you to shampoo Ms. Loyd's hair. Describe the procedure that would be necessary to help Ms. Loyd.

_____

_____

_____

Activity L *Head lice can be transmitted from one person to the next by direct contact or indirect contact. Place a "D" next to the methods of transmission that are direct, and an "I" next to the methods of transmission that are indirect.*

1. ____ Touching the hair of a person who has head lice

2. ____ Touching bedding or clothing (such as a hat) used by an infected person

3. ____ Using an infected person's brush or comb

4. ____ Resting your head on a pillow or the back of an upholstered chair used by an infected person

Activity M *Identify what is wrong with the following picture.*

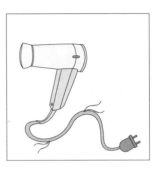

_____

_____

Activity N *Mark each statement as either "true" (T) or "false" (F). Correct the false statements.*

1. T F   If a person's hair is matted or tangled, it may need to be cut.

2. T F   It is not necessary to ask a person's permission before cutting his or her hair.

3. T F   To remove tangles from the hair, use a wide-tooth comb and start at the scalp, working down to the ends of the hair.

> Routine care is necessary to keep the hair clean and neat. For many people, the appearance of their hair affects how they feel about themselves. Respecting personal preference in products is important.

ASSISTING WITH SHAVING

Key Learning Points

- The tools and supplies used for shaving
- How to safely shave a man's face

Activity O *Select the single best answer for the following question.*

1. You notice that Mr. Smith's razor blade has become very dull, and you replace it. How should you dispose of the old razor blade?

   a. Dispose of it in a facility-approved waste container

   b. Dispose of it in a sharps container

   c. Leave it on Mr. Smith's over-bed table; the housekeeping staff will dispose of it

   d. Take it to the nurses' station

Activity P *Think About It! Briefly answer the following question in the space provided.*

Mrs. Robinson asks you to shave her armpits. How would you go about doing this?

_____

_____

_____

Activity Q *Mr. Flanders needs his face shaved. Some of the steps in the procedure for shaving a man's face are listed below. Write down the correct order of the steps in the boxes provided below.*

A. Shave the area between Mr. Flanders' nose and upper lip.

B. Place a towel across Mr. Flanders' shoulders and chest.

C. Fill the wash basin with warm water.

D. Shave Mr. Flanders' chin.

E. Apply shaving cream, gel, or soap to the beard.

F. Shave Mr. Flanders' neck.

G. Shave Mr. Flanders' cheeks.

H. Apply aftershave lotion, if Mr. Flanders requests it.

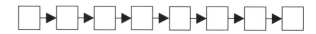

When shaving a person, always remember to wear gloves because a cut or a nick will put you at risk for exposure to bloodborne pathogens.

ASSISTING WITH THE APPLICATION OF MAKE-UP

Key Learning Points

- How the use of make-up can affect a person's sense of well being

Activity R *Think About It! Briefly answer the following question in the space provided.*

You have been assigned to care for Robert. You are quite surprised when Robert tells you he is expecting visitors and asks you if you would be willing to help him apply his make-up. How would you respond, and why?

_____

_____

_____

P	Q	T	Q	W	E	R	T	S
O	R	I	Z	G	D	D	A	S
D	A	N	D	R	U	F	F	F
I	S	E	T	O	Q	A	Z	W
A	D	A	Y	O	W	E	R	I
T	F	P	U	M	S	D	F	O
R	H	E	I	I	U	F	F	F
I	J	D	O	N	I	T	S	G
S	K	I	F	G	W	S	X	A
T	I	S	G	O	K	G	S	E

SUMMARY

Activity S *Use the clues to find words that are present in the grid of letters, either horizontally from left to right or vertically from top to bottom.*

Down

1. A doctor who specializes in the care of the feet
2. A fungal infection of the skin and nails, commonly known as "athlete's foot"
3. Activities related to maintaining a neat and attractive appearance, such as shampooing and styling the hair, shaving, and applying make-up

Across

1. Excessive itching and flaking of the scalp
2. The eggs of head lice, seen on the hair, near the scalp, in people with pediculosis capitis (head lice infestation)

CHAPTER 20

Basic Nutrition

FOOD AND HOW OUR BODIES USE IT

Key Learning Points

- The definition of the term *nutrition* and why our bodies need adequate nutrition
- The general types of nutrients and how the body uses them
- How MyPyramid can be used to help plan and provide better nutrition for a person

Activity A *Select the single best answer for each of the following questions.*

1. What is nutrition?
   a. The process of breaking down food into simple elements
   b. An essential element of food
   c. The unit of energy released by food inside our bodies
   d. The process of taking in and using food

2. Which one of the following nutrients provides us with maximum energy in terms of calories?
   a. Carbohydrates
   b. Proteins
   c. Fats
   d. Vitamins and minerals

3. What must be broken down into simple sugars before the body can use it?
   a. Fat
   b. Water
   c. Protein
   d. Starch

4. How do proteins help our bodies?
   a. They protect our organs and help us stay warm.
   b. They rebuild tissues that break down from normal use or as a result of illness or injury.
   c. They help prevent constipation.
   d. They harden our bones.

Activity B *Match the terms associated with the process of nutrition, given in Column A, with their explanations, given in Column B.*

Column A	Column B
____ 1. Ingestion	a. The transfer of nutrients from the digestive tract into the bloodstream
____ 2. Digestion	
____ 3. Absorption	b. The conversion of nutrients into energy in cells
____ 4. Metabolism	c. The intake of food
	d. The breaking down of food into simple elements

Activity C *Mark each statement as either "true" (T) or "false" (F). Correct the false statements.*

1. T F   The energy to power our bodies comes from water.

2. T F   Protein is found in foods such as milk and cheese, meat, poultry, fish, eggs, nuts, and dried peas and beans.

3. T F   Extra carbohydrates that are not used immediately as fuel are either stored in the liver or converted to fat and stored elsewhere in the body.

4. T F   Calcium helps the blood to clot and Vitamin K helps to build strong bones.

Activity D *Match the terms associated with types of nutrients, given in Column A, with their descriptions, given in Column B.*

Column A

_____ 1. Water

_____ 2. Fat

_____ 3. Minerals

_____ 4. Vitamins

_____ 5. Fiber

_____ 6. Carbohydrate

Column B

a. Can be dissolved in water as well as stored in the body

b. Accounts for approximately 50% to 60% of body weight

c. Provide structure within the body and regulate body process

d. Protects our organs and helps us to stay warm

e. The source of the body's most basic type of fuel, glucose

f. Prevents problems with bowel movements by adding bulk to feces

Activity E *Fill in the blanks using the words given in brackets.*

[fruit, vegetables, milk, meat and beans, grain]

1. Eat at least 3 oz of whole- _____ cereals, breads, crackers, rice, or pasta every day.

2. Choose fresh, frozen, canned, or dried _____ and be sure to eat 2 cups every day.

3. Eat 2½ cups of _____ every day, including carrots, sweet potatoes, spinach, and broccoli.

4. _____ are a good source of protein; be sure to choose low-fat or lean sources.

5. Go low-fat or fat-free when you choose _____, yogurt, and other dairy products.

> People who are receiving health care often have special needs as far as nutrition is concerned, but to be healthy, we all need to eat a variety of nutritious foods each day!

FACTORS THAT AFFECT FOOD CHOICES AND EATING HABITS

Key Learning Points

■ Factors that influence a person's food preferences

Activity F *Think About It! Briefly answer the following question in the space provided.*

Many factors influence the choices we make about food every day. List five factors that influence your food choices, and give an example of each from your own personal experience.

_____

_____

_____

_____

_____

SPECIAL DIETS

Key Learning Points

■ Common special diets

Activity G *Match the terms associated with types of diets, given in Column A, with their descriptions, given in Column B.*

Column A	Column B
____ 1. Regular "house" diet	a. Low in saturated fats and cholesterol
____ 2. Clear liquid diet	b. Contains limited amounts of carbohydrates
____ 3. Full liquid diet	c. A person may be allowed to have a small amount of salt, or none at all
____ 4. A soft diet	d. Well-balanced diet with no restrictions on specific foods or condiments
____ 5. A carbohydrate controlled diet	
____ 6. A sodium-restricted diet	e. Food that can be poured at room or body temperature
____ 7. A low cholesterol diet	f. Foods that are hard to chew or digest are removed
	g. Foods that can be poured at room temperature and can be seen through

Activity H *Mark each statement as either "true" (T) or "false" (F). Correct the false statements.*

1. T F Foods that are considered clear liquids include milk, vanilla ice cream, and juice.

2. T F A person on a sodium-restricted diet is not allowed to have salt at all.

3. T F Nutritional supplements are used to replace meals.

> Taking the time to learn about a person's medical condition and the reason a particular diet was ordered will make you a more effective member of the health care team.

MEAL TIME

Key Learning Points

- The importance of making meals attractive and the dining experience pleasant
- The steps that are taken to help prepare a person for meal time
- Ways that a nursing assistant may need to help a person during meal time
- The proper technique for feeding a person who cannot feed herself
- How the amount of solid food eaten is recorded

Activity I *Long-term care facilities that receive government funding must follow Omnibus Budget Reconciliation Act (OBRA) regulations pertaining to meals. Fill in the blanks using the words given in brackets.*

[attractive, individual, preference, religious, others, proper, health]

1. OBRA requires that meals meet the _____ nutritional needs of each resident.

2. Foods must be served at the _____ temperature.

3. Meals must be _____ to look at, and seasoned to the individual resident's _____.

4. Special diets, such as those followed for _____ or _____ reasons, must be provided for those residents who need them.

5. Dining in the company of _____ is also recommended.

Activity J *Think About It! Briefly answer the following question in the space provided.*

Many patients and residents have little or no appetite. List five things that can decrease a person's appetite. Then, list five things you can do to help increase a person's appetite.

_____

_____

_____

_____

_____

Activity K *Place an "X" next to the type of assistance a nursing assistant may be expected to provide at meal time.*

1. ___ Removing the cover from the tray

2. ___ Describing the foods and their location on the tray to the person

3. ___ Seasoning food according to your taste

4. ___ Serving dessert only when the person has made an effort to eat from the plate on his own

5. ___ Helping the person to open milk cartons and other packages

6. ___ Switching on the radio or television for the person to enjoy

7. ___ Giving the person his medication

Activity L *Match the following thickened liquid consistencies, given in Column A, with their descriptions, given in Column B.*

Column A

___ **1.** Honey

___ **2.** Nectar

___ **1.** Pudding

Column B

a. This consistency "plops" rather than pours and is eaten with a spoon.

b. When poured, the stream looks like a solid column, or it drizzles.

c. This consistency can be poured very easily. The stream has a ribbon-like appearance.

Activity M *You are assisting Mrs. Giamelli, who has very poor eyesight, with eating her dinner. You know that if you can describe the location of the food in terms of a clock face, Mrs. Giamelli will be able to eat fairly well on her own. Fill in the numbers on the clock face shown below and then write down how you would describe the location of the food on the plate to Mrs. Giamelli.*

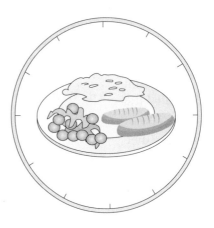

_____

_____

_____

Activity N *It is dinnertime at the long-term care facility and you are assisting Mr. Linkins with his meal. Some of the steps that are taken when assisting a person with a meal are given below. Write down the correct order of the steps in the boxes provided below.*

1. Ask Mr. Linkins if he would like to use a clothing protector.
2. Check the meal tray to make sure that it has Mr. Linkins' name on it and that it contains the correct diet for Mr. Linkins.
3. Wash Mr. Linkins' hands and face.
4. Assist Mr. Linkins with toileting.
5. Uncover the meal tray and tell Mr. Linkins what is on the tray.
6. Allow Mr. Linkins to assist with the eating process to the best of his ability.
7. Remove the tray and the clothing protector, if used.

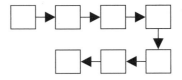

Activity O *The nurse has asked you to record the percentage of each food that Mr. Flannery eats during the meal. Mr. Flannery's meal tray before and after dinner is shown below. What would you record?*

1. ___ Chicken

2. ___ Mashed potatoes

3. ___ Salad

4. ___ Ice cream

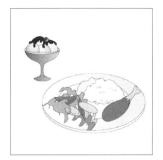 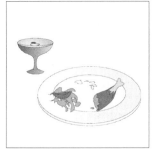

Activity P *Mark each statement as either "true" (T) or "false" (F). Correct the false statements.*

1. T F Wearing a clothing protector is a matter of personal choice; therefore, it is important to ask the resident if he wants to wear a clothing protector or not.

2. T F When assisting a person with a meal, it is important not to talk.

3. T F Assistive devices, such as specially made eating utensils, help a disabled person regain independence, which is important for self esteem.

Activity Q *Think About It! Briefly answer the following question in the space provided.*

After dinner, you notice that Mrs. Li did not touch her soup but ate all the noodles that you had served. List two reasons why talking with Mrs. Li about why she did not eat her soup would be useful. Then, write down what you would say to Mrs. Li to initiate the conversation.

_____

_____

_____

When our emotional needs are met, it is easier for us to meet our physical needs. Ensuring that meal time is pleasant can help improve a person's appetite.

OTHER WAYS OF PROVIDING FLUIDS AND NUTRITION

Key Learning Points

- Other ways of providing nutrition for people who are unable to take food by mouth

Activity R *Following are some terms related to fluids and nutrients. Fill in the blanks using the words given in brackets.*

[intravenous therapy, enteral nutrition, regurgitation, infusion pump, total parenteral nutrition]

1. To help avoid _____ and aspiration, the head of the bed is raised during enteral feeding.

2. _____ is not a source of complete nutrition, but it is useful when a person needs fluids.

3. Enteral feedings may be given at scheduled times or continuously by an _____.

4. In _____, nourishment is delivered directly into the bloodstream through a large catheter inserted into a large vein near the heart.

5. _____ involves placing food directly into the stomach or intestines, which eliminates the need for the person to chew or swallow.

Activity S *Descriptions of some feeding tubes are given below. The names of those feeding tubes are listed in jumbled form. Use the pictures and descriptions as clues to form correct words.*

1. A feeding tube that is inserted through the nose, down the throat, and into the stomach
2. A feeding tube that is inserted into the stomach through a surgical incision made in the abdomen
3. A feeding tube that is inserted into the jejunum through a surgical incision made in the abdomen

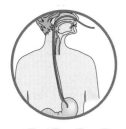

A T C A N S I O R S G

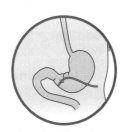

R S M G T Y A O S O T

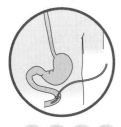

J S Y O U O E M T N J

FLUIDS AND HYDRATION

Key Learning Points

■ The fluid needs of the body and factors that affect the body's fluid balance
■ Methods used to measure and record fluid intake and output

Activity T *Think About It!* Briefly answer the following question in the space provided.

The nurse has told you that Mr. Spreewell's fluid balance must be closely monitored. Explain how you will assist in this task.

_____

_____

_____

Activity U *Use the clues on the next page to complete the crossword puzzle.*

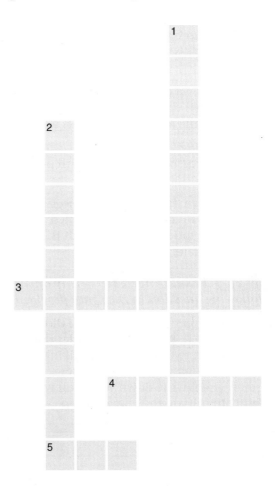

Across

3. A measuring device to measure fluid quantity
4. Occurs when there is too much fluid in the tissues of the body
5. Not allowed to have anything by mouth

Down

1. When the amount of fluid taken into the body equals the amount of fluid that leaves the body, a state of _____ occurs
2. Occurs when there is too little fluid in the tissues of the body

Activity V *Place an "X" next to the measures that a nursing assistant should take to encourage more fluid intake.*

1. ___ Serve room-temperature water
2. ___ Serve fluids that taste good
3. ___ Serve coffee, tea, and soda at the appropriate temperature
4. ___ Provide frequent oral hygiene
5. ___ Offer small amounts of a drink frequently throughout the day
6. ___ Offer large amounts of a drink three times daily, with meals
7. ___ Fill the pitcher regularly with fresh, cold water
8. ___ Know about the amount and type of fluids that should be offered
9. ___ Set an example by drinking fluids while providing patient or resident care

Activity W *Think About It! Briefly answer the following questions in the space provided.*

1. You have been asked to calculate fluid intake of the following residents. Write down the fluid intake of each resident in milliliters.

   a. Mr. Scott's meal tray contained a 12-ounce can of soda, an 8-ounce carton of milk, and 120 ml of water at the beginning of the meal. He finished his soda and milk but drank only half of the water.

   _____

   b. Ms. Sean's tray contained an 8-ounce glass of orange juice, 240 ml of coffee, and one 6-ounce container of ice cream. She drank half of the juice and all of the coffee, and she ate half the container of ice cream.

   _____

   c. Mrs. Ray's tray contained a 16-ounce glass of iced tea, an 8-ounce carton of milk, and 180 ml of broth. She drank three-fourths of the glass of tea and all of her milk, but no broth.

   _____

2. Convert the following measurements in ounces to milliliters.

   a. 8 ounces = _____
   b. 16 ounces = _____
   c. 12 ounces = _____
   d. 32 ounces = _____
   e. 4 ounces = _____
   f. 10 ounces = _____
   g. 5 ounces = _____

> Maintaining proper fluid balance is important for health. When you help your patients or residents meet their fluid needs, you are helping to keep them healthy.

SUMMARY

Activity X *Use the clues to complete the crossword puzzle.*

Across

5. The intake of food or fluids

Down

1. Substances in foods and fluids that the body uses to grow, to repair itself, and to carry out processes essential for living
2. A person who has a degree in nutrition
3. Transfer of nutrients from the digestive tract into the bloodstream
4. Loss of appetite

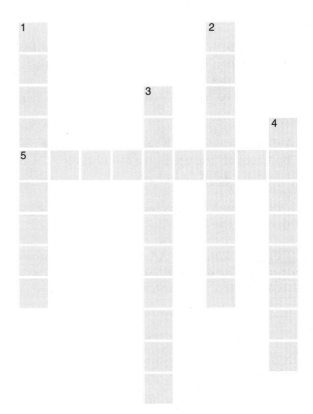

Assisting With Urinary and Bowel Elimination

ASSISTING WITH ELIMINATION

Key Learning Points

- Two methods the body uses to eliminate waste products
- Attitudes that people may have regarding the processes of urinary or bowel elimination
- Actions the nursing assistant can take to promote normal urinary and bowel elimination, and why normal urinary and bowel elimination is essential to health

Activity A *Mark each statement as either "true" (T) or "false" (F). Correct the false statements.*

1. T F The patient or resident who cannot get out of bed uses a bedside commode.

2. T F Hand rails may be attached alongside the toilet to make it easier for the person to sit down and get back up.

3. T F A bedpan is appropriate when a person cannot get out of bed.

4. T F Men who cannot get out of bed use a urinal for urinary elimination.

5. T F A person suffering from injury or disability would not use a fracture pan.

6. T F Devices for obtaining urine specimens include a specimen cup ("commode hat"), bedpan, and urinal.

Activity B *Place an "X" next to each of the following statements that is correct about elimination.*

1. ____ Most people consider elimination a very private activity.

2. ____ Regularly exercising and eating foods that contain fiber help promote regular bowel movements.

3. ____ The most comfortable position for using a bedpan is lying flat on one's back.

4. ____ Drinking plenty of fluids helps the kidneys work properly.

5. ____ The collection of midstream "clean catch" urine specimens prevents contamination by bacteria.

6. ____ Illness or disability usually has little or no effect on a person's normal elimination habits.

7. ____ A specimen container is properly labeled when the label contains the person's name, room number, date, and time.

8. ____ Urinalysis is a rarely used diagnostic tool in the health care setting.

Activity C *Think About It! Briefly answer the following question in the space provided.*

Nursing assistants help patients or residents with elimination as necessary. When giving such assistance, preserving a sense of dignity is important. Describe how the nursing assistant can help to preserve the patient's or resident's dignity when assisting with elimination.

_____

_____

_____

> As a nursing assistant, you will need to assist your patients or residents with elimination as necessary. A professional attitude will help to ease your patient's or resident's embarrassment when it comes to needing assistance with elimination.

URINARY ELIMINATION

Key Learning Points

- Terminology associated with urinary elimination and normal characteristics of urine
- Methods used to measure and record urinary output
- The use of urinary catheters and how to provide routine catheter care
- Problems associated with urinary elimination and methods the nursing assistant uses to assist people having those problems
- The underlying principles of bladder training

Activity D *Fill in the blanks using the words given in brackets.*

[urination, nocturia, micturition, hematuria, voiding, dysuria]

1. A slight red tinge to the urine may indicate _____, or blood in the urine.

2. Several terms used to define the process of passing urine from the body include _____, _____, and _____.

3. _____ is the need to get up more than once or twice during the night to urinate.

4. _____ is difficulty voiding that may be associated with pain.

Activity E *Think About It! Briefly answer the following question in the space provided.*

The nurse has asked you to keep a record of the amount of urine that each one of the following residents or patients passes each time he or she voids. How would you go about collecting and measuring the urine output in each of the following situations?

a. Mrs. Williams uses a regular toilet

_____

b. Mr. Johannsen uses a urinal

_____

c. Mrs. Snowden has a urinary catheter

_____

d. Mrs. Lipkins uses a bedside commode

_____

Activity F *Use the clues to complete the crossword puzzle.*

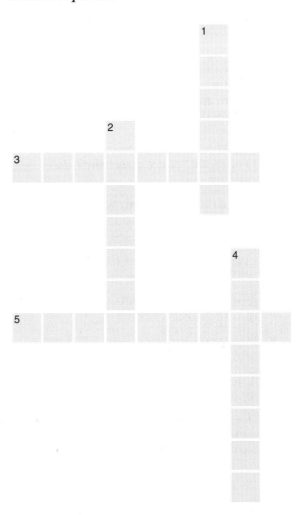

Across

3. Excessive urine output
5. Blood in the urine

Down

1. The state of voiding less than 100 mL of urine over the course of 24 hours
2. Discomfort or difficulty voiding
4. The state of voiding a very small amount of urine over a given period of time (e.g., voiding only 100 to 400 mL of urine over 24 hours)

Activity G *Look at the figures below. Then fill in the blanks using the words given in brackets.*

[Suprapubic, Straight, Indwelling]

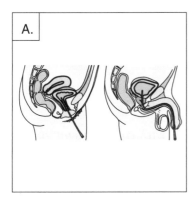

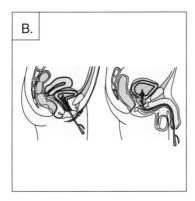

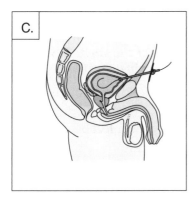

A. A _____ catheter is inserted to drain the bladder and then removed.

B. An _____ catheter is left inside the bladder to provide continuous urine drainage.

C. A _____ catheter is inserted surgically through an abdominal incision.

Activity H *Mark each statement as either "true" (T) or "false" (F). Correct the false statements.*

1. T F A urinary catheter is necessary for a person who is unable to urinate.

2. T F Health care–associated infections (HAIs) are not very common in people who have been catheterized.

3. T F Sterile technique helps to introduce infectious bacteria into the bladder.

Activity I *Select the single best answer for each of the following questions.*

1. A catheter is a tube that is inserted into the body for:
   a. Examining the contents of the small intestine
   b. Administering or removing fluids
   c. Supplying vitamins to the body
   d. Providing anesthesia

2. Which of the following catheters is also known as a retention or Foley catheter?
   a. Suprapubic catheter
   b. Indwelling catheter
   c. Ultrasonic catheter
   d. Straight catheter

Activity J *Mark each statement as either "true" (T) or "false" (F). Correct the false statements.*

1. T F Urinary incontinence can result from a bladder infection.

2. T F Urinary incontinence places a person at risk for skin problems.

3. T F Urinary incontinence is always permanent.

4. T F Childbirth, obesity, and loss of muscle tone as the result of aging can contribute to stress incontinence.

Activity K *Select the single best answer for each of the following questions.*

1. What is urge incontinence?

   a. The involuntary release of urine right after feeling a strong urge to void

   b. Another term used to indicate a urinary tract infection

   c. The inability of the bladder to empty during urination

   d. None of the above

2. What is functional incontinence?

   a. Incontinence that occurs in the absence of physical or nervous system problems affecting the urinary tract

   b. The state of being confused or disoriented

   c. A feeling of comfort experienced in a new environment

   d. The involuntary release of urine right after feeling a strong urge to void

3. Which of the following relates to overflow incontinence?

   a. It is a problem associated with water retention

   b. It is a problem that causes a person to dribble urine between visits to the bathroom

   c. It is a problem that causes the bladder muscle to spasm

   d. It is a problem that results from insufficient intake of water

Activity L *Fill in the blanks.*

1. _____ and _____ are worn under clothing to absorb moisture and keep it away from the body.

2. A _____ can be used to manage urinary incontinence in men.

Although caring for a person who is incontinent can be frustrating and emotionally draining, it is important to treat patients or residents who are incontinent with compassion. Having wet clothes or smelling like urine can be very embarrassing. In addition, being incontinent of urine places a person at risk for skin problems. When you help to keep a person who is incontinent clean and dry, you are protecting the person's physical health as well as her emotional health.

BOWEL ELIMINATION

Key Learning Points

- The process of bowel elimination and characteristics of normal stool
- Terms related to abnormal bowel function
- Types of enemas and their indications for use
- Proper technique for assisting with urinary and bowel elimination, obtaining urine and stool samples, providing catheter care, and administering enemas

Activity M *Fill in the blanks.*

1. _____ is a mixture of partially digested food and fluid.

2. The process of _____ moves chyme through the intestines.

3. _____ and _____ are natural by-products of digestion.

4. To _____ is to have a bowel movement.

Activity N *Mark each statement as either "true" (T) or "false" (F). Correct the false statement.*

1. T F The amount of food and fluids consumed does not affect a person's bowel patterns.

2. T F Enemas are often used to treat diarrhea.

3. T F Bacterial and viral infections are common causes of diarrhea.

4. T F Bowel movements vary from person to person.

5. T F Constipation, when not relieved, blocks the passage of normal stool, causing fecal impaction.

6. T F A finger is inserted into a person's rectum to check for fecal impaction.

Activity O *Select the single best answer for each of the following questions.*

1. Which of the following is a risk factor for constipation?

   a. Practicing good infection control techniques

   b. Exercising daily

   c. Eating little dietary fiber

   d. Administering an enema

2. Which of the following is a common method of bowel training?

  a. Offering the commode or bedpan at regular scheduled intervals

  b. Encouraging the person to eat less

  c. Using psychological methods to train the person

  d. None of the above

Activity P *Mark each statement as either "true" (T) or "false" (F). Correct the false statements.*

1. T F Diarrhea can cause dehydration, especially in young children and older adults.

2. T F Constipation develops when feces remain in the intestines for too long.

3. T F Regular and frequent use of laxatives is safe.

4. T F Stool softeners chemically stimulate the intestines to cause bowel movement.

5. T F A fecal impaction develops when diarrhea is not relieved.

6. T F Fecal (bowel) incontinence is the inability to hold one's feces, or the involuntary loss of feces from the bowel.

Activity Q *Think About It! Briefly answer the following questions in the space provided.*

Mrs. Joyce has a fecal impaction and requires an enema. Describe how to position and prepare her for this procedure.

_____

_____

_____

Activity R *Look at the following pictures and identify the different types of enemas.*

1. _____ A

2. _____ B

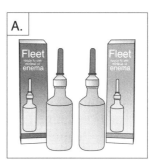

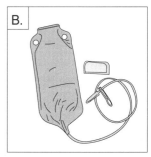

Activity S *Use the clues to complete the crossword puzzle.*

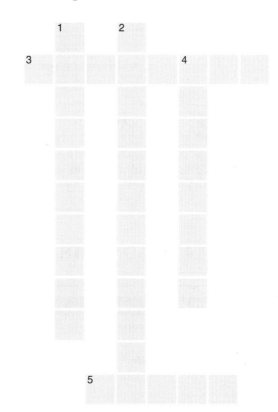

Across

3. A type of catheter that is inserted and removed immediately

5. The process of introducing fluid into the large intestine to remove stool from the rectum

Down

1. A pre-packaged, pre-mixed enema that usually contains a solution that irritates the intestinal mucosa to promote peristalsis

2. An enema containing mineral, olive, or cottonseed oil.

4. An enema that is prepared using castile soap and water

Activity T *Match the terms, given in Column A, with their descriptions, given in Column B.*

Column A

___ **1.** Cleansing enema

___ **2.** Oil retention enema

___ **3.** Commercial enema

___ **4.** Sim's

Column B

a. Used to help remove fecal impaction

b. Usually contains 120 ml of a solution that irritates the intestinal mucosa to promote peristalsis

c. Position that should be used to administer an enema

d. Used to empty the intestine of fecal material

> You can help your patients or residents to maintain normal bowel and urinary elimination by encouraging fluids, answering the call light promptly, and providing for the person's privacy and comfort.

CARING FOR A PERSON WITH AN OSTOMY

Key Learning Points

- How to provide routine stoma care

Activity U *Mark each statement as either "true" (T) or "false" (F). Correct the false statements.*

1. T F An ostomy is an alternate way of removing feces from the body.

2. T F When a person has an ostomy, the person passes feces through the anus and into a pouch called a stoma.

3. T F Diverticulitis is an inflammatory disease of the bowel.

4. T F A person with an ileostomy is quite prone to constipation.

5. T F A person with an ostomy created near the beginning of the large intestine will produce feces that are more solid and formed.

6. T F Because the skin around the ostomy comes into contact with feces, it must be kept clean to prevent irritation.

7. T F If the ostomy appliance is being changed while the person is in bed, the person should be positioned in either the Sim's OR the lateral position.

Activity V *Identify the type of ostomy shown in each of the figures.*

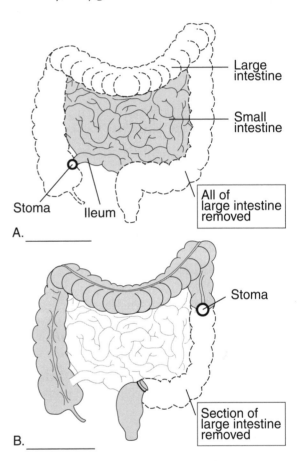

A. _____

B. _____

Activity W *Briefly answer the following question in the space provided.*

One of your residents, Mrs. Cheng, has been diagnosed with diverticulitis and will have to have a colostomy. Mrs. Cheng has always been a very modest and conservative lady. What can you do to help Mrs. Cheng adjust to her colostomy?

_____

_____

_____

Activity X *Some steps involved in providing stoma care are given below. After each step, write why it is done.*

1. Make sure that the bed is positioned at a comfortable working height.

_____

2. Fanfold the top linens to below the person's waist.

_____

3. Position the bed protector on the bed, alongside the person.

_____

4. Put on the gloves.

_____

5. Remove the ostomy appliance by holding the skin taut and gently pulling the appliance away, starting at the top. If the adhesive is making removal difficult, use warm water or the adhesive solvent to soften the adhesive.

_____

SUMMARY

Activity Y *Use the clues to find words that are present in the grid of letters, either horizontally from left to right, or vertically from top to bottom.*

Down

1. Involuntary wave-like muscular movements, such as those in the digestive system that move chyme (partially digested food) through the intestines
2. Voiding that is more frequent than usual
3. Voiding less than 100 mL of urine over 24 hours
4. Something hidden or invisible to the naked eye
5. A tube inserted into the body to administer or remove fluids

Q	A	Z	M	Q	P	A	S	Q
W	S	X	N	Z	M	P	D	A
E	D	C	H	Y	M	E	F	S
R	F	V	B	Q	A	R	G	W
T	G	O	V	W	S	I	H	F
Y	H	L	C	E	D	S	J	R
U	J	I	X	R	F	T	K	E
O	K	G	Z	T	G	A	L	Q
C	L	U	S	Y	H	L	Z	U
C	Z	R	A	C	T	S	X	E
U	R	I	N	A	T	I	O	N
L	E	A	K	T	L	S	I	C
T	T	U	I	H	B	D	K	Y
R	F	V	B	E	T	F	G	F
T	G	B	V	T	W	Z	X	B
W	U	R	G	E	N	C	Y	C
D	R	Q	R	R	T	Y	U	X
C	I	S	A	S	R	G	L	E
T	N	O	C	T	U	R	I	A
H	A	E	R	F	Y	U	I	S
B	E	D	P	A	N	C	F	A

Across

6. The liquid substance that results from digestion of food in the stomach
7. The process of passing urine from the body; also known as micturition and voiding
8. A device a man uses for defecation when he cannot get out of bed
9. The need to urinate immediately
10. The need to get up more than once or twice during the night to urinate

CHAPTER 22

Caring for People Who Are Terminally Ill

INTRODUCTION TO CARING FOR PEOPLE WHO ARE TERMINALLY ILL

Key Learning Points

- Terminal illness and examples of specific illnesses that are considered terminal

Activity A *Think About It! Briefly answer the following question in the space provided.*

List five diseases or conditions that are considered terminal.

_____

_____

_____

Activity B *Providing holistic care to patients and residents is always important, but even more so when caring for someone who is dying. Keeping this in mind, mark each statement as either "true" (T) or "false" (F). Correct the false statements.*

1. T F Focus on making the patient or resident comfortable and filling his or her last days with love and compassion.

2. T F Focus on the patient's or resident's physical as well as emotional and spiritual needs.

3. T F Avoid exploring your own feelings and emotions regarding death and dying.

4. T F A person who is dying may want to talk to you. Listen to whatever the patient or resident wants to say but remember to be judgmental.

> Caring for a terminally ill person can be very rewarding, but it can also be emotionally draining. When caring for a person who is terminally ill, recognize that you will also go through the grieving process as part of caring for the person, and make allowances for this.

STAGES OF GRIEF

Key Learning Points

- The stages of grief and their effects on the terminally ill person
- The effects of a terminal illness on the person's family

Activity C *Match the stages of grief given in Column A with their descriptions given in Column B.*

Column A	Column B
____ **1.** Denial	**a.** The person wants to makes a deal with someone he or she feels has control
____ **2.** Anger	

_____ **3.** Bargaining

_____ **4.** Depression

_____ **5.** Acceptance

over his or her fate (e.g., God, a health care provider).

b. The person will be sad and may have regrets about things he or she was not able to accomplish in his or her life.

c. The person refuses to accept the diagnosis or feels that a mistake has been made.

d. The person may become moody, withdrawn, unco-operative, or hostile.

e. The person completes unfinished business and says his or her goodbyes.

Activity D *Mark each statement as either "true" (T) or "false" (F). Correct the false statements.*

1. T F   As a nursing assistant, it is your duty to convince a terminally ill person that advances in medical technology can be of no help.

2. T F   You must allow a terminally ill person to experience a feeling of hope, without being unrealistic.

3. T F   When a family member of a terminally ill person directs her anger at you, you should take it personally.

4. T F   You should try to ignore a terminally ill person who wants to talk to you about death.

5. T F   Arranging for the assistance of clergy or other professionals experienced in grief counseling may be of great comfort to the patient and the family.

WILLS

Key Learning Points

- The role of a nursing assistant when a person wishes to make a will

Activity E *You are caring for Mr. Thomas, a terminally ill patient. Mr. Thomas expresses a desire to make a will. Briefly answer the following questions in the space provided.*

1. Do you think that this information needs to be relayed immediately to the nurse?

_____

2. Mr. Thomas asks you to sign his will as a witness. You are one of the benefactors of the will. What should you do under these circumstances?

_____

DYING WITH DIGNITY

Key Learning Points

- The terms "supportive care" and "palliative care" and how these types of care can be used to maintain a person's quality of life during the end-of-life period
- The role of hospice in the care of the terminally ill person
- Care concerns when providing for the needs of the person with a terminal illness

Activity F *Fill in the blanks using the words given in brackets.*

[supportive care, life-sustaining, palliative, hospice]

1. _____ entails offering treatments that will not prolong life, but will make a person more comfortable.

2. _____ agencies and facilities are organizations founded with the mission of offering the terminally ill person the best quality of life possible, and ensuring his or her comfort and dignity as death approaches.

3. _____ care focuses on relieving uncomfortable symptoms, not on curing the problem that is causing the symptoms.

4. _____ treatment tends to prolong life through respiratory ventilation, cardio-pulmonary resuscitation (CPR), and the placement of a feeding tube or intravenous (IV) line.

Activity G *Following are treatments that may be provided to a terminally ill person. Place an "SC" next to treatments that represent supportive care and an "LST" next to treatments that represent life-sustaining treatments.*

1. ____ Oxygen therapy

2. ____ Respiratory ventilation

3. ____ Placement of an IV line for provision of nutrition

4. ____ Nutritional supplementation

5. ____ Pain medication

6. ____ Grooming and hygiene

7. ____ Positioning assistance

8. ____ Cardiopulmonary resuscitation

EFFECTS OF CARING FOR THE TERMINALLY ILL ON THE CAREGIVER

Key Learning Points

■ How caring for terminally ill people can affect the nursing assistant

Activity H *Think About It! Briefly answer the following question in the space provided.*

You have been caring for Mrs. Ford, who is now in the last stage of cancer. As you watch her family suffer and grieve, you feel helpless and emotionally drained. How would you cope with this situation?

_____

_____

_____

SUMMARY

Activity I *Complete the crossword puzzle below using the following clues.*

Down

1. The stage in which the person will be sad and may have regrets about things he or she was not able to accomplish in life

2. The stage in which the person wants to "make a deal" with someone he or she feels has control over his or her fate

4. The stage in which the person comes to terms with the reality of his or her own impending death, and is finally at peace with this knowledge

6. A legal statement that expresses a person's wishes for the management of his or her affairs after death

Across

3. Mental anguish, specifically associated with loss

5. A desire for a positive occurrence or outcome

7. The stage in which the person refuses to accept the diagnosis or feels that a mistake has been made

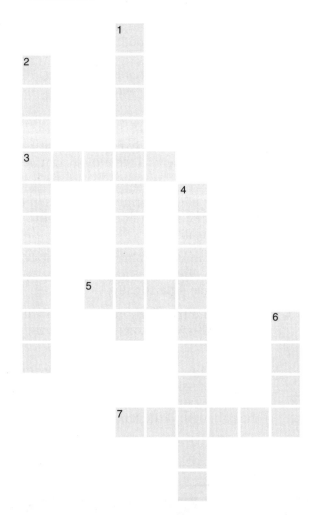

CHAPTER 23

Caring for People Who Are Dying

INTRODUCTION TO CARING FOR PEOPLE WHO ARE DYING

Key Learning Points

- How a nursing assistant's own feelings about death can affect the care given to a dying patient or resident
- The physical signs that frequently signal impending death

Activity A *Think About It! Briefly answer the following question in the space provided.*

As a nursing assistant, you will certainly find yourself in the position of caring for a patient or resident who is dying. Explore your own feelings and attitudes towards death. What have been your own personal experiences with death? In what way do you think this would affect the care you provide to your terminally ill patients or residents?

_____

_____

_____

Activity B *Write the words given in the brackets next to their descriptions.*

[cyanotic, Cheyne-Stokes respiration, biological death, brain dead]

1. _____ Mr. Tindall's vital body functions have stopped.

2. _____ Miss Martha's skin appears blue-tinged.

3. _____ Mrs. Tinowicz breathes in an irregular, shallow, and an alternating fast-slow pattern.

4. _____ Mr. Wolenski has been showing no brain activity for more than 24 hours.

Activity C *Select the single best answer for the following questions.*

1. Which of the following is a physical sign of impending death?
   a. Increased pain
   b. Increased thirst
   c. Irregular, shallow breathing
   d. Increased urine output

2. Which of the following happens when circulation fails?
   a. The blood pressure rises
   b. The pulse becomes rapid and weak
   c. The skin feels warm
   d. The body temperature falls

3. Which of the following generally does NOT result from nervous system changes?
   a. Decreased muscle tone
   b. Blurred vision
   c. Loss of sensation in arms and legs
   d. Diminished hearing

Activity D *Match the body functions given in Column A with their signs of failure given in Column B.*

Column A

____ **1.** Circulation

____ **2.** Respiration

____ **3.** Digestion

____ **4.** Nervous system

Column B

a. A person may experience nausea, vomiting, abdominal swelling, fecal impaction, or bowel incontinence

b. A person's blood pressure drops and the pulse becomes rapid and weak

c. A person may lose sensation in his arms or legs, and pain may diminish

d. A person may take very irregular, shallow breaths, in an alternating fast–slow pattern

CARING FOR A DYING PERSON

Key Learning Points

- Ways in which the nursing assistant can provide comfort for the dying person
- How cultural and religious influences can affect how the dying person views death

Activity E *Place an "X" next to the statements that reflect behavior that may be an unconscious effort on the nursing assistant's part to avoid a person who is dying.*

1. ____ The nursing assistant does not check in on the dying person as often as he checks in on his other patients or residents.

2. ____ The nursing assistant provides only the necessary care and then leaves the person's room quickly, afraid that if he stays, the person will want to talk about death.

3. ____ The nursing assistant shows an interest in the person and allows the person to talk about death.

4. ____ The nursing assistant expresses concerns such as, "I'm afraid I'll cry if my resident dies."

5. ____ The nursing assistant becomes attached to his patient or resident and feels concerned about the person's death.

6. ____ The nursing assistant acts overly cheerful when around the dying person.

Activity F *The following sentences are related to providing holistic care to a dying person. Observe the figure and fill in the blanks in the sentences below using the words given in brackets.*

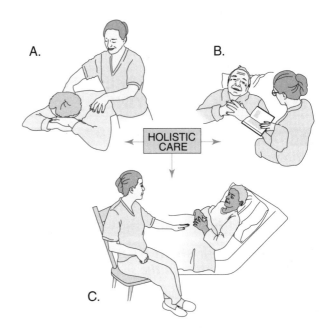

[physical, back massage, spiritual, emotional]

1. By taking care of the dying person's _____ and _____ needs, the nursing assistant provides holistic care.

2. A _____ can help a person to rest and feel better.

3. By reading aloud from a holy book that has special meaning for the person, the nursing assistant would be helping the person to meet his or her _____ needs.

Activity G *Place an "X" next to the activities that would help a nursing assistant meet a dying person's physical needs.*

1. ___ Providing frequent skin care to a patient or resident

2. ___ Listening when the patient or resident wants to talk

3. ___ Providing frequent oral care to a patient or resident

4. ___ Repositioning the person frequently

5. ___ Letting the patient or resident cry

6. ___ Asking a counselor to speak to the patient or resident about death

Activity H *Select the single best answer for each of the following questions.*

1. To make communication more effective, what kind of questions should you ask the dying person if she loses the ability to speak clearly?

   a. Open-ended questions

   b. "Fill in the blanks" questions

   c. "Yes or No" questions

   d. Multiple choice questions

2. How would you respond if a family member expresses a wish to assist in providing physical care to the dying person?

   a. Encourage the family member by suggesting ways in which he or she can help.

   b. Assume that the family member will not be able to provide care to a dying person, as he or she has no formal training.

   c. Ask the family member to wait until you have finished caring for the dying person.

   d. Just say "I will have to ask the nurse about this."

3. Which of the following actions would let a person know that she is cared for and is not alone?

   a. Gently holding the person's hand or touching her shoulder when you are speaking to her

   b. Gently smoothing the person's hair after you have finished straightening the bed linens

   c. Comforting the person with a back massage

   d. All of the above

Activity I *Match the terms given in Column A with their descriptions given in Column B.*

Column A

___ 1. Spirituality

___ 2. Reincarnation

___ 3. Afterlife

Column B

a. The idea that a person's soul will live again on Earth in the form of an animal or human being yet to be born

b. A state of being where the dead meet again with loved ones who have passed on before them

c. A belief that a higher being offers hope and peace

> Providing holistic care is as important at the end of life as it is at any other time. You must take steps to prevent any discomfort you may have with the subject of death from compromising your ability to care for people who are dying.

CARE OF THE FAMILY

Key Learning Points

- The different ways in which family members may show grief
- Ways that a nursing assistant can help the family of a dying person

Activity J *Select the single best answer for each of the following questions.*

1. Mr. Potter is terminally ill. His family is outside his room, looking tired and worried. When you approach them and ask if they need anything, Mr. Potter's daughter snaps at you, saying, "How dare you ask us that! You don't know the kind of grief we are going through. Leave us alone!" How would you respond?

   a. You would snap back at Mr. Potter's daughter.

   b. You would walk away without saying a word, and ignore them for the rest of the day.

   c. You would continue to be polite and not take Mr. Potter's daughter's words personally.

   d. You would insist that they have some refreshments, whether they would like to or not.

2. You are walking past Mrs. Green's room, when you hear loud voices coming from inside the room. When you look inside, you see that a few family members are arguing heatedly and seem to be on the verge of starting a fight. What would you do?

   a. Notify the nurse immediately

   b. Enter the room and ask the family members to calm down

   c. Stand in between those who are arguing, in an attempt to prevent a fight from occurring.

   d. Assume that it is a family matter that does not concern you, and carry on with your duties.

Activity K *A nursing assistant can help comfort the family of a dying person by way of simple kindnesses. Fill in the blanks using the words given in brackets.*

[help, basic needs, talk, competent, good communication, compassionate]

1. Ensure _____ between the family members and the health care team.

2. Encourage family members to _____ to the dying person and to _____ with the person's care.

3. Ensure that the family members' _____ are met.

4. Often, the most comforting thing to family members is knowing that their loved one is receiving _____, _____ care.

> Ensuring good communication between the health care team and the family members, meeting the family members' basic needs, and being available to provide care for the person who is dying are all ways that you can comfort the family.

POSTMORTEM CARE

Key Learning Points

- The various responsibilities that a nursing assistant may have following the death of a patient or resident

Activity L *Mark each statement as either "true" (T) or "false" (F). Correct the false statements.*

1. T F   Postmortem care is the care of a person's body before the person's death.

2. T F   Postmortem care is necessary to prevent skin damage and discoloration.

3. T F   Rigor mortis is the stiffening of the muscles that usually develops within 2 to 4 hours of death.

4. T F   It is easy to position the body in proper alignment after rigor mortis occurs.

5. T F   An autopsy is an examination of the person's organs and tissues after the person has died.

Activity M *The figure below shows the contents of the postmortem care kit. Identify the items and write their names in the corresponding spaces below.*

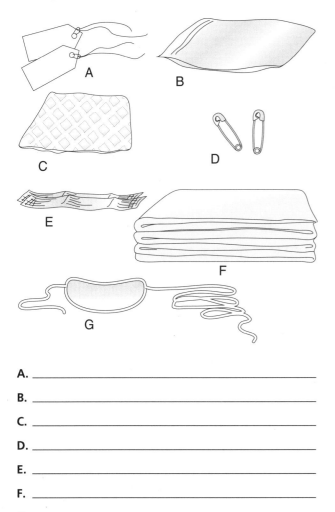

A. _____

B. _____

C. _____

D. _____

E. _____

F. _____

G. _____

Activity N *Select the single best answer for the following question.*

1. When preparing a person's body for the family to view after death, we do all of the following EXCEPT:

   a. Change the soiled bed linens

   b. Cover the person's face with a sheet

   c. Straighten up the room

   d. Collect the person's belongings

SUMMARY

Activity O *Words shown in the picture have been jumbled. Use the clues to form correct words using the letters given in the picture.*

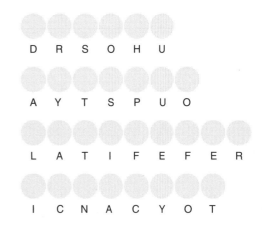

D R S O H U

A Y T S P U O

L A T I F E F E R

I C N A C Y O T

1. A covering used to wrap the body of a person who has died
2. Examination of a person's organs and tissues after the person has died, done to confirm or identify the cause of the person's death
3. A state of being where the dead meet again with loved ones who have passed on before them
4. Adjective used to describe skin, lips, or nail beds that have a blue or gray tinge

CHAPTER 24

Basic Body Structure and Function

INTRODUCTION TO BASIC BODY STRUCTURE AND FUNCTION

Key Learning Points

■ The definition of the terms *anatomy* and *physiology*

Activity A *Fill in the blanks using the words given in the brackets.*

[anatomy, physiology, disease, health care team]

1. The _____ plays an important role in helping people to achieve their best possible level of functioning.

2. _____ is the study of how the body parts work.

3. Changes in a person's normal anatomy or physiology can lead to _____ or disability.

4. _____ is the study of what body parts look like, where they are located, how big they are, and how they connect to other body parts.

HOW IS THE BODY ORGANIZED?

Key Learning Points

■ The basic organizational levels of the body

Activity B *Match the terms given in Column A with their descriptions given in Column B.*

Column A

_____ 1. Cell membrane

_____ 2. Nucleus

_____ 3. Organelles

_____ 4. Cytoplasm

Column B

a. Jelly-like substance of a cell where the organelles float

b. Structures inside of the cell that help the cell to make the energy it needs to stay alive and rid itself of waste products

c. The cell's "brain"; contains all of the information the cell needs to do its job, grow, and reproduce

d. Surrounds the cytoplasm and gives the cell its shape

Activity C *All living things share the same basic levels of organization. Take a look at the following figure. Write the correct order of the levels of organization by filling in the boxes below.*

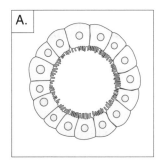

A.

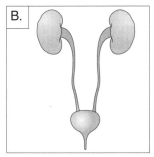

B.

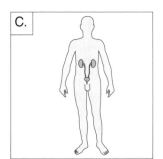

C.

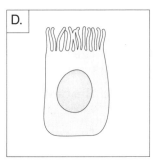

D.

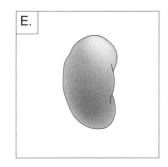

E.

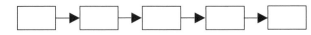

Activity D *Look at the following figure. Label the figure using the words given in brackets.*

[rough endoplasmic reticulum, Golgi apparatus, smooth endoplasmic reticulum, centrioles, mitochondrion]

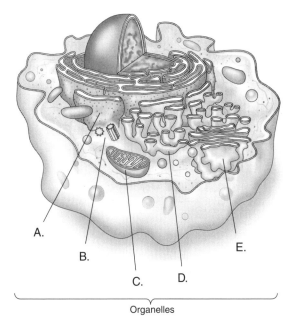

A.

B.

C.

D.

E.

Organelles

A. _____

B. _____

C. _____

D. _____

E. _____

Activity E *Match the types of tissues given in Column A with their functions given in Column B.*

Column A

_____ **1.** Epithelial tissue

_____ **2.** Connective tissue

_____ **3.** Muscle tissue

_____ **4.** Nervous tissue

Column B

a. Conducts information

b. Produces movement

c. Supports and forms the framework for all parts of the body

d. Covers the outside of the body, lines its internal structures, and forms glands

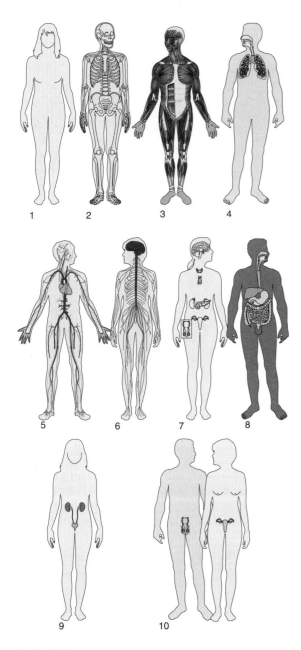

7. _____

8. _____

9. _____

10. _____

Activity G *Match the organ systems given in Column A with their corresponding organs given in Column B.*

Column A

____ **1.** The integumen-tary system

____ **2.** The skeletal system

____ **3.** The muscular system

____ **4.** The respiratory system

____ **5.** The cardio-vascular system

____ **6.** The nervous system

____ **7.** The endocrine system

____ **8.** The digestive system

____ **9.** The urinary system

____ **10.** The reproductive system

Column B

a. The lungs and the airways

b. The blood, the heart, and the blood vessels

c. The bones

d. The skin and its glands, the hair, and the nails

e. The muscles

f. The kidneys, the bladder, the ureters, and the urethra

g. The sex organs (i.e. ovaries, testes)

h. The brain, spinal cord, and nerves

i. The glands throughout the body that produce hormones

j. The teeth, sali-vary glands, tongue, esopha-gus, stomach, small intestine, large intestine, liver, pancreas, and gallbladder

Activity F *An organ system is a group of organs that work together to perform a specific function for the body. Human beings have ten main organ systems. Identify the organ systems shown in the figures above.*

1. _____

2. _____

3. _____

4. _____

5. _____

6. _____

HEALTH AND DISEASE

Key Learning Points

- The definition of the term *homeostasis* and examples of how the body maintains the balance necessary for life
- How the body's inability to maintain homeostasis affects a person's health
- The categories of disease and some factors that may put a person at risk for developing a certain disease

Activity H *Think About It! Briefly answer the following question in the space provided.*

You are playing tennis with a friend. As you run back and forth on the court, you start breathing harder and your heart rate increases. Soon, you begin to sweat and feel thirsty. Describe the changes your body is making to maintain homeostasis, or a state of internal balance.

_____

_____

_____

Activity I *Mark each statement as either "true" (T) or "false" (F). Correct the false statements.*

1. T F   A person's living conditions and health habits do not play a major role in a person's overall health.

2. T F   A person who has a chronic disease, such as diabetes or high blood pressure, is at increased risk for developing another disease.

3. T F   Some types of cancer, diabetes, and heart disease can be inherited.

4. T F   A person's emotional health does not directly affect his or her physical health.

Activity J *List at least five factors that can put a person at risk for disease, or negatively affect his or her ability to recover from disease.*

1. _____

2. _____

3. _____

4. _____

5. _____

Activity K *The following sentences are related to common categories of diseases. Fill in the blanks using the words given in brackets.*

[Degenerative diseases, Metabolic (endocrine) disorders, Immune disorders, Psychiatric disorders]

1. _____, such as diabetes, occur when the body is unable to metabolize or absorb certain nutrients.

2. _____, such as depression, affect a person's ability to function normally.

3. _____, such as AIDS, reduce the immune system's ability to fight off infection.

4. _____, such as osteoporosis and muscular dystrophy, occur when the tissues of the body wear out or break down.

All of the organ systems constantly work together to maintain a state of balance or homeostasis. A disease occurs when the structure or function of an organ or an organ system is abnormal. Being aware of the factors that put a person at risk for disease will allow you to provide better care for your patients or residents because you will have a better understanding of each person's special needs.

SUMMARY

Activity L   *Use the clues to find words that are present in the grid of letters, either horizontally from left to right or vertically from top to bottom.*

Down

1. A group of cells similar in structure and specialized to perform a specific function
2. Impaired physical or emotional function
3. The jelly-like substance within a cell within which the organelles float
4. Structures inside of the cell that help the cell to make the energy it needs to stay alive and to rid itself of waste products

Across

1. A condition that occurs when the structure or function of an organ or an organ system is abnormal
2. The basic unit of life
3. The study of what body parts look like, where they are located, how big they are, and how they connect to other body parts
4. A group of tissues functioning together for a similar purpose
5. The cell's "brain"; it contains all of the information the cell needs in order to do its job, grow, and reproduce

Q	W	T	E	T	D	E	Q	U
A	S	I	R	T	I	F	A	J
D	I	S	E	A	S	E	Z	M
Q	U	S	X	O	A	Q	W	I
A	J	U	E	L	B	A	Y	W
Z	M	E	D	P	I	X	H	C
W	I	T	C	E	L	L	N	V
S	K	H	H	M	I	U	Y	C
X	O	A	N	A	T	O	M	Y
E	L	W	E	R	Y	L	E	T
D	P	O	D	F	G	P	D	O
C	O	R	G	A	N	O	C	P
R	A	G	N	V	C	O	C	L
F	H	A	U	R	W	A	R	A
V	J	N	U	C	L	E	U	S
Y	W	E	Y	W	E	L	E	M
H	C	L	H	C	D	P	D	H
N	V	L	N	V	C	O	C	N
U	R	E	U	R	Q	A	R	U
J	N	S	J	N	F	H	F	J

CHAPTER 25

The Integumentary System

INTRODUCTION TO THE INTEGUMENTARY SYSTEM

Key Learning Points

- Changes in a person's normal skin color that can indicate a serious health problem

Activity A *Match the terms, given in Column A, with their definitions, given in Column B.*

Column A

_____ **1.** Jaundice

_____ **2.** Pallor

_____ **3.** Flushing

_____ **4.** Cyanosis

Column B

a. A paleness of skin

b. A blue or gray discoloration of the skin, lips, and nail beds

c. A yellow discoloration of the skin and the whites of the eyes

d. A redness of skin

As the body's most visible organ system, the integumentary system can provide clues to a person's overall health. Changes in a person's skin tone or the development of a rash may signal an internal problem, such as liver disease, a heart or lung problem, or an infection.

STRUCTURE OF THE INTEGUMENTARY SYSTEM

Key Learning Points

- The layers of the skin
- The accessory structures of the skin

Activity B *Match the terms, given in Column A, with their definitions, given in Column B.*

Column A

_____ **1.** Keratin

_____ **2.** Melanin

_____ **3.** Sebum

_____ **4.** Eccrine gland

_____ **5.** Apocrine gland

Column B

a. Produces a thin, watery fluid

b. Found mostly in the skin of the armpits (axillae) and the perineum

c. A substance that causes cells to thicken and become resistant to water

d. A dark pigment that gives our skin, hair, and eyes color

e. An oily substance that lubricates the skin and helps to prevent it from drying out

Activity C *A figure of the skin is shown below. Label the figure using the words given in brackets.*

[hair follicle, dermis, epidermis, melanin-producing cells, sweat gland, subcutaneous tissue]

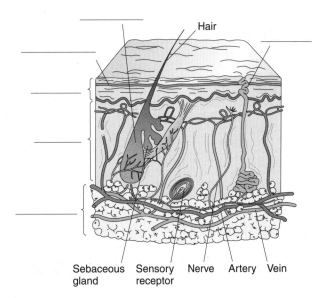

Sebaceous gland Sensory receptor Nerve Artery Vein

Activity D *Mark each statement as either "true" (T) or "false" (F). Correct the false statements.*

1. T F The epidermis is the outer layer of the skin.

2. T F The epidermis contains blood vessels and nerve cells.

3. T F The dermis is the deepest layer of the skin.

4. T F The blood vessels and nerves that supply the skin originate in the subcutaneous tissue and send branches into the dermis.

5. T F The sebum is slightly basic.

6. T F Melanin gives the hair its color.

7. T F Nails are made of special skin cells that have been hardened by the presence of keratin.

FUNCTION OF THE INTEGUMENTARY SYSTEM

Key Learning Points

■ The major functions of the integumentary system

Activity E *Place an "X" next to the function(s) of the body's integumentary system.*

1. ____ It offers a physical form of protection against microbes, chemicals, and other agents that could harm the body.

2. ____ It helps to maintain the body's fluid balance.

3. ____ It helps to regulate the body's temperature.

4. ____ It kills bacteria that invade our body.

5. ____ It absorbs fluid to maintain fluid balance.

6. ____ It eliminates small amounts of waste material.

Activity F *Look at the figures given below. Then fill in the blanks using the words given in brackets.*

[low, high, dilate, constrict, less, more]

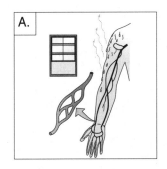 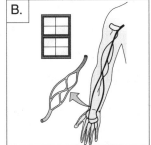

The skin plays an important role in maintaining the body's temperature within the proper range. When the internal temperature is _____, the blood vessels in the skin _____, causing _____ blood to pass near the surface of the skin, allowing heat to escape into the environment. When the internal temperature is too _____, the blood vessels in the skin _____, causing _____ blood to pass near the surface of the skin, keeping the heat inside of the body.

THE EFFECTS OF AGING ON THE INTEGUMENTARY SYSTEM

Key Learning Points

- How normal aging processes affect the integumentary system

Activity G *Mark each statement as either "true" (T) or "false" (F). Correct the false statements.*

1. **T F** Wrinkles, gray hair, and "age spots" are all very visible signs of a skin disease.

2. **T F** "Age spots" (sometimes called "liver spots") are caused by deposits of bile in certain areas.

3. **T F** Wrinkles form due to the loss of collagen and the thinning of adipose (fatty) tissue in the subcutaneous layer.

4. **T F** Brown hair is caused by the loss of melanin from the hair.

Activity H *Think About It! Briefly answer the following question in the space provided.*

Mrs. Diehl is 92 years old. What special precautions would you take to protect her skin when you are assisting her with routine activities such as bathing, transferring, and grooming? Why are these precautions necessary?

_____

_____

_____

DISORDERS OF THE INTEGUMENTARY SYSTEM

Key Learning Points

- How pressure ulcers are formed and what conditions may increase a patient's or resident's risk of developing a pressure ulcer
- How the nursing assistant helps to prevent residents and patients from developing pressure ulcers

- The different types of wounds that a patient or resident might have
- The nursing assistant's duties regarding wound care
- Terms used to describe skin lesions

Activity I *Place an "X" next to the statements that describe conditions that can lead to the development of a pressure ulcer.*

1. ____ When a part of a person's body presses against a surface, such as a mattress

2. ____ When a person sleeps on wrinkled bed linens or an object in the bed for a long period

3. ____ When a person sits on a bedpan for a long period

4. ____ When a person wears a splint or brace that presses against the skin

5. ____ When a person has a new rash on his or her body

Activity J *Look at the figures and mark the pressure points where pressure ulcers are likely to form.*

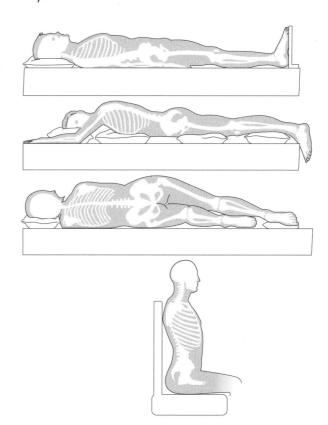

Activity K *Some of the events that lead to the development of a pressure ulcer are listed below. Write down the correct order of the steps in the boxes provided below.*

1. Lack of blood flow to the tissue deprives the tissue of oxygen and nutrients.
2. Tissue death, called necrosis, occurs as a result of a lack of oxygen.
3. The weight of the person's body squeezes the soft tissue between the bony prominence and the surface the person is resting on.
4. The necrotic (dead) skin and underlying tissues peel off or break open, creating an open sore.
5. The flow of blood to the tissue is disrupted.

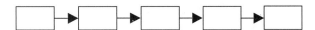

Activity L *Think About It! Briefly answer the following question in the space provided.*

Mr. Vincente, a home health care client, is 72 years old. He has congestive heart failure. Because it is difficult for him to walk and he tires very easily, Mr. Vincente usually moves from the bed to his easy chair in front of the television in the morning and stays there all day, getting up only occasionally to go to the bathroom. Because Mr. Vincente is a widower and he doesn't have much interest in cooking, he eats mostly microwave dinners and prepackaged snacks. Mr. Vincente lives in the southern United States, where it gets very hot and humid in the summer, and his house is not air-conditioned. What risk factors for the development of a pressure ulcer does Mr. Vincente have?

_____

_____

_____

_____

_____

Activity M *The four stages of a developing pressure ulcer are shown below. Look at the picture and write down the correct order of the stages in the boxes provided below.*

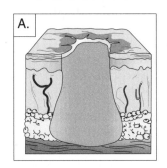

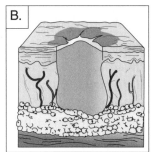

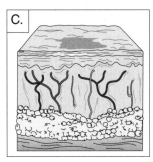

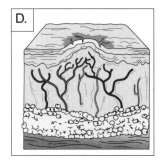

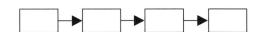

Activity N *As a nursing assistant, there are many things you can do to help keep a person's skin healthy. Briefly describe what the nursing assistant is doing to keep the person's skin healthy in each of the figures below.*

A. _____

B. _____

C. _____

D. _____

E. _____

F. _____

G. _____

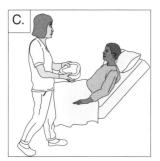

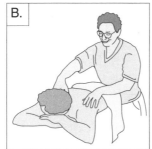

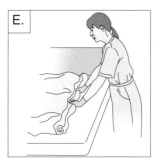

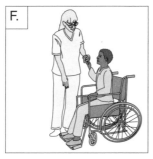

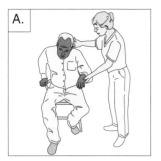

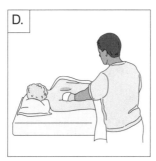

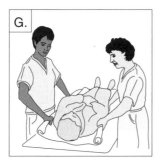

Activity O *Match the specialty beds, given in Column A, with their descriptions, given in Column B.*

Column A

____ **1.** An air fluidized bed

____ **2.** An alternating pressure bed

____ **3.** An XPRT Pulmonary Therapy Surface

Column B

a. Offers rotational percussion and vibration therapies

b. Supports the person on a fabric-covered layer of tiny ceramic beads

c. Supports the person on a series of compartments that fill with air and then deflate on a rotating basis

Prevention of pressure ulcers is extremely important, because pressure ulcers are very painful, difficult to treat, and potentially fatal. You will do many things to prevent your patients or residents from developing pressure ulcers, including repositioning, observing, providing good skin and perineal care, changing wet and soiled linens promptly, and encouraging exercise.

Activity P *Match the different types of wound healing, given in Column A, with their descriptions, given in Column B.*

Column A	Column B
____ **1.** First-intention wound healing	**a.** Wound is left open for a period of time to make sure that an infection is not going to occur, then the wound edges are cleaned and closed with sutures or staples
____ **2.** Second-intention wound healing	
____ **3.** Third-intention wound healing	
	b. Wound is closed surgically with sutures or staples
	c. Wound is cleaned, rinsed and left open to heal from the inside out

Activity Q *Think About It! Briefly answer the following question in the space provided.*

You are caring for Mr. Smith, who has a wound drain that is connected to a collection device. You know that you should check the collection device frequently. What observations about the drainage in the collection device would you report to the nurse immediately?

_____

_____

_____

Activity R *Some of the steps in the procedure for using a Montgomery tie, as shown in the figure, are listed below. Write down the correct order of the steps in the boxes provided below.*

a. The adhesive strip of the Montgomery tie is applied to the person's skin alongside the dressing.

b. The dressing is placed on the wound.

c. The ties are tied together over the dressing, to hold it in place.

d. When it is time to change the dressing, the ties are untied, the dressing is replaced, and then the ties are retied.

e. Another Montgomery tie is placed in the same way on the other side of the dressing.

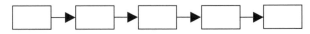

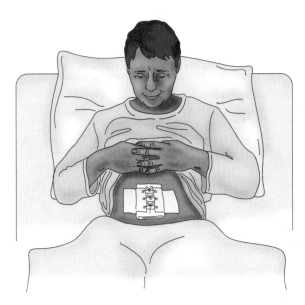

Activity S *Match the types of burns, given in Column A, with their descriptions, given in Column B.*

Column A	Column B
____ **1.** First-degree burns	**a.** Involve the epidermis and dermis, the subcutaneous layer, and often the underlying muscles and bones as well
____ **2.** Second-degree burns	
____ **3.** Third-degree burns	
	b. Cause injury to the outermost layer of the skin, the epidermis
	c. Penetrate into the dermis of the skin

Activity T *Use the clues to complete the crossword puzzle.*

Across

4. A vesicle that contains pus, a thick, yellowish fluid
6. An abrasion, or a scraping away of the surface of the skin

Down

1. A small, flat, reddened lesion
2. A group of lesions
3. A general term for inflammation of the skin
4. A small, raised, firm, lesion
5. A general term used to describe any break in the skin
7. Skin disorder caused by the chicken-pox virus

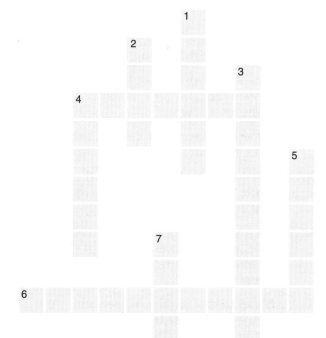

SUMMARY

Activity U *Words shown in the picture have been jumbled. Use the clues to form correct words using the letters given in the picture.*

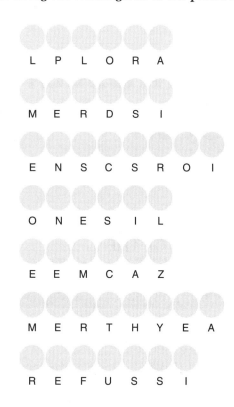

L P L O R A

M E R D S I

E N S C S R O I

O N E S I L

E E M C A Z

M E R T H Y E A

R E F U S S I

1. Paleness of the skin
2. The deepest layer of skin, where sensory receptors, blood vessels, nerves, glands, and hair follicles are found
3. Tissue death as a result of a lack of oxygen
4. A general term used to describe any break in the skin
5. A type of chronic dermatitis that is usually accompanied by severe itching, scaling, and crusting of the surface of the skin
6. Redness of the skin
7. A crack in the skin

CHAPTER 26

The Musculoskeletal System

STRUCTURE OF THE MUSCULOSKELETAL SYSTEM

Key Learning Points

- The major parts of the musculoskeletal system
- The four types of bones found in the skeletal system
- Terms used to describe joint movement
- The three types of muscles found in the muscular system

Activity A *Mark each statement as either "true" (T) or "false" (F). Correct the false statements.*

1. T F Long bones consist of a shaft, called the epiphyses, and two rounded ends, called the diaphysis.

2. T F The range of motion of a joint is the complete extent of movement that the joint is normally capable of without causing pain.

3. T F The skeleton gives structure and shape to the body, and protects key vital organs, such as the heart and the brain, from injury.

4. T F Synovial fluid, a tough, fibrous substance, fills in the space between the bones in a slightly movable joint and acts as a shock absorber.

5. T F Skeletal muscle is involuntary muscle.

Activity B *Place an "X" next to the statements that correctly describe a bone.*

1. _____ Bones are strong enough to support and protect the body and yet light enough to allow movement.

2. _____ Bones are classified according to their joint structure.

3. _____ The outside of the bone is hard and solid while the inside of the bone is sponge-like and airy.

4. _____ Thin strands of bone form a net-like structure, and the spaces in between the thin strands of bone are filled with bone marrow.

5. _____ Bones do not require oxygen and nutrients because they are not made of living cells.

FUNCTION OF THE MUSCULOSKELETAL SYSTEM

Key Learning Points

- The main functions of the musculoskeletal system

Activity C *Mark each statement as either "true" (T) or "false" (F). Correct the false statements.*

1. T F   The skull surrounds and protects the brain, while the rib cage surrounds and protects the lungs and heart.

2. T F   Sodium, an important mineral that keeps the bones strong and helps the cardiac muscle to function properly, is stored in the bones.

3. T F   The muscles of the back, neck, shoulders, and abdomen help us to maintain an upright posture.

4. T F   Contraction of the skeletal muscles helps us to maintain a constant body temperature by cooling us down.

5. T F   Contracting a muscle causes it to shorten, drawing the origin and insertion points closer to each other, resulting in movement.

6. T F   The bones function as a factory for the production of blood cells.

THE EFFECTS OF AGING ON THE MUSCULOSKELETAL SYSTEM

Key Learning Points

- How normal aging processes affect the musculoskeletal system

Activity D *Think About It! Briefly answer the following question in the space provided.*

The normal process of aging causes significant changes in the musculoskeletal system. List three normal age-related changes that affect the musculoskeletal system. Then describe how each of these changes can affect the elderly people in your care, especially if other factors are present that make these changes occur at a much faster rate.

_____

_____

_____

_____

_____

Many of the people you will care for will have problems with mobility as a result of aging or a musculoskeletal disorder. Many of your daily duties are related to preventing complications of immobility, relieving musculoskeletal discomfort, and helping your patients or residents to retain or regain musculoskeletal function.

DISORDERS OF THE MUSCULOSKELETAL SYSTEM

Key Learning Points

- Disorders that can affect the musculoskeletal system

Activity E *Think About It! Briefly answer the following question in the space provided.*

Mrs. Bradford has osteoporosis. List four special considerations that you will have when caring for Mrs. Bradford.

_____

_____

_____

Activity F *There are three common types of arthritis you may see in the health care setting. Fill in the table below, which summarizes these three types of arthritis, using the words given in brackets.*

[tear, autoimmune, women (*used two times*) crystals, elderly, wear, uric, middle age, men (*used two times*), young]

	OSTEOARTHRITIS	RHEUMATOID ARTHRITIS	GOUT
Cause	A degenerative disorder that is the result of normal _____ and _____ on the joint	Thought to be an _____ disorder, occurring when the immune system attacks the body's own tissues	A metabolic disorder that is caused by a build-up of _____ acid, leading to the formation of _____ in the joints
Most Likely to Affect	_____ people; both genders	_____ people, _____ more often than _____	People older than _____; _____ more often than _____

Activity G *Fill in the blanks using the words given in brackets.*

[myasthenia gravis, total joint replacement, abduction, dowager's hump, estrogen, phantom pain, prosthetic, cast]

1. A _____ involves removing the ends of the bones in the affected joint and replacing them with parts made from metal and plastic.

2. A _____ device may allow a person who has had a limb amputated to regain mobility, function, and a more normal appearance.

3. Patients who have had hip replacement surgery need to use a special wedge-shaped pillow, called an _____ pillow, which goes between the legs and attaches to each leg with Velcro fasteners.

4. _____ may be experienced by a person who has had a body part amputated and is caused by the healing of the nerves that were cut during the surgery.

5. _____, a hormone, helps to prevent bone loss in women.

6. Crumbling of the bones of the spinal column causes the upper back to curve into the deformity known as a _____.

7. In _____, the muscle's ability to respond to commands from the nervous system is affected.

8. A _____ is a method of external fixation, or fixation that is achieved without surgery.

Activity H *Place an "X" next to the risk factors that can increase a person's risk for developing osteoporosis.*

1. ____ Menopause

2. ____ White race

3. ____ Excess estrogen

4. ____ "Small bones"

5. ____ Smoking

6. ____ Inactivity or immobility

7. ____ Diseases of the thyroid and adrenal glands

8. ____ Lifting weights

9. ____ A diet that is high in calcium, vitamin D, and protein

10. ____ Excessive use of steroids

Activity I *Think About It! Briefly answer the following question in the space provided.*

Mr. Whitman recently had hip replacement surgery. What special considerations do you need to keep in mind when caring for Mr. Whitman?

_____

_____

_____

Activity J *Mark each statement as either "true" (T) or "false" (F). Correct the false statements.*

1. T F Osteoporosis is most common in older men.

2. T F While gout can affect any joint, the big toe is most commonly affected.

3. T F In rheumatoid arthritis, the person dies because the muscles that allow him to breathe eventually become too weak to perform this vital function.

4. T F Fixation is the word used to describe the process of bringing the broken ends of the bone into alignment.

5. T F The notation "ORIF" on a person's chart means that the person has had surgery to achieve an "Open Reduction, Internal Fixation."

6. T F Osteoporosis, or excessive loss of bone tissue, is a normal age-related change.

7. T F The bones most commonly affected by osteoporosis are the bones of the spine, the pelvis, and the long bones in the arms and legs.

8. T F In an older person, fractures take longer to heal and they may heal improperly.

9. T F Complications from diabetes can lead to the need for amputation of the foot or toe.

Activity K *Following are some steps in the development of osteoarthritis. Write down the correct order of the steps by filling in the boxes below.*

A. The cycle repeats until the cartilage has been worn down to the point where bone is actually rubbing against bone as the joint moves.
B. The joint becomes swollen, stiff, and very painful.
C. The rough area becomes inflamed, and bony deposits build up.

D. The bony deposits rub against the cartilage, causing even more damage.
E. Due to normal use of the joint, the smooth cartilage on the ends of the bones becomes rough.

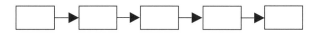

Activity L *A few common types of fractures are depicted. Use the clues provided in the pictures to complete the crossword puzzle.*

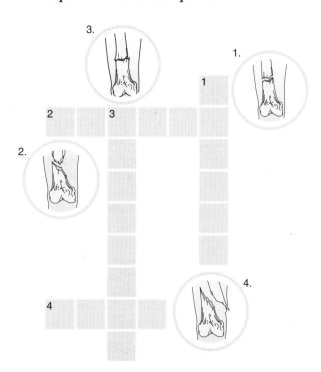

Now, write the name of the fracture next to its description below.

1. _____ The broken ends of the bone do not protrude through the skin

2. _____ Carries a very high risk of infection

3. _____ Common in children, because their bones are quite flexible

4. _____ Often seen in people who have fallen or jumped from a great height

5. _____ Often seen when a bone has been crushed under great weight

6. _____ Common when the bone has been subjected to a twisting force

Activity M *There are several different ways to treat fractures. Match each treatment, given in Column A, with its description, given in Column B.*

Column A

_____ 1. Closed reduction

_____ 2. External fixation

_____ 3. Internal fixation

_____ 4. Open reduction

_____ 5. Traction

Column B

a. A cast made of fiberglass or plaster of Paris is applied to keep the bone in proper alignment until healing occurs

b. Metal plates, screws, rods, pins or wires are used to hold the broken ends of the bone in place until the bone is healed

c. The doctor lines up the ends of the bone by pushing them back into place

d. Used to keep the broken ends of the bone in alignment until the fracture can be permanently repaired

e. The bone is surgically exposed so that the doctor can line up the ends of the broken bones

GENERAL CARE MEASURES

Key Learning Points

- Methods used to maintain joint function in the health care setting
- How to help a person perform range-of-motion exercises

Activity N *Select the single best answer for each of the following questions.*

1. When assisting a person with range-of-motion exercises, what should you do?

   a. Follow the care plan or the instructions given to you by the nurse or physical therapist exactly

   b. Move through the exercises in a systematic way

   c. Avoid pushing the joint past its point of resistance

   d. All of the above

2. What complication does performing range-of-motion exercises help to prevent?

   a. Contractures

   b. Permanent muscle weakness

   c. Brittle bones

   d. All of the above

Activity O *Mark each statement as either "true" (T) or "false" (F). Correct the false statements.*

1. T F   Range-of-motion exercises are done to preserve joint and muscle function in a person who has limited use of his musculoskeletal system.

2. T F   A nursing assistant might perform active range-of-motion exercises for a person who is in a coma.

Disorders of the musculoskeletal system are usually painful. Pain can make it difficult for a person to relax, rest, or sleep. Several of the things you do everyday for your patients or residents will help to relieve or prevent pain, such as giving back massages, applying heat or cold, and assisting with range-of-motion exercises. In addition, when you notice and report a patient's or resident's pain, you are making a very important contribution to that person's quality of life.

SUMMARY

Activity P *Use the clues to complete the crossword puzzle.*

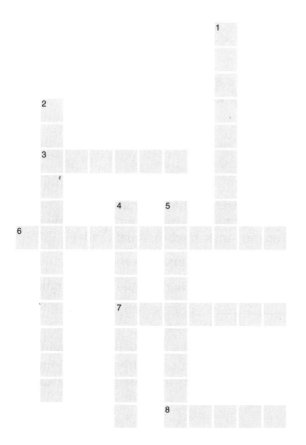

Across

3. A band of connective tissue that attaches a skeletal muscle to a bone
6. A broad flat sheet of tendon that attaches one skeletal muscle to another
7. The loss of muscle size and strength
8. The end of the amputated limb that is left after surgery

Down

1. Strong bands of fibrous tissue that cross over the joint capsule, attaching one bone to another and stabilizing the joint
2. The excessive loss of bone tissue
4. Found in flat bones and the ends of the long bones
5. Inflammation of the joints, usually associated with pain and stiffness

CHAPTER 27

The Respiratory System

STRUCTURE OF THE RESPIRATORY SYSTEM

Key Learning Points

■ The main parts of the respiratory system

Activity A *A figure of the respiratory system is shown below. Label the figure using the words given in brackets. Then, write each part next to its description in the numbered list.*

[pharynx, lower respiratory tract, larynx, bronchiole, bronchus, upper respiratory tract, diaphragm, lungs, trachea, nasal cavity]

1. _____ The inside of the nose

2. _____ The main organs of respiration

3. _____ Connects each lung to the trachea

4. _____ Strong muscle that separates the chest cavity from the abdominal cavity and assists in ventilation

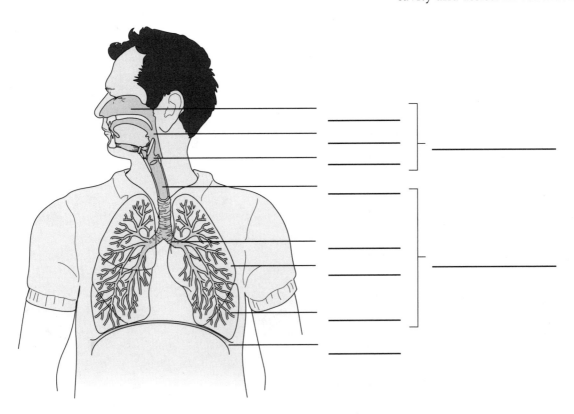

5. _____ Tiniest branches of the bronchi

6. _____ Responsible for speech (also called the "voice box")

7. _____ Passage that carries air from the pharynx down into the chest toward the lungs (also called the "windpipe")

8. _____ The throat region

Activity B *Select the single best answer for each of the following questions.*

1. What does the lower respiratory tract consist of?
   a. The oral cavity
   b. The nasal cavity, pharynx, and larynx
   c. The trachea, bronchi, bronchioles, and lungs
   d. All of the above

2. The respiratory tract is lined with a mucous membrane. What is the role of the blood vessels in the mucous membrane that lines the nasal cavity?
   a. The blood vessels transfer body heat to the air, warming it up to a comfortable temperature
   b. The blood vessels prevent dirt, dust, and microbes from entering lungs
   c. The blood vessels pick up moisture from the warm and moist nasal cavity
   d. The blood vessels protect the delicate lung tissue

3. Both the nasal and oral cavities open into the pharynx. How is this "sharing of space" advantageous?
   a. It allows us to breathe and swallow at the same time without choking
   b. It allows us to breathe through the mouth, as well as through the nose
   c. It prevents air from entering the digestive tract
   d. It prevents food from entering the respiratory tract

4. What is the name of the structure that covers the opening of the larynx and snaps shut when we swallow?
   a. The alveolus
   b. The pharynx
   c. The pleura
   d. The epiglottis

5. What supports the trachea and keeps it open?
   a. "C"-shaped rings of cartilage
   b. The windpipe
   c. Cilia
   d. Bronchioles

6. What are alveoli?
   a. Grape-like clusters of tiny air sacs where gas exchange occurs
   b. The smallest branches of the airway
   c. Tiny hair-like structures that line the trachea and bronchi
   d. The divisions of the lung

Activity C *Mark each statement as either "true" (T) or "false" (F). Correct the false statements.*

1. T F The airway consists of a series of passages that increase in diameter as they approach the lungs.

2. T F The cilia constantly move, moving mucus upward toward the pharynx so that it can be coughed up.

3. T F An inflammation of the larynx, or laryngitis, usually affects a person's ability to talk.

4. T F Each bronchus is surrounded by a network of tiny blood vessels where gas exchange occurs.

5. T F The lungs are divided into sections called pleura.

FUNCTION OF THE RESPIRATORY SYSTEM

Key Learning Points

■ The main functions of the respiratory system

Activity D *Fill in the blanks using the words given in brackets.*

[chemoreceptors, alveolus, intercostal muscles, inhalation, medulla, diaphragm, exhalation]

1. Ventilation has two phases: _____ and _____.

2. The _____ is a strong, dome-shaped muscle that separates the chest cavity from the abdominal cavity.

3. The _____, which are located between the ribs, help with the respiratory effort.

4. The rate and depth of breathing is controlled mainly by the central nervous system, in the part of the brain called the _____.

5. Special cells, called _____, located in the medulla and in some of the major arteries, monitor the amount of carbon dioxide and oxygen in the blood.

6. Carbon dioxide moves from the blood into the _____, and is removed from the body when we exhale.

THE EFFECTS OF AGING ON THE RESPIRATORY SYSTEM

Key Learning Points

■ How normal aging processes affect the respiratory system

Activity E *Think About It! Briefly answer the following questions in the spaces provided.*

1. Toxic substances, such as pollutants in the air and tobacco smoke, have a very harmful effect on the respiratory system. Describe two ways that these toxic substances harm the respiratory system. Then list two things you can do to help keep your respiratory system functioning properly well into old age.

_____

_____

_____

2. List two risk factors that put older people at greater risk for respiratory infections than younger people.

_____

_____

_____

DISORDERS OF THE RESPIRATORY SYSTEM

Key Learning Points

■ The disorders that can affect the respiratory system

Activity F *Select the single best answer for each of the following questions.*

1. Mrs. Wells has pneumonia. What might be a nursing assistant's job responsibility when caring for Mrs. Wells?

   a. To administer oxygen therapy to help Mrs. Wells to breathe

   b. To determine which microbe is causing the pneumonia

   c. To give Mrs. Wells her antibiotics

   d. To collect a sputum specimen for analysis

2. Which of the following conditions is associated with a productive cough?

   a. Bronchitis

   b. Influenza

   c. Pneumonia

   d. Emphysema

3. Why is it important for staff and residents of long-term care facilities to receive an annual "flu shot"?

   a. Because influenza virus can cause serious complications in older people

   b. Because infection with the influenza virus can lead to a serious liver disorder

   c. Because the influenza virus can lead to an extremely severe form of asthma

   d. Because infection with the influenza virus causes the fragile walls of the alveoli to break

4. Which of the following are signs and symptoms of influenza?

   a. Fever, pain when breathing, cyanosis, and a productive cough

   b. Sore throat, dry cough, stuffy nose, headache, body aches, weakness, and fever

   c. Vomiting, diarrhea, and loss of appetite

   d. Wheezing and difficulty breathing

5. Why does a person find an asthma attack very frightening?

   a. Because the airways can narrow to the point that breathing becomes almost impossible

   b. Because the person may have a seizure

   c. Because the treatment for asthma is very painful

   d. Because the person must take supplemental oxygen to carry out even the simplest activities of daily living

6. Which of the following can trigger an asthma attack?

   a. Stress

   b. Exercise

   c. Cold weather

   d. All of the above

7. Which lung disorders are described by the term *chronic obstructive pulmonary disease* (COPD)?

   a. Pneumothorax and hemothorax

   b. Chronic bronchitis and bronchitis

   c. Emphysema and chronic bronchitis

   d. Bronchitis and asthma

Activity G *Fill in the blanks using the words given in brackets.*

[pleura, barrel chest, cyanosis, bronchodilators, bronchitis, sputum, hemoptysis]

1. _____ refers to the bluish skin resulting because of decreased oxygen levels in the blood.

2. _____ consists of mucus and other respiratory secretions that are coughed up from the lungs, bronchi, and trachea.

3. The _____ is the membrane that lines the chest cavity and covers the lungs.

4. _____ may cause a dry, non-productive cough that sounds like a "bark."

5. _____ are used to treat asthma. They stop the muscle spasms responsible for the narrowing of the airways during an asthma attack.

6. _____, often seen in people with emphysema, is caused by years of having extra air trapped in the lung tissue, which causes the chest cavity to enlarge over time.

7. _____ refers to sputum that contains blood.

Activity H *Mark each statement as either "true" (T) or "false" (F). Correct the false statements.*

1. T F A productive cough is one in which a person coughs up phlegm.

2. T F Pleurisy is an inflammation of the pleura, the membrane that lines the chest cavity and covers the lungs.

3. T F Pleurisy often accompanies lower respiratory tract infections such as bronchitis.

4. T F Both bacterial and viral bronchitis can lead to pneumonia if the bronchial infection is not treated promptly and properly.

5. T F Influenza can be caused by various types of viruses, and usually only affects the upper respiratory tract.

6. T F Elderly people and very young children who get the flu are at minimal risk for developing serious complications, such as an extremely severe form of pneumonia.

7. T F An acute asthma attack cannot be treated with inhaled drugs.

8. T F The leading cause of chronic obstructive pulmonary disease (COPD) is exposure to asbestos and coal dust.

Activity I *Chronic obstructive pulmonary disease (COPD) is a general term used to describe two related lung disorders, emphysema and chronic bronchitis. Fill in the table below, which summarizes these two types of COPD, using the words given in brackets.*

[shallow, rapid, inhaling tobacco smoke (*used two times*), oxygen, bronchioles, catch, alveoli, mucus (*used two times*), infection (*used two times*), toxin, bronchi, air (*used two times*), fluid, breath, productive, infections, supplemental oxygen (*used two times*), tightness]

	EMPHYSEMA	CHRONIC BRONCHITIS
Leading cause	_____	_____
How the condition causes problems	When a _____ is inhaled, it damages the thin walls of the _____, causing them to break. Because the lung tissue is damaged, it is no longer "springy," and _____ gets trapped in the large, damaged alveoli. The trapped air cannot be exhaled and exchanged for new _____-rich air. In addition, excess _____ can collect in the damaged alveoli, creating an excellent place for _____-causing microbes to collect and multiply.	Long-term irritation of the _____ and _____ leads to the production of thick _____, which blocks the airways. _____ cannot pass freely through the airways. In addition, _____-causing microbes can collect in the _____ and multiply, leading to infection.
Signs and symptoms	Problems getting a proper _____. _____ and _____ breathing. Must stop to _____ a breath when talking or engaging in physical activity.	Nagging, _____ cough. _____ in the chest. Frequent respiratory tract _____.
Supportive therapy	_____	_____

Activity J *Place an "X" next to statements that are true about cancers that affect the respiratory tract.*

1. ____ Cancer of the lungs and airway is the most common cause of cancer-related death in the United States.

2. ____ Cancer only affects the lower respiratory tract.

3. ____ Radiologic studies, bronchoscopy, and surgery are methods used to diagnose cancer.

4. ____ Treatment of cancer may lead to physical disfigurement.

5. ____ After lung surgery, drains are inserted in the person's chest cavity.

6. ____ Treatment of lung cancer may involve surgical removal of all or part of the lung.

7. ____ Bronchoscopy carries the most risk for the person and is associated with the most discomfort.

8. ____ Radiologic studies involve chest x-rays, computed tomography (CT) scans, and magnetic resonance imaging (MRI) scans.

Activity K *Pneumothorax and hemothorax are often complications of chest trauma. Place a "P" next to the phrases that relate to pneumothorax and an "H" next to the phrases that relate to hemothorax.*

1. ___ Occurs when air builds up in the space between the lungs and the chest wall

2. ___ Occurs when blood builds up in the space between the lungs and the chest wall

3. ___ Can be caused by a penetrating chest wound that results in air being drawn into the chest cavity through the wound

4. ___ Can be caused by internal bleeding that can be caused by an injury to the chest or a rupture in the lung tissue

RESPIRATORY THERAPY

Key Learning Points

■ How oxygen therapy is used to assist a person with respiration
■ The guidelines that a nursing assistant should follow when caring for patients or residents receiving oxygen therapy

Activity L *Mr. Cheyney, a resident at the long-term care facility where you work, has chronic obstructive pulmonary disease (COPD). Many people on the health care team are involved in helping Mr. Cheyney to achieve satisfactory respiration. Place an "NA" next to phrases that describe actions that you, a nursing assistant, can take to help Mr. Cheyney with his respiration. Place an "RT/N" next to actions that the respiratory therapist or nurse will take to help Mr. Cheyney.*

1. ___ Checks the flow meter frequently to make sure that Mr. Cheyney is receiving the proper amount of oxygen

2. ___ Listens to Mr. Cheyney's breath sounds and looks at certain measurements to evaluate Mr. Cheyney's respiratory function

3. ___ Provides frequent oral care to relieve dryness of the nose and mouth and to reduce the number of microbes in Mr. Cheyney's mouth

4. ___ Helps to develop a treatment plan for Mr. Cheyney

5. ___ Sets up and adjusts Mr. Cheyney's oxygen therapy

6. ___ Watches for signs of skin irritation around Mr. Cheyney's ears, over his cheeks, and around his nostrils

Activity M *Select the single best answer for each of the following questions.*

1. Why is moisture often added to the supplemental oxygen?
   a. The moisture helps the oxygen to smell more pleasant
   b. The moisture helps to reduce the risk of fire
   c. The moisture increases the oxygen content of the air
   d. The moisture makes the oxygen less drying to the person's nose and mouth

2. Why should portable oxygen tanks be moved with caution?
   a. Because moving the tank can result in the readings of the gauge going below 85%
   b. Because moving the tank can affect the supply of oxygen
   c. Because moving the tank could result in injury if the tank is accidentally knocked over and the valve at the top breaks
   d. Because moving the tank puts the person at risk for falling

3. Which source of supplemental oxygen is often used in the home health care setting?
   a. Pressurized tank
   b. Wall-mounted delivery system
   c. Oxygen concentrator
   d. Humidity bottle

4. What is an endotracheal tube?

   a. A tube inserted through the nose or mouth and extending to the trachea, where a balloon cuff on the end holds it in place and prevents secretions that drain from the mouth from entering the respiratory tract

   b. A tube inserted in a surgically created opening in the neck that opens into the trachea

   c. A soft rubber tube that is inserted into the person's nose extending back toward the throat, providing an opening that air can flow through

   d. A tube that stops the tongue from falling back into the throat, keeping the airway open

5. What should you do while taking care of a person with an endotracheal tube?

   a. Check on the person frequently to help him feel more secure

   b. Avoid providing frequent oral care to minimize the risk of aspiration

   c. Change the person's diet to full liquids because he cannot chew

   d. Keep the call light out of the person's reach

6. Which of the following patients may need to have a permanent tracheostomy?

   a. Mrs. Jones, who has liver cancer

   b. Mr. Dunlap, who will be on a mechanical ventilator for at least 3 days

   c. Mr. Robeson, who is a quadriplegic and unable to breathe without the aid of a mechanical ventilator

   d. Ms. Ingersoll, who has laryngitis

7. Which of the following is a potential complication of suctioning?

   a. Paralysis

   b. Hypoxia

   c. Displacement of the tube through coughing

   d. All of the above

Activity N *Mark each statement as either "true" (T) or "false" (F). Correct the false statements.*

1. T F A reading of less than 85% on the pulse oximeter is a sign that the person's tissues may not be receiving enough oxygen.

2. T F Oxygen is considered a drug and requires a doctor's order to be used.

3. T F Supplemental oxygen is about 20% oxygen and the rest is nitrogen.

4. T F Oxygen is usually delivered to the patient or resident at a rate of 2 to 15 liters per minute.

5. T F Receiving too much oxygen is better than receiving too little oxygen.

6. T F If a nursing assistant notices that the setting on a resident's flow meter does not match the amount of oxygen that has been ordered, he should adjust the setting so that it matches what is stated on the nursing care plan.

Activity O *Match the terms associated with the respiratory therapy, given in Column A, with their descriptions, given in Column B.*

Column A

____ 1. Flow meter

____ 2. Pulse oximeter

____ 3. Wall-mounted delivery system

____ 4. Pressurized tank

____ 5. Oxygen concentrator

____ 6. Nasal cannula

____ 7. Facemask

____ 8. Nasopharyngeal airway

____ 9. Oropharyngeal airway

Column B

a. A device that filters nitrogen from room air, leaving pure oxygen

b. A device made of soft, molded plastic material that delivers oxygen through the mouth and nose

c. A device that sets the flow rate

d. A hard plastic device inserted into a person's mouth to keep the airway open

e. Contains oxygen under pressure

f. A device used to monitor the oxygen content of the blood

g. Oxygen is pumped into the person's room from a central location, and a valve and flow meter are inserted into the wall to access the oxygen

h. Prongs of soft plastic tubing that are inserted into the nostrils

i. A soft rubber tube that is inserted into a person's nose to provide an opening for air to flow through

Activity P *Think About It! Briefly answer the following question in the space provided.*

Mr. Cross, a patient in the hospital where you work, is receiving oxygen therapy. The respiratory therapist has set up and adjusted Mr. Cross' oxygen therapy and attached a pulse oximeter to Mr. Cross' fingertip. A humidity bottle is being used as part of Mr. Cross' oxygen therapy. Summarize your role in taking care of Mr. Cross.

_____

_____

_____

Activity Q *Think About It! Briefly answer the following question in the space provided.*

Supplemental oxygen is often delivered through a nasal cannula or a facemask. List three advantages and three disadvantages of using a nasal cannula to administer oxygen. Then, list two advantages and two disadvantages of using a facemask.

_____

_____

_____

_____

_____

_____

_____

_____

Activity R *Think About It! Briefly answer the following question in the space provided.*

A mechanical ventilator performs the function of breathing for a person who cannot breathe on his own. List five situations where a person might require mechanical ventilation.

_____

_____

_____

Activity S *Being intubated with an endotracheal tube can be very uncomfortable and frightening for the patient or resident. Place an "X" next to reasons why using an endotracheal tube is uncomfortable and frightening for the patient or resident.*

1. ____ The endotracheal tube travels through the larynx, making it impossible for the person to talk.

2. ____ The person cannot sit up while the endotracheal tube is in place.

3. ____ The endotracheal tube makes it impossible for the person to take food or fluids through the mouth.

4. ____ The endotracheal tube can result in gagging and choking.

5. ____ The person may have to be restrained to prevent her from pulling out the tube.

A nursing assistant's main responsibility in caring for any patient or resident with a respiratory problem is that of observation. Because you are the one who will spend the most time with your patients or residents, you will be the one who will have the best opportunity to observe signs that a person may be having problems with ventilation or gas exchange.

GENERAL CARE MEASURES

Key Learning Points

■ Other methods used to help a person who is having trouble with respiration

Activity T *Place an "X" next to the actions that are within a nursing assistant's scope of practice.*

1. ___ Observing for signs of problems with ventilation or gas exchange

2. ___ Positioning the person in the Fowler's or semi-Fowler's position to make breathing easier

3. ___ Providing frequent oral care

4. ___ Increasing the oxygen flow rate as necessary

5. ___ Exchanging a patient's or resident's empty oxygen tank for a full one

6. ___ Encouraging the patient or resident to drink plenty of fluids

7. ___ Telling patients or residents who smoke to stop

Activity U *Think About It! Briefly answer the following question in the space provided.*

Mr. Taylor has asthma. He tends to use the call light frequently and asks for seemingly trivial things. What might be the reason behind this behavior? What should you do?

_____

_____

_____

_____

_____

> When caring for a person with a respiratory disorder, you provide holistic care when you help the person to feel safe and secure. Think about how frightening it would be not to be able to breathe easily on your own!

SUMMARY

Activity V *Use the clues to find words that are present in the grid of letters, either horizontally from left to right or vertically from top to bottom.*

N	A	S	A	A	L	S	F	Z
A	S	T	H	M	A	X	C	B
S	T	R	Q	R	R	Z	A	R
A	H	A	A	F	Y	C	S	O
L	S	C	Z	V	N	A	X	N
C	I	H	E	G	X	Y	B	C
A	T	E	C	B	Y	H	B	H
V	I	A	L	V	E	O	L	I
I	G	I	U	S	D	F	B	U
T	N	G	N	D	D	F	Q	H
Y	Y	N	G	Z	A	F	M	A
D	R	Y	S	P	U	T	U	M
I	A	R	N	N	J	L	C	A
S	H	A	F	E	G	H	U	T
O	P	L	E	U	R	I	S	Y
N	N	S	A	M	L	S	F	Z
A	E	T	H	O	A	X	C	B
S	U	R	Q	T	R	Z	A	R
A	M	A	A	H	Y	C	S	O
L	O	C	Z	O	N	A	X	N
C	N	H	E	R	X	Y	B	C
A	I	E	C	A	Y	H	B	H
I	A	T	S	X	J	K	V	D

Down

1. The inside of the nose
2. Part of the respiratory airway; also known as "the voice box"
3. The passage that carries air from the larynx down into the chest toward the lungs
4. Passageways that carry air from the trachea to the lungs
5. The primary organs for respiration
6. A slippery, sticky substance that is secreted by special cells and serves to keep the surfaces of mucous membranes moist
7. Inflammation of the lung tissue
8. Air builds up in the space between the lungs and the chest wall

Across

9. Inflammation of the pleura, the membrane that lines the chest cavity and covers the lungs
10. A condition that affects the bronchi and bronchioles of the lungs
11. Grape-like clusters of tiny air sacs in the lungs, where gas exchange takes place
12. Mucus and other respiratory secretions that are coughed up from the lungs, bronchi, and trachea

The Cardiovascular System

STRUCTURE OF THE CARDIOVASCULAR SYSTEM

Key Learning Points

■ The major parts of the cardiovascular system

Activity A *Select the single best answer for each of the following questions.*

1. The two main components of blood are:
   a. The arteries and veins
   b. The lymphatic system and the conduction system
   c. The plasma and the blood cells
   d. The heart and the heart valves

2. What is plasma?
   a. Blood cells
   b. The liquid part of the blood
   c. The walls of the blood vessels
   d. Tiny cells that are thinner at the edges

3. Why are the red blood cells red?
   a. Because hemoglobin turns bright red when combined with oxygen
   b. Because they are manufactured in the red bone marrow
   c. Because of the presence of plasma proteins
   d. Because lymph capillaries absorb fluid from the surrounding tissues

4. How many white blood cells does the blood of a healthy person contain per cubic millimeter?
   a. Approximately 5 million white blood cells
   b. 5,000 to 8,000 white blood cells
   c. 5,000 to 10,000 white blood cells
   d. Approximately 150,000 to 450,000 white blood cells

5. What is hemostasis?
   a. The process of allowing the blood vessels to constrict or dilate according to the body's needs
   b. The process that stops the flow of blood from the circulatory system by forming a clot
   c. The process of transferring substances in and out of the blood
   d. The process of returning the fluid that leaks into the tissues to the bloodstream

6. What is the inner layer of a blood vessel called?
   a. The tunica intima
   b. The tunica media
   c. The tunica externa
   d. None of the above

7. What are lymph nodes?

   a. Masses of lymphatic tissue that "clean" the lymph by removing bacteria and other large particles

   b. Lymph capillaries that join together to form larger vessels

   c. Fluids that enter the lymph capillaries

   d. Chemicals that stimulate the production of certain white blood cells (T cells) in the event of an infection

8. What is valvular insufficiency?

   a. A condition that occurs when the body draws on "extra" blood from the spleen during times of massive blood loss

   b. A condition that occurs when lymph capillaries absorb excess fluid from the surrounding tissues

   c. A condition that occurs when damaged valves are unable to create a seal when they close, allowing blood to flow "backwards"

   d. A condition that occurs when the flow of oxygen-rich blood to the tissues of the heart is disrupted

Activity B *Match the terms, given in Column A, with their definitions, given in Column B.*

Column A

___ 1. Plasma

___ 2. Red blood cells

___ 3. White blood cells

___ 4. Thrombocytes

___ 5. Capillary bed

___ 6. Sinoatrial node

Column B

a. Blood cells that fight infection

b. Sets the pace for heart contraction

c. The liquid portion of the blood

d. Network of small vessels that connect the arterioles and the venules

e. Blood cells responsible for hemostasis

f. Blood cells that carry oxygen

Activity C *Mark each statement as either "true" (T) or "false" (F). Correct the false statements.*

1. T F Cardio means "heart," and vascular means "blood."

2. T F As the blood circulates through the body, giving off oxygen and taking on carbon dioxide, the number of oxygen molecules on the hemoglobin molecule decreases, and the blood becomes bright red in color.

3. T F Red blood cells are manufactured in the red bone marrow and are continuously replaced as old ones wear out.

4. T F The tunica intima is the tough outer layer of the blood vessel.

5. T F A thin film of fluid between the epicardium and the outer layer of the pericardium allows the pericardial layers to slide smoothly against each other each time the heart pumps.

6. T F The thymus gland helps to filter blood and break down worn-out red blood cells.

7. T F Because the atria must send the blood much further with each contraction, they are larger than the ventricles, and have thicker, more muscular walls.

Activity D *Words shown in the picture have been jumbled. Use the clues to form correct words using the letters given in the picture.*

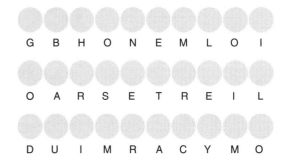

G B H O N E M L O I

O A R S E T R E I L

D U I M R A C Y M O

1. The protein found on red blood cells that allow them to carry oxygen

2. The smallest arteries

3. The muscular middle layer of the heart, which allows the heart to pump

Activity E *Following are some terms related to the cardiovascular system. Specify one function of each term in relation to its role in the cardiovascular system.*

1. Albumin ———————————————

2. Fibrinogen —————————————

3. Globulins ——————————————

4. Erythrocytes —————————————

5. Leukocytes —————————————

6. Platelets ——————————————

7. Lymphatic system ———————————

Activity F *Blood vessels include arteries and veins. Place an "A" next to statements related to arteries and a "V" next to statements related to veins.*

1. ___ Carry blood to the heart

2. ___ Contain more smooth muscle

3. ___ Carry blood away from the heart

4. ___ Contain valves, which help blood to flow back to the heart

5. ___ Receive blood that is being pumped from the heart under great force and pressure

6. ___ Assisted by contraction of nearby skeletal muscles

Activity G *A figure of the heart is shown below. Label the figure using the words given in brackets.*

[pulmonary veins, myocardium, aorta, right ventricle, superior vena cava, left atrium, pulmonary artery, mitral (bicuspid) valve, tricuspid valve, right atrium, left ventricle, pulmonary valve, septum]

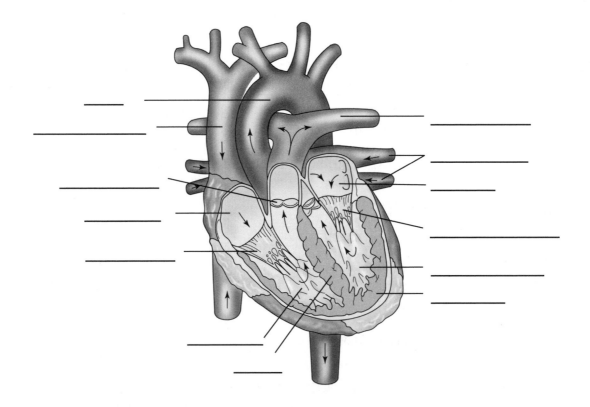

Activity H *Fill in the blanks using the words given in brackets.*

[aortic, rheumatic fever, valves, pulmonary, mitral, conduction system, tricuspid]

1. _____ are flaps of tissue that snap shut after the blood passes through to prevent backflow.

2. The _____ valve separates the right atrium from the right ventricle.

3. The _____ valve separates the left atrium from the left ventricle.

4. The _____ valve is located where the pulmonary artery leaves the right ventricle.

5. The _____ valve is located where the aorta leaves the left ventricle.

6. A type of infection called _____ can cause the valves to become thickened and scarred.

7. The electrical impulse travels through the myocardium via a special pathway called the _____.

FUNCTION OF THE CARDIOVASCULAR SYSTEM

Key Learning Points

- The major functions of the cardiovascular system

Activity I *Think About It! Briefly answer the following question in the space provided.*

List and describe three functions of the cardiovascular system.

_____

_____

_____

Activity J *Match the terms, given in Column A, with their definitions, given in Column B.*

Column A

____ 1. Circulation

____ 2. Pulmonary circulation

____ 3. Systemic circulation

____ 4. Systole

____ 5. Diastole

____ 6. Cardiac cycle

Column B

a. Contraction of the myocardium, sending blood out of the heart

b. Sequence of atrial diastole and ventricular systole

c. Continuous movement of the blood

d. Relaxation of the myocardium, during which the chambers fill with blood

e. Pumping of blood by the right side of the heart to the lungs

f. Pumping of newly oxygenated blood by the left side of the heart to the rest of the body

Activity K *Circulation involves two circuits, the pulmonary circulation and the systemic circulation. In the pulmonary circulation, the blood is pumped to the lungs to pick up a fresh load of oxygen. In the systemic circulation, the newly oxygenated blood is pumped to the rest of the body. The steps in this process are given below, along with a figure showing the pattern of circulation. Following these steps, draw arrows on the figure showing the path of the blood.*

PULMONARY CIRCULATION

1. The superior vena cava and the inferior vena cava empty into the right atrium of the heart.

2. The right atrium pumps the oxygen-poor blood into the right ventricle.

3. The right ventricle pumps the oxygen-poor blood into the pulmonary artery, which branches into the right and left pulmonary arteries.

4. The blood moves through the capillary beds surrounding the alveoli in the lungs, picking up a fresh load of oxygen.

5. The newly oxygenated blood enters the pulmonary veins, which return the blood to the left atrium of the heart.

SYSTEMIC CIRCULATION

6. The left atrium pumps the oxygen-rich blood into the left ventricle.
7. The left ventricle pumps the oxygen-rich blood into the aorta.
8. The aorta branches into the arteries that carry blood to the rest of the body. The blood releases its oxygen.
9. The veins of the body, carrying oxygen-poor blood, empty into the superior vena cava and the inferior vena cava, so that the process can begin again.

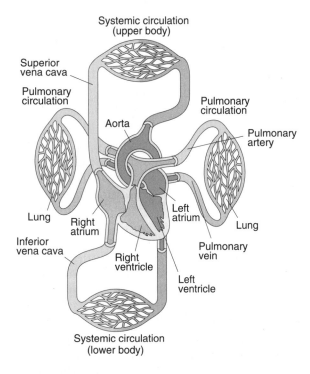

Systemic circulation
(upper body)

Superior
vena cava

Pulmonary
circulation

Aorta

Pulmonary
circulation

Pulmonary
artery

Lung

Right
atrium

Left
atrium

Lung

Inferior
vena cava

Right
ventricle

Pulmonary
vein

Left
ventricle

Systemic circulation
(lower body)

Activity L *Mark each statement as either "true" (T) or "false" (F). Correct the false statements.*

1. **T F** The orderly sequence of systole and diastole is crucial for maximizing the amount of blood that is pumped throughout the body each time the heart contracts.

2. **T F** While taking an apical pulse with a stethoscope, the first sound ("lubb") is the sound of the pulmonary and aortic valves closing during ventricular diastole.

3. **T F** The cardiovascular system plays a role in temperature regulation.

4. **T F** The cardiovascular system helps to allow microbes to gain access to the body.

THE EFFECTS OF AGING ON THE CARDIOVASCULAR SYSTEM

Key Learning Points

- How aging affects the cardiovascular system
- How exercise and a healthy life style can diminish the effects of aging on the cardiovascular system

Activity M *Think About It! Briefly answer the following question in the space provided.*

List four factors that may cause the cardiovascular system to age faster.

_____

_____

_____

Activity N *Select the single best answer for each of the following questions.*

1. How does smoking affect the cardiovascular system?
   a. Smoking increases oxygen supply to the heart.
   b. Smoking causes the blood vessels to dilate.
   c. Smoking causes the arterioles and capillaries to constrict, depriving tissues of vital blood flow.
   d. Smoking decreases the number of blood cells.

2. What affects the ability of the heart to contract forcefully?
   a. Changes in the tissues of the heart, such as a loss of muscle tone and a loss of elasticity
   b. The body's needs for oxygen and nutrients
   c. The body's ability to control blood pressure and flow
   d. The body's ability to maintain adequate blood flow to the brain

Activity O *Think About It! Briefly answer the following question in the space provided.*

Mr. Clark is 65 years old and has had a history of a cardiovascular disease. This morning, he got out of bed quickly because he overslept, and he felt lightheaded and dizzy. Explain how Mr. Clark's symptoms of lightheadedness and dizziness on rising could be related to his cardiovascular condition.

_____

_____

_____

> When the effects of aging are combined with a lifetime of unhealthy habits or a chronic disease, the effect on cardiovascular function can be major!

DISORDERS OF THE CARDIOVASCULAR SYSTEM

Key Learning Points

- Various disorders that affect the cardiovascular system

Activity P *Place an "X" next to the factors that can cause anemia.*

1. ____ Decreased number of red blood cells

2. ____ Slow chronic blood loss

3. ____ Diets that are high in iron or certain B vitamins

4. ____ Impaired red blood cell production

Activity Q *Select the single best answer for each of the following questions.*

1. What can occur when the blood clots too easily?

   a. A clot can form in a small blood vessel causing the flow of blood to be impaired, depriving the tissues of oxygen and nutrients

   b. Fibrinogen production is impaired

   c. A small bump can cause a large bruise; a more severe injury can result in a fatal hemorrhage

   d. The platelet count is low

2. Why is a balloon angioplasty performed?

   a. To stimulate the heart muscle to contract

   b. To bypass the blocked arteries and reestablish blood flow

   c. To widen a narrowed portion of an artery to improve blood flow

   d. To replace a damaged valve

3. What happens in congestive heart failure?

   a. The blood backs up in the lungs because the left ventricle's ability to pump the blood into the systemic circulation is impaired.

   b. The blood backs up in the venous system because the right ventricle's ability to pump the blood into the pulmonary circulation is impaired.

   c. The veins in the legs and abdomen become swollen, and fluid may leak into the tissues, causing significant edema and skin breakdown.

   d. One or more of the coronary arteries becomes completely blocked, preventing blood from reaching the parts of the heart that are fed by the affected arteries.

4. How is heart block treated?

   a. By performing a coronary artery bypass

   b. By implanting a pacemaker, an electrical device that stimulates the heart to contract

   c. By measuring and monitoring fluid intake and output

   d. By conducting balloon angioplasty

Activity R *Mark each statement as either "true" (T) or "false" (F). Correct the false statements.*

1. T F In disorders such as sickle cell anemia, red blood cells are unable to carry oxygen because of their abnormal shape.

2. T F Leukemia can result from cancer of the heart.

3. T F Smoking, eating a diet low in cholesterol and saturated fat, and a lack of physical activity can increase a person's chances of developing atherosclerosis.

4. T F Disorders that cause the ventricles to lose muscle tone and become large and flabby can cause angina pectoris.

5. T F Heart failure is a common type of dysrhthmia.

Activity S *Match the terms, given in Column A, with their descriptions, given in Column B.*

Column A

____ 1. Anemia

____ 2. Sickle cell anemia

____ 3. Leukemia

____ 4. Embolus

____ 5. Atherosclerosis

____ 6. Venous thrombosis

____ 7. Venous ulcers

Column B

a. Excessive production of white blood cells

b. Group of disorders affecting the red blood cells

c. Increases risk for pulmonary embolism

d. A blood clot that moves from one place to another

e. Sores as a result of poor circulation

f. Production of abnormally shaped red blood cells

g. Narrowing of the inside of the arteries due to plaque build-up

Activity T *Fill in the blanks using the words given in brackets.*

[claudication, thrombi, congenital, heart failure, bone marrow, anticoagulants, hemoglobin]

1. A disorder that affects the _____, where blood cells are made, can cause a decrease in the number of circulating red blood cells, leading to anemia.

2. The body needs iron in order to make _____.

3. Blood clots, called _____, can also break loose and travel to other parts of the body such as the brain, lungs, or heart.

4. People who have blood that clots too easily may need to take drugs called _____ or "blood thinners" to help keep clots from forming where they are not needed.

5. Pain and cramping, called _____, occurs because the muscles are not receiving enough oxygen.

6. Most heart disorders in children are _____, which means that they were "present at birth."

7. _____ occurs when the heart is unable to pump enough blood to meet the body's needs.

Activity U *Think About It! Briefly answer the following question in the space provided.*

Atherosclerosis causes blocking of the arteries. Depending on which arteries are affected, atherosclerosis can have serious consequences. List the possible consequence of atherosclerosis when it involves each of the following arteries.

1. Atherosclerosis of the arteries that supply the brain

_____

2. Atherosclerosis of the arteries that supply the heart

_____

3. Atherosclerosis of the arteries that supply the kidneys

_____

4. Atherosclerosis of the arteries that supply the legs

_____

Activity V *Place an "X" next to cardiac risk factors that CANNOT be changed.*

1. ____ Poorly controlled hypertension

2. ____ Increasing age

3. ____ A diet high in saturated fat and cholesterol

4. ____ Physical inactivity

5. ____ Gender

6. ____ Heredity

7. ____ Obesity

8. ____ "Apple"-shaped body type

9. ____ Smoking

DIAGNOSIS OF CARDIOVASCULAR DISORDERS

Key Learning Points
- Diagnostic tests that are often used to diagnose disorders of the cardiovascular system

Activity W *Match the diagnostic tests, given in Column A, with their descriptions, given in Column B.*

Column A	Column B
____ 1. Electro-cardiography	a. An electrocardiogram (EKG) is obtained during exercise
____ 2. Stress test	b. Sound waves are used to check the blood flow in the large arteries and veins of the arms and legs
____ 3. Echocardio-graphy	c. The electrical activity of the heart is traced and recorded on paper
____ 4. Doppler ultrasound	d. Commonly known as "x-rays"
____ 5. Radiography	e. Sound waves are bounced against the body to produce an image

SUMMARY

Activity X *Use the clues to complete the crossword puzzle.*

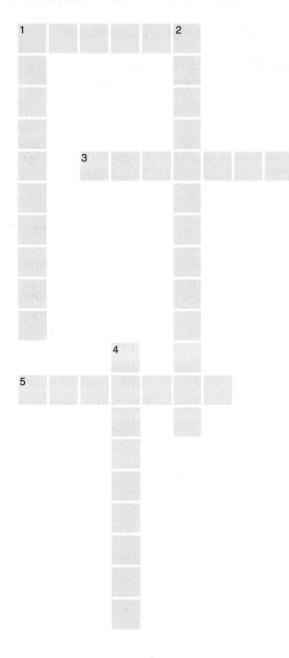

Across

1. A part of the lymphatic system that helps to filter blood and break down worn-out red blood cells.
3. A blood clot that breaks loose and travels to other parts of the body, such as the brain, lungs, or heart.
5. A plasma protein that plays a role in moving fluid in and out of the bloodstream.

Down

1. A small mass of special tissue in the heart called the _____ node sets the pace for contraction by generating an electrical impulse.
2. _____ should not be handled with bare hands as it can be absorbed through the skin.
4. People with venous thrombosis are at risk for _____ embolism.

CHAPTER 29

The Nervous System

STRUCTURE OF THE NERVOUS SYSTEM

Key Learning Points

■ The structures that make up the two main divisions of the nervous system

Activity A *Place a "C" next to the structures that are a part of the central nervous system, and a "P" next to the structures that are a part of the peripheral nervous system.*

1. ____ Cerebellum

2. ____ Sensory nerves

3. ____ Diencephalon

4. ____ Motor nerves

5. ____ Brain stem

6. ____ Cerebrum

7. ____ Cranial nerves

Activity B *Mark each statement as either "true" (T) or "false" (F). Correct the false statements.*

1. T F A neuron is a cell that can send and receive information.

2. T F The axon is a long extension from the cell body that receives information.

3. T F The cerebrum is the smallest part of the brain.

4. T F The brain, a large, soft mass of nervous tissue, is where information is processed and instructions are issued.

5. T F The brain stem plays a role in balance.

Activity C *Match the terms, given in Column A, with their descriptions, given in Column B.*

Column A	Column B
____ 1. Cranial nerves	a. This system receives information, processes it, and issues instructions
____ 2. Sensory nerves	b. These nerves carry commands from the brain, down the spinal cord and out to the muscles and organs of the body
____ 3. Motor nerves	
____ 4. Peripheral nervous system	c. These nerves are connected directly to the brain
____ 5. Central nervous system	d. These nerves carry information from the internal organs and the outside world to the spinal cord
	e. This system is the line of communication between the central nervous system and the rest of the body

Activity D *A neuron is a cell that can send and receive information. Label the figure below using the words given in brackets.*

[dendrites, cell body, axon, synapse, myelin]

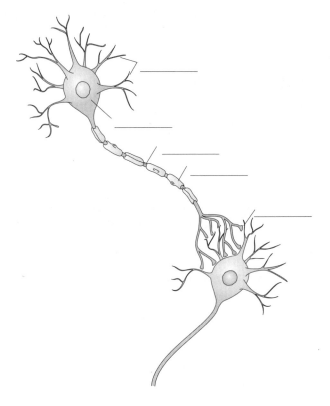

FUNCTION OF THE NERVOUS SYSTEM

Key Learning Points

■ Main functions of the nervous system

Activity E *Fill in the blanks using the words given in brackets.*

[think, taste, create, feel, hear, smell, see, move]

The nervous system allows us to experience the world around us. Without our nervous systems, we would not be able to experience the
_____ and _____ of a ripe peach,
_____ a beautiful piece of music,
_____ a loved one's face, or _____
the soft fur of a favorite pet. We would not be able to _____, _____, or
_____.

THE EFFECTS OF AGING ON THE NERVOUS SYSTEM

Key Learning Points

■ How aging affects the nervous system

Activity F *Think About It! Briefly answer the following question in the space provided.*

Due to changes that occur with aging, older people tend to have slowed conduction times. Write down what slowed conduction times put an older person at risk for, and why. Then write down three ways you can help to minimize this risk.

_____

_____

_____

_____

_____

DISORDERS OF THE NERVOUS SYSTEM

Key Learning Points

■ Various disorders that affect the nervous system

Activity G *Use the clues to complete the crossword puzzle.*

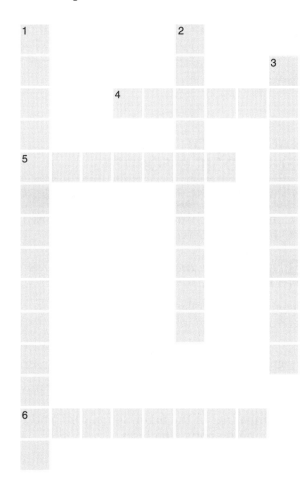

Across

4. A disorder that occurs when blood flow to a part of the brain is completely blocked, causing the tissue to die

5. General term for a group of disorders that affect a person's ability to communicate with others

6. A disorder characterized by chronic seizure activity

Down

1. These can result in tetraplegia

2. A progressive neurologic disorder that is characterized by tremor and weakness in the muscles and a shuffling gait

3. This can lead to epilepsy, memory problems, or behavioral problems

Activity H *Mark each statement as either "true" (T) or "false" (F). Correct the false statements.*

1. T F Transient ischemic attacks (TIAs) are permanent episodes of dysfunction that are caused by decreased blood flow (ischemia) to the brain.

2. T F A stroke occurs when blood flow to a part of the brain is completely blocked, causing the tissue to die.

3. T F Parkinson's disease is a progressive disease, which means that it gets better with time.

4. T F People in the late stages of amyotrophic lateral sclerosis (ALS, Lou Gehrig's disease) are totally paralyzed, yet their minds remain sharp.

5. T F Multiple sclerosis (MS) usually affects the central nervous system first, and then moves outward toward the nerves in the hands, feet, and eyes.

Activity I *Think About It! Briefly answer the following question in the space provided.*

Mrs. Ingram has Parkinson's disease. Using the word "TRAP", list the 4 main effects of Parkinson's disease.

_____

_____

_____

_____

Activity J *Think About It! Briefly answer the following questions in the spaces provided.*

List three risk factors that increase a person's chances of having a stroke.

1. _____

2. _____

3. _____

List two of the most common disabilities resulting from stroke and define them.

1. _____

2. _____

Look at the picture below. Why is the device shown in the picture being used for a person who has had a stroke?

_____

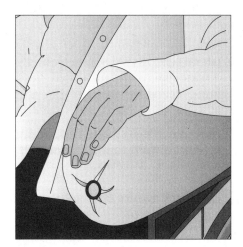

For a person who has survived a stroke or a devastating spinal cord injury, the emotional effects can be harder to overcome than the physical ones. Loss of control over one's own body and the accompanying loss of independence can be very devastating for a patient or resident.

DIAGNOSIS OF NEUROLOGIC DISORDERS

Key Learning Points

- Common diagnostic procedures that are used to help detect nervous system disorders

Activity K *Fill in the blanks using the words given in brackets.*

[imaging studies, diagnostic tests, electroencephalography]

1. _____ are often ordered for people with signs and symptoms of a neurologic disorder.

2. _____, such as computed tomography (CT) scans, allow doctors to see physical abnormalities of the brain, spinal cord, and surrounding bony structures.

3. _____ is used to monitor the electrical activity of the brain.

SUMMARY

Activity L *Descriptions of some parts of the nervous system are given below. The names of those parts are listed in jumbled form. Use the pictures and descriptions to form correct words.*

1. A cell that can send and receive information
2. The three layers of connective tissue that cover and protect the brain and spinal cord
3. The largest part of the brain; involved with voluntary motor control, speech, and processing of sensory input
4. Coordinates the brain's commands to the muscles and plays a role in balance
5. A fatty, white substance that protects the axon and helps to speed the conduction of nerve impulses along the axon
6. The gap between the axon of one neuron and the dendrites of the next

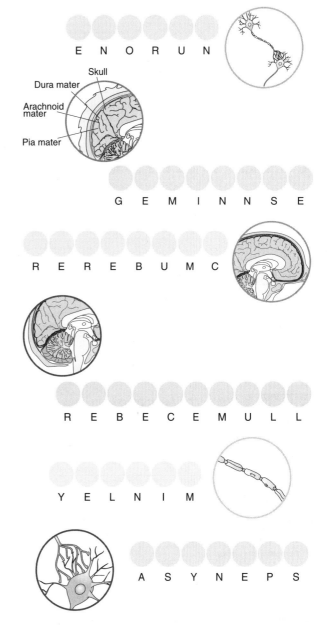

E   N   O   R   U   N

Skull
Dura mater
Arachnoid mater
Pia mater

G   E   M   I   N   N   S   E

R   E   R   E   B   U   M   C

R   E   B   E   C   E   M   U   L   L

Y   E   L   N   I   M

A   S   Y   N   E   P   S

CHAPTER 30

The Sensory System

STRUCTURE OF THE SENSORY SYSTEM

Key Learning Points

- The main function of the sensory system
- The two main divisions of the sensory system

Activity A *Fill in the blanks using the words given in brackets.*

[stimulus, sensory receptors, special sense, general sense]

1. _____ are cells or groups of cells associated with a sensory nerve.

2. The sensory receptors pick up information, called a _____, and translate it into a nerve impulse.

3. The sensory receptors that are responsible for _____ are found throughout the body.

4. The sensory receptors that are responsible for _____ are located in the specific sense organs.

GENERAL SENSE

Key Learning Points

- The body's general senses

Activity B *Briefly answer the following question in the space provided below:*

General sense is responsible for our sense of touch, position, and pain. For each of these, describe one way in which it helps protect the body from harm.

_____

_____

_____

_____

TASTE AND SMELL

Key Learning Points

- How we experience taste and smell
- How aging affects a person's senses of taste and smell

Activity C *Select the single best answer for each of the following questions.*

1. Which special cells detect chemicals in the food we eat, the beverages we drink, and the air we breathe?

   a. Chemoreceptors
   b. Tactile receptors
   c. Auditory receptors
   d. Motor receptors

2. We have thousands of taste buds, and each taste bud consists of about 100 chemo-receptors, plus some supporting cells. Where are they located?

   a. In the nasal cavity

   b. On the tongue

   c. In the skin

   d. In the ears

3. The receptors that allow us to smell are stimulated by chemicals that have been dissolved in fluid. What is this fluid?

   a. Saliva

   b. Tears

   c. Mucus

   d. Aqueous humor

Activity D *Mark each statement as either "true" (T) or "false" (F). Correct the false statements.*

1. T F   As we get older, the number of chemoreceptors on the tongue and on the roof of the nasal cavity decreases.

2. T F   As a result of aging, the senses of taste and smell become more intense, leading to an overall increase in appetite.

3. T F   To make up for a diminished sense of taste and smell, older people often season their food more heavily than younger people.

4. T F   There are no dangers associated with a diminished ability to taste or smell, as we hardly rely on these senses to keep us safe.

SIGHT

Key Learning Points

- How we experience sight
- The effects of aging on the eye
- Disorders that can affect the eye
- How to care for eyeglasses, contact lenses, and artificial eyes
- Special considerations that are taken when caring for a blind person

Activity E *Use the clues to complete the crossword puzzle.*

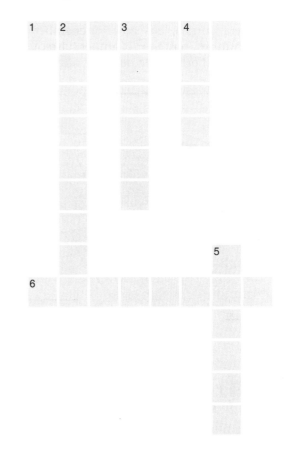

Across

1. The layer of the eye that contains the blood vessels that supply blood to the retina and other parts of the eye

6. A disorder where there is gradual yellowing and hardening of the lens of the eye

Down

2. Farsightedness, when people have trouble seeing objects that are close to them

3. The innermost layer of the eye that contains receptors, called rods and cones, which turn light into nerve impulses

4. The colored part of the eye that controls the amount of light that enters the eye through the pupil

5. The tough outer layer of the eye, made of connective tissue

Activity F *The following picture shows the structure of the eye. Label the picture using the words given in brackets.*

[pupil, sclera, cornea, lens, anterior chamber (aqueous humor), posterior chamber (vitreous humor), ciliary body, optic nerve, conjunctiva]

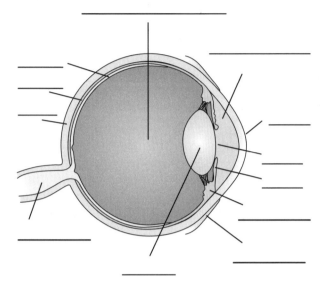

Activity G *Place an "X" next to the changes that occur in the eye due to aging.*

1. ____ The number of receptors in the retina decreases, and the lens becomes more opaque (cloudy).

2. ____ The irregular curve of the cornea bends the light rays in funny ways, which results in a blurred, distorted image.

3. ____ The iris becomes more rigid, which means that it takes longer for a person's eyes to adjust when she moves from a bright area to a dim one, or vice versa.

4. ____ There is a decrease in tear production, which leads to dryness and irritation of the eyes.

5. ____ The eyeball elongates, causing a condition called myopia.

Activity H *Match the disorders of the eye, given in Column A, with their descriptions, given in Column B.*

Column A

____ **1.** Macular degeneration

____ **2.** Conjunctivitis

____ **3.** Cataracts

____ **4.** Glaucoma

____ **5.** Diabetic retinopathy

Column B

a. An infection and inflammation of the conjunctiva, the clear membrane that lines the inside of the eyelids and covers most of the surface of the eye

b. Deposits build up in the middle of the retina, damaging the receptors in the area and interfering with the person's ability to see

c. A disorder of the eye that occurs when the pressure within the eye is increased to dangerous levels

d. A complication of diabetes that can lead to blindness

e. The gradual yellowing and hardening of the lens of the eye

Activity I *Think About It! Briefly answer the following question in the space provided.*

Miss Scott, a resident at the nursing home where you work, is blind. List three guidelines that a nursing assistant should keep in mind when helping Miss Scott.

_____

_____

_____

Activity J *The following sentences are related to helping a person care for eyeglasses, contact lenses, or an artificial eye. Fill in the blanks using the words given in brackets.*

[contact lens, prosthetic eye, cleaning, soaking, eyeglasses]

1. Clean _____ with a cloth and a special solution made specifically for that purpose, or with warm water.

2. A _____ is made of molded plastic and fits directly on the eyeball.

3. The types of _____ and _____ solutions that are used with contact lenses vary according to the type of lens.

4. A person who has had an eye removed may choose to wear a _____, which is made of ceramic or plastic and is usually designed to be very close in appearance to the person's own eye.

> Always handle your patients' or residents' eyeglasses, contact lenses, and artificial eyes with care. These items are expensive and difficult to replace. In addition, improper handling of contact lenses or prosthetic eyes can lead to infection of the eye.

HEARING AND BALANCE

Key Learning Points

- How we experience sound
- The effects of aging on the ear
- Disorders that can affect the ear
- Techniques for communicating with a hearing-impaired person
- Proper technique for inserting and removing an in-the-ear hearing aid

Activity K *Some of the steps that allow us to hear sounds are listed below. Write down the correct order of the steps in the boxes provided below.*

1. The tympanic membrane vibrations are passed to the first bone of the middle ear.
2. The malleus sends vibrations to the incus, and then to the stapes.

3. Sounds travel in the form of sound waves, which are captured by the pinna and sent down the external auditory canal.
4. The stapes rests against the oval window, a membrane at the opening of the cochlea.
5. As the sound waves travel down the external auditory canal, they come in contact with the tympanic membrane, causing it to vibrate.
6. When the stapes vibrates, it causes the oval window to vibrate, sending the vibrations through the fluid inside the cochlea.
7. The moving fluid stimulates the receptors inside the cochlea, which then sends nerve impulses via the cochlear nerve to the brain.
8. The brain interprets these nerve impulses as sound.

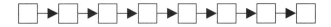

Activity L *Mark each statement as either "true" (T) or "false" (F). Correct the false statements.*

1. T F Motion sickness occurs when the messages your ears are sending to your brain about your body's position do not match the messages your eyes are sending to your brain about your body's position.

2. T F Unlike other organs, the ear is not prone to age-related changes.

3. T F Many older people with presbycusis are mistakenly labeled "confused" or "disoriented" by family members, friends, or health care professionals.

4. T F When speaking with an elderly person with presbycusis, it is helpful to speak as loudly as possible using a higher tone of voice.

Activity M *Select the single best answer for each of the following questions.*

1. Which of the following statements is true about otitis media?

   a. It is common in people who swim frequently.

   b. It is an infection of the middle ear that is common in young children.

   c. It occurs when the insides of the ears get wet during showering or bathing.

   d. It causes a person to have difficulty telling the difference between similar-sounding high-pitched sounds, like "th" and "s."

2. Which of the following statements best describes Ménière's disease?

   a. It occurs when fluid builds up in the middle ear.

   b. It is a disease of the inner ear, named after the French doctor who first described it.

   c. It occurs when people lose their hearing gradually later in life.

   d. Conversations can be difficult to follow, especially when many people are talking at once or there is a lot of background noise.

3. Which of the following statements is true regarding sensorineural hearing loss?

   a. It occurs when something prevents sound waves from reaching the receptors in the cochlea.

   b. It causes a change in the stapes, preventing it from moving properly.

   c. It occurs when the receptors are unable to receive stimuli or transmit nerve impulses.

   d. To correct it, the doctor makes a small slit in the eardrum and inserts a tube to equalize the pressure.

Activity N *Place an "X" next to the figure(s) that show good ways to communicate with a person who is hearing-impaired. Then, write down what communication method is being used. If the communication method shown is incorrect, write down the correct communication method.*

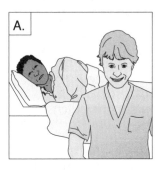

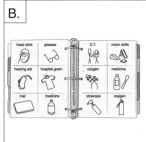

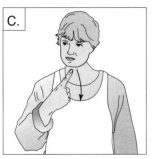

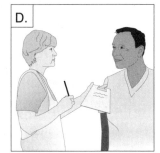

1. ____ A. _____

2. ____ B. _____

3. ____ C. _____

4. ____ D. _____

Activity O *Mark each statement as either "true" (T) or "false" (F). Correct the false statements.*

1. T F All people with hearing loss can benefit from a hearing aid.

1. T F Hearing aids must not be exposed to extreme heat or cold, moisture, or hairspray.

1. T F Hearing aids need to be removed and cleaned weekly.

SUMMARY

Activity P *Some vocabulary words from this chapter are given below in jumbled form. Use the clues and the pictures to form correct words.*

1. A system used by a blind person to read that uses letters made from combinations of raised dots

2. The gradual yellowing and hardening of the lens of the eye

3. A form of hearing loss as a result of the inability of the stapes to move properly

4. Receptors found in the skin that are stimulated when something comes in contact with the surface of the body and presses on them, causing them to change shape

5. Dizziness

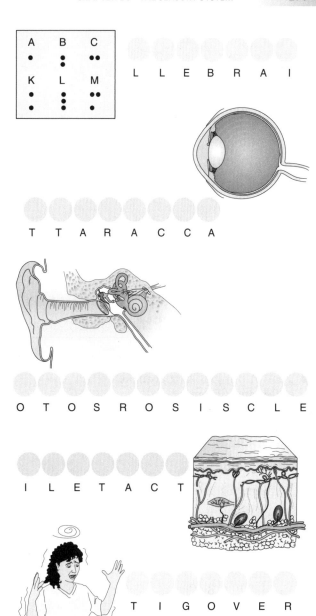

L L E B R A I

T T A R A C C A

O T O S R O S I S C L E

I L E T A C T

T I G O V E R

The Endocrine System

STRUCTURE OF THE ENDOCRINE SYSTEM

Key Learning Points

■ The various glands that make up the endocrine system

Activity A *Place an "X" next to the glands that are part of the endocrine system.*

1. ____ Pituitary gland

2. ____ Pineal gland

3. ____ Salivary gland

4. ____ Thyroid gland

5. ____ Sweat gland

6. ____ Thymus gland

7. ____ Adrenal gland

8. ____ Sex gland

Activity B *The figure shows the human endocrine system. Label the figure using the words given in brackets.*

[pineal gland, ovaries, thyroid gland, parathyroid gland, pancreas, pituitary gland, thymus, adrenal glands, testis]

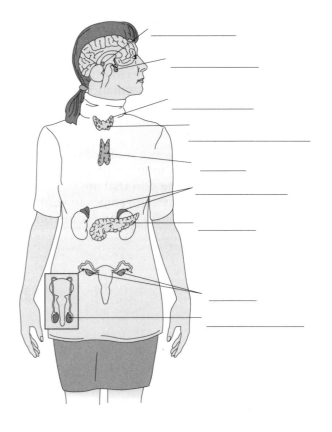

FUNCTIONS OF THE ENDOCRINE SYSTEM

Key Learning Points

■ The main function of the endocrine system
■ The feedback mechanism that controls the endocrine system
■ The hormones produced by the different glands of the endocrine system

Activity C *Some of the steps in the feedback system are listed below. Write down the correct order of the steps in the boxes provided below.*

1. The amount of hormone (or some other related substance) reaches a certain level in the body.
2. The gland begins to produce its hormone
3. The gland stops the production of the hormone.
4. The internal environment of the body changes.
5. The gland continues to produce the hormone.

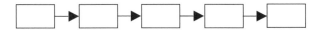

Activity D *Think About It! Briefly answer the following question in the space provided.*

Which gland is considered the "master" gland of the endocrine system, and why?

_____

_____

_____

Activity E *Match the organs of the body, given in Column A, with the hormones that control their functions, given in Column B.*

Column A

____ 1. Ovaries

____ 2. Uterus

____ 3. Kidneys

____ 4. Breast

____ 5. Long bone

Column B

a. Antidiuretic hormone (ADH)

b. Growth hormone

c. Prolactin

d. Oxytocin

f. Gonadotropins

Activity F *Match the hormones, given in Column A, with their specific functions, given in Column B.*

Column A

____ 1. Thyroxine

____ 2. Thymosin

____ 3. Melatonin

____ 4. Parathyroid hormone (PTH)

____ 5. Calcitonin

Column B

a. Suppresses the body's inflammatory response

b. Limits fluid loss from the body

c. Lowers blood glucose levels

____ 6. Insulin

____ 7. Glucagon

____ 8. Epinephrine

____ 9. Glucocorticoids

____ 10. Mineralocorticoids

____ 11. Oxytocin

____ 12. Prolactin

____ 13. Antidiuretic hormone (ADH)

d. Stimulates production of T cells

e. Regulates sodium and potassium

f. Decreases blood calcium levels

g. Increases blood calcium levels

h. Stimulates milk production by the breasts

i. Regulates the sleep-awake cycle

j. Raises blood glucose levels

k. Regulates metabolism

l. Stimulates fight or flight response

m. Stimulates uterine contractions

Activity G *Label the figure using the words given in brackets. Then use the same words to fill in the blanks in the sentences below.*

[adrenal gland, kidney, medulla, cortex]

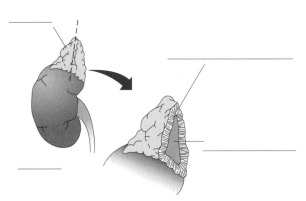

The _____ consists of two parts.
The _____ is the outer portion, while the _____ is the inner portion.
The adrenal glands are located on the top of the _____.

Activity H *Match the hormones produced by the adrenal glands, given in Column A, with their specific functions, given in Column B.*

Column A

_____ **1.** Epinephrine and norepinephrine

_____ **2.** Glucocorticoids

_____ **3.** Mineralocorticoids

_____ **4.** Androgens

Column B

a. They help the body to maintain a reserve of glucose (sugar) that can be used in times of stress

b. They help to regulate the level of certain minerals in the body, particularly sodium and potassium

c. They are converted by the body into the sex hormones *testosterone* (in men) and *estradiol* (in women)

d. They help the heart and lungs deliver more oxygen and nutrients to the muscles, preparing the body for "flight or fight"

Activity I *Think About It! Briefly answer the following questions in the spaces provided.*

1. Mrs. Selma is an asthma patient. She is kept on hydrocortisone medication. Why is Mrs. Selma prescribed the hydrocortisone medication?

_____

_____

_____

2. Why is the pancreas called both an endocrine gland and an exocrine gland?

_____

_____

_____

3. Mr. Patel has goiter. What are the factors that can cause goiter?

_____

_____

_____

Activity J *Insulin helps us to regulate our blood glucose levels. Some of the steps involved in regulating blood glucose levels are listed below. Write down the correct order of the steps in the boxes provided below.*

1. Mr. Dawson has lunch because he is feeling hungry.

2. Mr. Dawson's pancreas releases insulin into the bloodstream.

3. The level of glucose in Mr. Dawson's blood rises.

4. Extra glucose is converted into glycogen or fat.

5. Insulin moves glucose from the bloodstream into the cells, where it can be used as energy.

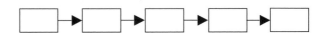

Activity K *Mark each statement as either "true" (T) or "false" (F). Correct the false statements.*

1. T F Aldosterone helps the kidneys to reabsorb sodium and secrete potassium.

2. T F Glucagon is responsible for lowering blood glucose levels.

3. T F The gonads secrete the hormones that result in the onset of puberty and that regulate reproduction.

4. T F Calcitonin is one of the hormones that helps to maintain calcium levels in the bloodstream.

THE EFFECT OF AGING ON THE ENDOCRINE SYSTEM

Key Learning Points

- How the aging process affects the endocrine system

Activity L *Think About It! Briefly answer the following question in the space provided.*

List a normal effect of aging on the endocrine system in women, and in men.

_____

_____

_____

DISORDERS OF THE ENDOCRINE SYSTEM

Key Learning Points

- How too little or too much of the various hormones can affect homeostasis
- The special care needs of people who have endocrine system disorders

Activity M *Match the endocrine disorders, given in Column A, with their characteristics, given in Column B.*

Column A

_____ 1. Pituitary dwarfism

_____ 2. Pituitary gigantism

_____ 3. Acromegaly

Column B

a. Mr. Merlino is 65 years old and has excessive growth of the bones of the hands, feet, and face

b. Mark is 18 years old and much shorter than average, but still well proportioned

c. Tim is 17 years old and much taller than average, but still well proportioned

Activity N *Place an "X" next to the phrases that describe signs and symptoms of hyperthyroidism, and a "Y" next to the phrases that describe signs and symptoms of hypothyroidism.*

1. ____ Mr. Johnson consumes more food than average, but he still loses weight considerably.

2. ____ Mrs. Mina's food intake is low but she still gains weight.

3. ____ Mr. Roberts is always cold.

4. ____ Mr. Drake perspires a great deal.

5. ____ Mr. Watson has difficulty sleeping.

Activity O *Mark each statement as either "true" (T) or "false" (F). Correct the false statements.*

1. T F Diabetes mellitus can occur in people of all ages and races, but people of Native American or African descent are affected most often.

2. T F Type 1 diabetes mellitus is more common but much less severe than type 2 diabetes mellitus.

3. T F Type 1 diabetes mellitus is the form of diabetes that most often affects older adults.

4. T F A person with type 1 diabetes must receive daily injections of insulin.

5. T F Too much insulin causes hypoglycemia, a dangerous drop in blood glucose levels.

6. T F Too little insulin results in hyperglycemia, or too much glucose in the bloodstream.

7. T F Hypoglycemia can lead to a state called diabetic coma in people with diabetes.

8. T F Type 2 diabetes commonly occurs in overweight adults.

9. T F In people with type 2 diabetes the pancreas still produces some insulin, but the cells of the body are unable to respond to the insulin.

10. T F Type 2 diabetes is treated through diet, exercise, and the use of oral medications to increase the effectiveness of insulin.

11. T F Controlling the diet is the only way to treat type 2 diabetes.

Activity P *Think About It! Briefly answer the following question in the space provided.*

1. You are caring for Tanya, who has type 1 diabetes. Tanya receives two insulin injections each day.

    a. Why is it important to serve meals and snacks to Tanya at the scheduled time?

    _____

    _____

    _____

    b. What precautions should you take when you are checking Tanya's glucose level using the "finger stick" method?

    _____

    _____

    _____

2. You are caring for Mr. Ronald, a resident with type 1 diabetes. Mr. Ronald has atherosclerosis, a common complication of diabetes. He also has an infection on his toe that has become worse over the past 2 weeks and shows no signs of healing.

    a. Why was Mr. Ronald at increased risk for developing atherosclerosis as a result of his diabetes?

    _____

    _____

    _____

    b. How does diabetes affect a person's ability to heal and fight infection?

    _____

    _____

    _____

> Diabetes is the most common of all endocrine gland disorders and is the seventh leading cause of death among the elderly.

SUMMARY

Activity Q *Words shown in the picture have been jumbled. Use the clues to form correct words using the letters given in the picture.*

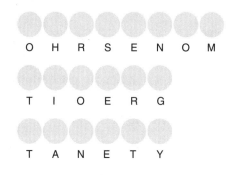

O H R S E N O M

T I O E R G

T A N E T Y

1. Chemicals that act on cells to produce a response
2. Enlargement of the thyroid gland
3. A condition that occurs when the body's calcium level drops too low; characterized by cramping of the skeletal muscles and an irregular heart beat

CHAPTER 32

The Digestive System

STRUCTURE OF THE DIGESTIVE SYSTEM

Key Learning Points

■ The organs that are part of the digestive system

Activity A *The figure shows the human digestive system. Label the organs that form a part of the digestive system using the words given in brackets.*

[ascending colon, pharynx, mouth, small intestine, rectum, jejunum, salivary glands, esophagus, transverse colon, stomach, descending colon, pancreas, gallbladder, large intestine, liver, duodenum, sigmoid colon, ileum, anus]

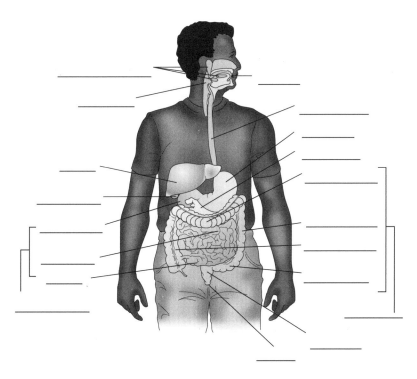

Activity B *Look at the figure and fill in the blanks in the sentences below using the words given in the figure.*

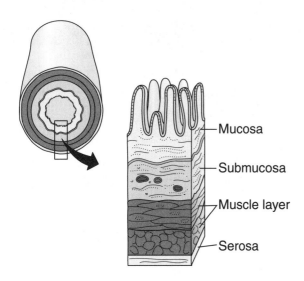

1. The _____ contains smooth muscle that is under involuntary control and helps move food through the system.

2. The _____ contains blood vessels and nerves.

3. The _____, a mucous membrane, lines the digestive tract and helps to trap disease-causing microbes.

4. The _____ is a tough outer layer of connective tissue.

Activity C *Think About It! Briefly answer the following question in the space provided.*

What is the purpose of the mucous membrane that lines the digestive tract? (BONUS: List another organ system that is lined with a mucous membrane).

_____

_____

_____

Activity D *Match the digestive organs, given in Column A, with their functions, given in Column B.*

Column A

____ **1.** Teeth and tongue

____ **2.** Esophagus

____ **3.** Appendix

____ **4.** Liver

____ **5.** Gallbladder

____ **6.** Pancreas

Column B

a. Stores bile produced by the liver that is not secreted directly into the duodenum

b. Produces and secretes bile into the duodenum, produces clotting factors and helps to clear our blood of toxins, such as alcohol and drugs

c. Accessory organs that assist with chewing and swallowing food

d. Produces substances that aid in digestion, as well as insulin and glucagon

e. The mucus secreted by this organ, as well as the action of its muscle layer, helps to move food downward and into the stomach

f. Has no known function

Activity E *The small intestine is shown below. Label the figure using the words given in brackets.*

[duodenum, ileum, jejunum]

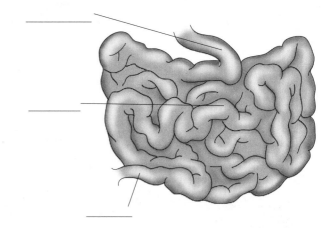

Activity F *Fill in the blanks using the words given in brackets.*

[pylorus, 20, hiatus, abdominal, pancreas, fundus, pyloric sphincter, gallbladder, esophageal sphincter, 4½, saliva, chest, colon, liver]

1. The esophagus passes through the _____ cavity, behind the heart and enters the _____ cavity at the _____, an opening in the diaphragm.

2. The _____ is the upper region of the stomach.

3. Food enters the stomach through the _____, which keeps the food from going back up the esophagus.

4. The _____ is the bottom region of the stomach. Food leaves the stomach through the _____, which prevents the food from returning to the stomach once it enters the small intestine.

5. The large intestine, also called the _____, is _____ feet long.

6. _____ is a substance that helps with chewing and swallowing by moistening the food.

7. The _____ is a large organ located just underneath the diaphragm that produces and secretes bile.

8. The small intestine is about _____ feet long.

9. The _____ is located behind the stomach, in the curve of the duodenum.

10. The _____ is a small pouch that is attached to the liver where bile is stored.

Activity G *The large intestine is shown below. Label the figures using the words given in brackets.*

[descending colon, cecum, ascending colon, appendix, anus, sigmoid colon, ileocecal valve, transverse colon, rectum]

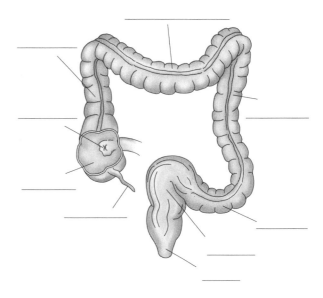

FUNCTION OF THE DIGESTIVE SYSTEM

Key Learning Points

■ The function of the organs of the digestive system

Activity H *The digestive system processes the food that we eat. Write the names of the organs or parts of organs that are responsible for each action listed, using the words given in brackets. Then write down the correct order of the events of digestion in the boxes below.*

[salivary glands, rectum, large intestine, stomach, jejunum, teeth, villi, duodenum]

1. _____ Absorption of nutrients begins.

2. _____ Bacteria act on the chyme to produce vitamin K and some B vitamins. Water is also absorbed into the bloodstream.

3. _____ The chyme mixes with bile (secreted by the liver) and digestive enzymes secreted by the pancreas.

4. _____ Chemical substances in our saliva start to work on the smaller pieces of food, breaking them down through chemical digestion.

5. _____ Through peristaltic action, food is mixed with hydrochloric acid, creating a liquid substance called chyme.

6. _____ As the feces (waste products of digestion) collect over a period of time, the urge to defecate (have a bowel movement) occurs.

7. _____ Mechanical digestion helps in the physical breakdown of food by mastication.

8. _____ Most absorption of nutrients takes place here.

□ → □ → □ → □
↓
□ ← □ ← □ ← □

Activity I *The small intestine is shown below. Label the figure using the words given in brackets. Then briefly describe how the small intestine is able to absorb nutrients from chyme.*

[submucosa, villi, mucosa]

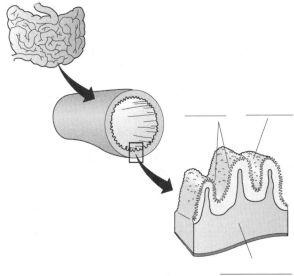

_____

How does the small intestine absorb nutrients from chyme?

_____

_____

_____

Activity J *Mark each statement as either "true" (T) or "false" (F). Correct the false statements.*

1. T F   The physical breaking up of food by mastication is called chemical digestion.

2. T F   The process of breaking down food through the use of enzymes is called chemical digestion.

3. T F   The peristaltic action of the stomach helps to mix the food with the acid and enzymes, forming feces.

4. T F   Once the chyme reaches the duodenum of the small intestine, absorption of nutrients begins.

5. T F   Bacteria that live in the large intestine act on the chyme to produce vitamin K and some B vitamins, which are absorbed by the body.

Activity K *Think About It! Briefly answer the following questions in the spaces provided.*

1. In a healthy person, how does liquid chyme take on the soft, moist, semi-solid consistency of normal feces as it reaches the end of the large intestine?

_____

_____

2. When does a person feel the need to defecate?

_____

_____

EFFECTS OF AGING ON THE DIGESTIVE SYSTEM

Key Learning Points

■ The effects of aging on the digestive system

Activity L *Match the age-related changes, given in Column A, with their effects on the digestive system, given in Column B.*

Column A

_____ 1. Missing or painful teeth and a decrease in the production of saliva

_____ 2. The production of saliva, stomach acid, and digestive enzymes slows

_____ 3. The movement of food through the digestive tract may be slower

Column B

a. Can put the older person at risk for constipation

b. Increases an older person's risk of choking

c. Makes chemical digestion less efficient

Activity M *Think About It! Briefly answer the following questions in the spaces provided.*

1. Mr. O'Brien is one of your residents. His partial dentures were broken after being dropped during a linen change. His remaining natural teeth do not allow him to chew as well. What precautions must you take when Mr. O'Brien is eating?

_____

_____

_____

2. Mrs. Loman is 87 years old. How does the aging process increase Mrs. Loman's risk for constipation? What will you do to help lower this risk?

_____

_____

_____

> ● Like all of the body's organ systems, the digestive system is affected by the process of aging. When you observe and report that one of your elderly patients or residents is having trouble eating, has had a change in his or her bowel elimination pattern, or has symptoms of a digestive disorder, you play an important part in helping to keep your patient or resident healthy and comfortable.

DISORDERS OF THE DIGESTIVE SYSTEM

Key Learning Points

■ Common digestive disorders and their symptoms

Activity N *Think About It! Briefly answer the following questions in the spaces provided.*

1. What is an ulcer? What are the factors that can increase a person's chances of developing an ulcer? Write the common complaints a person with an ulcer may have.

_____

_____

_____

_____

2. Which digestive disorder can cause the feces to be pale and "clay-colored"? Why do the feces appear this way? Also write some of the common symptoms in a person with this digestive disorder and commonly used methods of treating it.

_____

_____

_____

_____

Activity O *Identify the disorder shown in Figure A. Then label the areas where this disorder can occur in Figure B, using the words given in brackets.*

[inguinal, femoral, hiatal, umbilical]

The digestive disorder shown in Figure A is a _____.

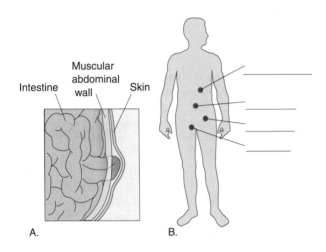

A.   B.

Activity P *Match the digestive disorders, given in Column A, with their descriptions, given in Column B.*

Column A

____ **1.** Gastric ulcer

____ **2.** Duodenal ulcer

____ **3.** Penetrating ulcer

____ **4.** Inguinal hernia

____ **5.** Femoral hernia

____ **6.** Umbilical hernia

____ **7.** Hiatal hernia

____ **8.** Strangulated hernia

Column B

a. Occurs most commonly in men when a loop of intestine bulges through the abdominal wall in the groin area

b. Occurs around the naval (belly button)

c. Occurs if the muscle tightens around the trapped tissue, cutting off its blood supply

d. Wearing away of the protective mucosa that lines the stomach

e. Occurs when part of the stomach passes through the hiatus, the opening in the diaphragm that allows the esophagus to pass into the abdominal cavity

f. Wearing away of the protective mucosa that lines the duodenum

g. Occurs most commonly in women when a loop of intestine bulges through the abdominal wall in the groin area

h. A life-threatening condition that affects all of the layers of the stomach or duodenum wall, not just the mucosa

DIAGNOSIS OF DIGESTIVE DISORDERS

Key Learning Points

■ Some of the tools used to diagnose digestive disorders

Activity Q *Think About It! Briefly answer the following question in the space provided.*

One of your residents, Mrs. Lewis, often complains after meals that whatever she ate "didn't agree with her." Usually, when you ask her what is wrong, she tells you that she has "heartburn" or "indigestion," but not to worry, because it will go away soon. Today, however, Mrs. Lewis tells you that her heartburn is "really bad," and she looks a little paler than usual. What should you do?

_____

_____

_____

Activity R *Fill in the blanks using the words given in brackets.*

[magnetic resonance imaging (MRI) scans, x-rays, stool, mouth, endoscopy, computed tomography (CT) scans, anus, barium]

1. An example of a simple test for a digestive complaint is laboratory analysis of a _____ sample.

2. _____ involves using a special instrument to look inside the digestive tract and obtain tissue or fluids for analysis.

3. The endoscope is passed through a person's _____ to view the upper digestive tract or the _____ to view the lower digestive tract.

4. Imaging studies, such as _____, _____ and _____ allow the doctor to view the organs of the digestive system without actually entering the body.

5. _____ is a liquid that coats the mucosa of the digestive tract, and makes the organs appear sharper and brighter when x-rayed.

> A person who is about to have a diagnostic procedure to evaluate her digestive system may have special care needs prior to the test. The nurse will let you know of any special instructions, which should be followed carefully.

SUMMARY

Activity S *Some vocabulary words from this chapter are given below in jumbled form. Use the clues and the pictures to form correct words.*

1. A long narrow tube that serves mainly as a passageway for food to get from the pharynx to the stomach
2. Folds in the lining of the stomach that allow the stomach capacity to increase
3. Another word for mastication

4. A disorder that occurs when an internal organ bulges through a weakness in the muscular wall of the abdominal cavity
5. A liquid that coats the mucosa of the digestive tract, making the organs appear sharper and brighter when x-rayed

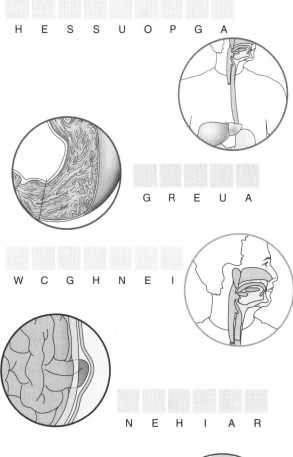

H E S S U O P G A

G R E U A

W C G H N E I

N E H I A R

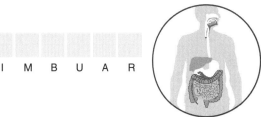

I M B U A R

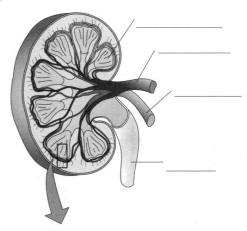

The Urinary System

STRUCTURE OF THE URINARY SYSTEM

Key Learning Points

■ The organs that are part of the urinary system

Activity A *The figure shows the human urinary system. Label the figure using the words given in brackets. Then, next to each label, briefly describe the function of the organ.*

[bladder, kidney, ureter, urethra]

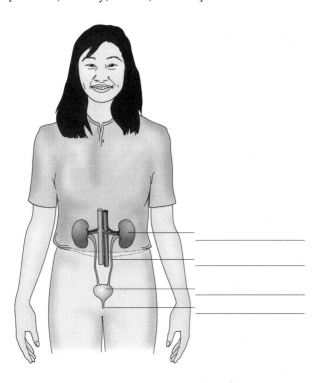

Activity B *Figures A and B show cross-sections of the kidney and a nephron. Label the figures using the words given in brackets. Then, write down the correct order of the steps describing how the kidneys produce urine in the boxes provided on the next page.*

[tubule, renal pyramid, efferent arteriole, afferent arteriole, renal artery, Bowman's capsule, renal vein, ureter, glomerulus]

A. Kidney

B. Nephron

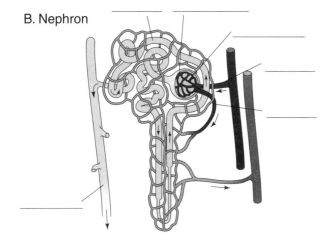

1. The blood passes through a series of arteries that get smaller and smaller, until it reaches the capillary bed of the glomerulus.
2. Filtrate passes through the small capillaries surrounding the tubules of the nephron, which reabsorb useful substances such as water, nutrients, and minerals from the filtrate.
3. Because the blood is under high pressure, a lot of the liquid in the blood squeezes through the semi-permeable walls of the capillaries in the glomerulus, taking the wastes and nutrients that are dissolved in it with it. This is the filtrate.
4. The filtrate that reaches the end of the tubules is urine.
5. Urine from each nephron is emptied into a collecting area, called the renal pelvis. From the renal pelvis, the urine flows into the ureters.
6. The blood enters the kidneys through the renal arteries under great pressure.
7. The blood enters the glomerulus through a vessel called the afferent arteriole.
8. The filtered blood leaves the glomerulus through the efferent arteriole. The filtrate enters the Bowman's capsule.

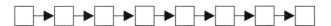

Activity C *Mark each statement as either "true" (T) or "false" (F). Correct the false statements.*

1. T F   The kidneys are located toward the back of the upper abdominal cavity, one on either side of the spinal column.

2. T F   The job of the kidneys is to remove solid waste from the body.

3. T F   The urethra is approximately 10 to 13 inches (25 to 32 cm) long, and carries urine from the kidneys to the bladder.

4. T F   The smooth muscle in the walls of the ureters keeps urine from flowing back into the ureters after it has emptied into the bladder.

Activity D *Fill in the blanks using the words given in brackets.*

[wide, 1 to 1.5 liters, half hour, Bowman's capsule, aorta, 160 to 180 liters, nephron]

1. The blood flow through the renal arteries, which are branches of the _____, is so efficient, that the kidneys are able to filter all of the body's blood every _____.

2. The ureters are _____ at the top where they connect to the renal pelvis, but they quickly become very narrow where they enter the bladder.

3. Each _____ consists of a glomerulus and a series of tubules. The glomerulus is a capillary bed, enclosed within a structure called _____.

4. The kidneys produce _____ of filtrate each day, but only about _____ is excreted from the body in the form of urine.

FUNCTION OF THE URINARY SYSTEM

Key Learning Points

■ The primary function of each organ of the urinary system

Activity E *Think About It! Briefly answer the following question in the space provided.*

When does a person feel the urge to urinate? What happens when you feel the urge to urinate and you delay urination for an extended period?

_____

_____

_____

Activity F *Fill in the blanks using the words given in brackets.*

[acid, 1 to 14, 1 pint (470 mL), 200 to 300, 7]

1. A moderately full bladder usually contains about _____ of urine.

2. When about _____ mL of urine collects in the bladder, the internal sphincter opens and allows urine to flood the upper segment of the urethra.

3. _____ is a normal by-product of cellular metabolism.

4. Human blood is slightly above a _____ on the pH scale, which ranges from _____.

Activity G *Mark each statement as either "true" (T) or "false" (F). Correct the false statements.*

1. T F   The urinary system maintains the level of urine in the body.

2. T F   Too little fluid in the body can lead to dehydration.

3. T F   The urinary system regulates the levels of minerals such as vitamin A, vitamin B, and vitamin D by either saving them or releasing them through urine.

THE EFFECTS OF AGING ON THE URINARY SYSTEM

Key Learning Points

■ The effects of aging on the urinary system

Activity H *Match the age-related changes that occur in the urinary system, given in Column A, with their descriptions, given in Column B.*

Column A	Column B
____ 1. Less efficient filtration	a. May result in episodes of overflow incontinence
____ 2. Decreased muscle tone	b. Decrease in the kidneys' ability to filter waste products from the bloodstream
____ 3. Enlargement of a man's prostate gland	c. Most common in older women who have had children or are obese; may contribute to stress incontinence

Although it is important for everyone to drink plenty of water and other fluids, it is especially important for older people. Drinking plenty of fluids helps the kidneys to work properly and regular urination flushes harmful bacteria from the bladder, helping to prevent urinary tract infections.

DISORDERS OF THE URINARY SYSTEM

Key Learning Points

■ Various disorders that can affect the urinary system

Activity I *Match the terms, given in Column A, with their descriptions, given in Column B.*

Column A

____ 1. Urethritis

____ 2. Cystitis

____ 3. Pyelonephritis

____ 4. Hematuria

____ 5. Acute renal failure

____ 6. Chronic renal failure

____ 7. Oliguria

____ 8. Anuria

Column B

a. Infection of the kidney

b. Results from a medical or surgical emergency that causes a decrease in the amount of blood flow through the kidneys

c. Results from a gradual loss of functioning nephrons

d. Infection of the bladder

e. Microbes responsible for sexually transmitted infections (STIs) such as gonorrhea, herpes, and chlamydia are common causes of this infection in men

f. Blood in the urine

g. The absence of urine

h. Scant amounts of urine, less than 400 ml in 24 hours

Activity J *Think About It! Briefly answer the following question in the space provided.*

Why is it important to wipe from the front to the back when providing perineal care for a woman?

_____

_____

_____

Activity K *Think About It! Briefly answer the following question in the space provided.*

List three signs and symptoms that could indicate a urinary tract infection.

_____

_____

_____

Activity L *Mark each statement as either "true" (T) or "false" (F). Correct the false statements.*

1. T F   When waste products in the form of mineral salts become very concentrated in the urine, they start to group together, forming kidney stones.

2. T F   In older people, symptoms of urinary tract infections always include urinary frequency, burning, and cramping.

3. T F   The most common causes of acute renal failure are hypertension and diabetes.

4. T F   Factors that may increase an older person's risk of developing kidney stones include immobility, not drinking enough fluids, and infections of the urinary system.

5. T F   In lithotripsy, the kidney stone is removed through a surgical incision.

6. T F   Signs of renal failure may include dehydration, swelling, hypertension, or oliguria followed by anuria.

7. T F   Later in chronic renal failure when the kidneys are unable to eliminate excess fluid, a person's body may swell from the build-up of fluids.

8. T F   Usually early in acute renal failure, because the kidneys cannot reabsorb filtrate back into the bloodstream, the person may become constipated.

9. T F   A person with a neurogenic bladder may have an underactive bladder that is spastic, or highly sensitive to stimulation.

Activity M *Think About It! Briefly answer the following question in the space provided.*

Mrs. Grande has been ignoring pain in her upper back region. One day, she suddenly panicked after finding traces of blood in her urine, accompanied by an increase in pain when she was voiding. What could be causing Mrs. Grande's symptoms?

_____

_____

_____

Activity N *Identify the urinary diversions shown in each of the figures.*

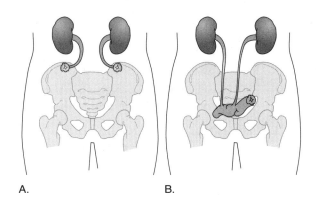

A.   B.

A. _____

B. _____

Activity O *Think About It! Briefly answer the following question in the space provided.*

Mrs. O'Donnell has a urostomy. List three things a nursing assistant should keep in mind when caring for Mrs. O'Donnell.

_____

_____

_____

Activity P *Fill in the blanks using the words given in brackets.*

[spina bifida, hemodialysis, bladder, bladder cancer, peritoneal, dialysis shunt]

1. During _____, the person's blood is drawn intravenously, passed through a machine with filters and solutions that clean the blood of waste, and then returned to the person's body through another vessel.

2. During _____ dialysis, solutions that absorb waste products are instilled into a person's abdominal cavity so that waste products can be absorbed into the solution through the membrane lining the abdominal cavity.

3. Do not place a blood pressure cuff on an arm that has a _____.

4. Tumors of the _____ are common among people who have smoked cigarettes.

5. _____ is a common reason for a person to have a ureterostomy or urostomy.

6. Birth defects such as _____ can result in a person having a urinary diversion procedure done.

DIAGNOSIS OF URINARY DISORDERS

Key Learning Points

■ Common diagnostic procedures that may be used to detect and diagnose urinary system disorders

Activity Q *Match the types of tests used to diagnose disorders of the urinary system, given in Column A, with their descriptions, given in Column B.*

Column A

_____ **1.** Urinalysis

_____ **2.** CT scans, MRI scans, and x-rays

_____ **3.** Cytoscopy

_____ **4.** Ureteroscopy

Column B

a. A small, lighted scope is inserted through the urethra and used to view the inside of the bladder

b. A small, lighted scope is inserted through the urethra and used to view the inside of the ureters

c. Can allow a doctor to see tumors and other abnormalities of the urinary system

d. The urine is examined under a microscope and by chemical means

Activity R *Think About It! Briefly answer the following question in the space provided.*

As a nursing assistant, what should you remember when you are involved in helping a patient or resident to prepare for a diagnostic test used to evaluate the urinary system?

_____

_____

_____

SUMMARY

Activity S *Some vocabulary words from this chapter are given below in jumbled form. Use the clues and the pictures to form correct words.*

1. Related to, involving, or located in the region of the kidneys

2. The liquid that forms the basis for urine

3. Infection of the bladder

4. A procedure that is done to remove waste products and fluids from the body when a person's kidneys fail and can no longer perform this task

5. The basic functional unit of the kidney; consists of a glomerulus and a series of tubules

N L R A E

T A T R E I L F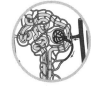

T I S Y T I S C

L D I A I S Y S

H N E N P O R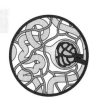

The Reproductive System

REPRODUCTION

Key Learning Points

■ The main function of the reproductive system

Activity A *Mark each statement as either "true" (T) or "false" (F). Correct the false statements.*

1. T F   One of the main functions of the reproductive system in both males and females is to produce and transport sex cells.

2. T F   Each of us receives blood from our parents that determines how we develop and what we look like physically.

3. T F   The organs that make up the reproductive system are the same in men and women.

Activity B *Fill in the blanks using the words given in brackets.*

[sperm, gametes, 46, sex, reproduction, conception, egg, genes, ovum, 23, chromosomes]

1. _____ is the process by which a living thing makes more living things like itself.

2. Each species has a set number of _____, or _____.

3. Human beings have _____ chromosomes.

4. The father and the mother each contribute _____ chromosomes.

5. The special cells contributed by each parent that contain half of the normal number of chromosomes are called _____ cells, or _____.

6. The male sex cell is called a _____ cell.

7. The female sex cell is called an _____, or _____.

8. When the sperm joins the egg, forming a cell that contains the complete number of chromosomes, _____ occurs.

THE FEMALE REPRODUCTIVE SYSTEM

Key Learning Points

■ The organs that make up the female reproductive system
■ The normal function of the female reproductive system
■ The effects of aging on the female reproductive system
■ The disorders that may affect the female reproductive system
■ Diagnostic tests commonly used to detect disorders of the female reproductive system

Activity C *A figure of the female reproductive system is shown below. Label the figure using the words given in brackets.*

[fallopian tube, cervix, uterus, ovary, vagina, fimbriae]

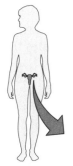

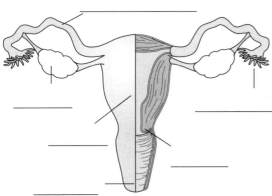

Activity D *Fill in the blanks using the words given in brackets.*

[oviducts, fimbriae, uterus, womb, fallopian tubes, prolactin, endometrium, ovulation, orifice, labia, vagina, clitoris, uterine tubes, lactation, ovaries]

1. The _____ are two small, almond-shaped organs located deep inside the abdomen on either side of the uterus.

2. _____ is the release of a ripe, mature egg from the ovaries each month.

3. The _____, also called _____ or _____, are slender tubes about 4 to 5 inches long that transport the egg from the ovary to the uterus.

4. The open ends of the fallopian tubes nearest the ovaries have small, fringe-like projections called _____.

5. The _____, sometimes referred to as the _____, is a hollow, pear-shaped organ.

6. The inner cavity of the uterus is shaped like a capital "T" and is lined with tissue called _____.

7. The _____ is a muscular tube about three inches long that connects the uterus to the outside of the body.

8. The vaginal opening, also called the vaginal _____, is where the vagina opens to the outside of the body.

9. The _____, or "lips," are folds of tissue that surround the vaginal opening.

10. The _____ is located at the upper folds of the internal labia and helps to initiate a woman's sexual arousal.

11. When the breast is stimulated by the hormone _____, the glandular tissue of the breasts produces milk, a process known as _____.

Activity E *A figure of the female breast is shown below. Label the figure using the words given in brackets.*

[fat, glandular tissue, duct, muscle]

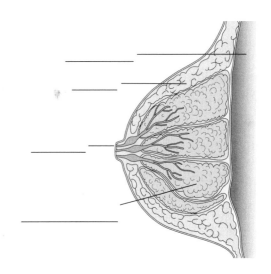

Activity F *Mark each statement as either "true" (T) or "false" (F). Correct the false statements.*

1. T F   When a baby girl develops and grows to be an adolescent; her ovaries produce the eggs used for reproduction.

2. T F   The uterus has three sections: the fundus, the body, and the cervix.

3. T F   The mucous membrane that lines the vagina serves to lubricate the vagina during sexual intercourse and protect the body from infection.

4. T F   The term *womb* is used to describe the vaginal opening, labia, and clitoris.

Activity G *Select the single best answer for each of the following questions.*

1. What helps the egg move from the ovary to the uterus?

   a. Fimbriae

   b. Cilia

   c. Peristalsis

   d. All of the above

2. Which statement about the cervix is true?

   a. It is where the vagina opens to the outside of the body

   b. It has an opening 10 cm in diameter that allows menstrual blood to leave the body each month

   c. It is the lower, narrow portion of the uterus

   d. All of the above

Activity H *Each month during a woman's reproductive years, her body prepares itself to become pregnant. Write down the correct order of the steps a woman's body takes to prepare for pregnancy in the boxes provided below.*

1. The empty follicle (corpus luteum) continues to produce estrogen, and it also begins to produce progesterone.

2. Each month during a woman's reproductive years the pituitary gland releases follicle-stimulating hormone (FSH).

3. The lining of the uterus (the endometrium) thickens, creating a soft, nourishing environment for a fertilized egg, should one arrive.

4. One egg-containing follicle continues to grow and mature, and the others die off.

5. The fertilized egg begins to divide, forming the cells and tissues that will eventually become a new human being.

6. The FSH causes about 20 eggs in the ovaries to begin to grow and mature and stimulates the follicles to produce estrogen.

7. Estrogen and progesterone initiate a process called implantation.

8. When the egg has matured, luteinizing hormone (LH), released by the pituitary gland, causes the follicle to burst, releasing the egg from the ovary (ovulation).

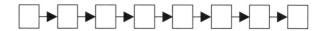

Activity I *Mark each statement as either "true" (T) or "false" (F). Correct the false statements.*

1. T F   Many women in their late 30s and early 40s often have difficulty becoming pregnant.

2. T F   Menopause occurs in most women sometime between the ages of 50 and 60 years and is caused by the loss of ovary function due to age.

3. T F   After the onset of menopause, the reproductive organs do not function and shrink to the size they were before puberty.

4. T F   Hormone replacement therapy can help to minimize some of the more annoying "side effects" of menopause, such as hot flashes.

Activity J *Match the disorders of the female reproductive system, given in Column A, with their descriptions, given in Column B.*

Column A

____ **1.** Amenorrhea

____ **2.** Dysmenor-rhea

____ **3.** Menorrhagia

____ **4.** Infertility

____ **5.** Cystocele

____ **6.** Cysts

____ **7.** Fibroids

____ **8.** Cervical cancer

____ **9.** Rectocele

____ **10.** Endometrial cancer

____ **11.** Ovarian cancer

____ **12.** Breast cancer

Column B

a. Can form on the ovaries after ovulation, causing intense pain

b. The inability to become pregnant or to carry a pregnancy to full term

c. Painful menstruation

d. Excessive bleeding during a menstrual period

e. The absence of menstrual flow in a girl who has not begun to menstruate by the age of 16 years or in a woman who has had previous menstrual periods

f. Type of pelvic organ prolapse in which the bladder pushes into the anterior vaginal wall

g. The most commonly occurring cancer in women; can develop in women with relatives having the same disorder (especially a mother or sister), or in womaen who have no family history of the disease

h. Most commonly occurs in women between the ages of 40 and 65 years and is a leading cause of cancer death for women

i. Is more common among women between the ages of 30 and 50 years and can be caused by a sexually transmitted viral infection

j. Cancer of the lining of the uterus

k. Also called myomas

l. Type of pelvic organ prolapse in which the rectum pushes into the posterior vaginal wall

Activity K *Think About It! Briefly answer the following questions in the spaces provided.*

1. Look at the figure below. What is the woman doing? Why is it important for women to do this each month?

_____

_____

_____

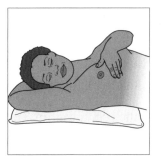

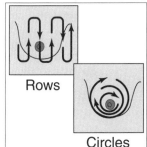

Rows

Circles

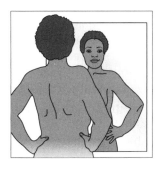

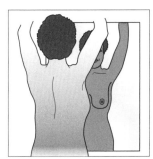

2. What are some of the emotions that a person who is being evaluated for a disorder involving the reproductive system may have? Describe ways that a nursing assistant can help a person who is being prepared for a diagnostic procedure involving the reproductive system.

_____

_____

_____

_____

_____

_____

Activity L *Match the diagnostic procedures used to screen for female reproductive disorders, given in Column A, with their descriptions, given in Column B.*

Column A

_____ **1.** Pap test

_____ **2.** Biopsy

_____ **3.** Dilation and curettage (D&C)

_____ **4.** Imaging studies

_____ **5.** Ultrasonography

_____ **6.** Mammography

Column B

a. Can be used to reveal tumors or cysts on the ovaries and in other structures of the female reproductive tract

b. An x-ray of breast tissue that can detect breast tumors at a very early stage

c. Routinely performed to detect changes in the cervix that may indicate early cervical cancer

d. A tissue sample is obtained and examined under a microscope for cancerous cells

e. Can allow a doctor to see tumors or scar tissue that may be blocking the fallopian tubes

f. A surgical procedure in which the cervix is made wider and tissue is scraped from the inside of the cervix and the uterus

Activity M *Mark each statement as either "true" (T) or "false" (F). Correct the false statements.*

1. T F A mastectomy may be performed on a woman who has been diagnosed with certain types of ovarian cancer.

2. T F A hysterectomy that is performed through the vagina by cutting around the cervix is called a total vaginal hysterectomy (TVH).

3. T F During a hysterectomy, the woman's fallopian tubes and ovaries are always removed along with her uterus.

THE MALE REPRODUCTIVE SYSTEM

Key Learning Points

- The organs that make up the male reproductive system
- The normal function of the male reproductive system
- The effects of aging on the male reproductive system
- The disorders that may affect the male reproductive system
- Diagnostic tests commonly used to detect disorders of the male reproductive system

Activity N *A figure of the male reproductive system is shown below. Label the figure using the words given in brackets.*

[prostate gland, vas deferens, urinary bladder, testis, epididymis, penis, urethra, seminal vesicle]

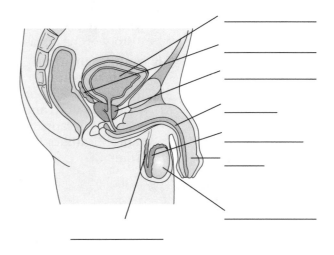

Activity O *Fill in the blanks using the words given in brackets.*

[testosterone, epididymis, penis, impotence, prostate gland, vas deferens, constantly, ejaculation, glans penis, interstitial cell-stimulating hormone, testicles, flagellum]

1. The _____ are two walnut-like organs located in the scrotum, a loose, bag-like sac of skin that is suspended outside of the body, between the thighs.

2. After the sperm cells leave the testes, they move into the _____, a series of coiled tubes.

3. The sperm cell is the only human body cell that has a _____.

4. From the epididymis, the sperm cell moves into the _____, a passageway that transports the sperm cell to the urethra.

5. Semen and urine leave the man's body through the _____.

6. If a male has not been circumcised, a loose fold of skin called the foreskin covers the _____.

7. The mature male reproductive system produces sperm cells _____.

8. Sperm cells are deposited in the female reproductive tract through the process of _____.

9. The pituitary gland secretes _____, which stimulates the testicles to produce _____.

10. As a man ages, the _____ tends to enlarge, making urination difficult.

11. _____ is the inability to achieve or maintain an erection long enough to engage in sexual activity.

Activity P *Think About It! Briefly answer the following question in the space provided.*

List two important functions of the testicles.

_____

_____

_____

Activity Q *Select the single best answer for each of the following questions.*

1. What happens in the epididymis?
   a. The sperm cells mix with fluid to produce semen
   b. The sperm cells mature and gain the ability to swim
   c. The sperm cells leave the man's body
   d. Fertilization of the egg takes place

2. Which gland produces the fluid that mixes with sperm cells to form semen?
   a. The testis
   b. The urinary bladder
   c. The prostate gland
   d. The epididymis

Activity R *Match the types of cancer that can affect the male reproductive system, given in Column A, with their descriptions, given in Column B.*

Column A	Column B
____ 1. Testicular cancer	a. Signs may include lesions on the penis
____ 2. Prostate cancer	b. Usually affects young to middle-aged adult men and can easily spread to other parts of the body through the lymphatic system before it is detected
____ 3. Penile cancer	c. Most commonly occurs in men older than 50 years; typically grows slowly and has a good cure rate with early detection

SEXUALLY TRANSMITTED INFECTIONS

Key Learning Points

■ Sexually transmitted infections (STIs) that may affect the male or female reproductive systems

Activity S *Match the sexually transmitted infections, given in Column A, with their descriptions, given in Column B.*

Column A

____ **1.** Herpes simplex

____ **2.** Gonorrhea

____ **3.** Chlamydia

____ **4.** Genital (venereal) warts

____ **5.** Syphilis

____ **6.** AIDS

____ **7.** Pelvic inflammatory disease (PID)

Column B

a. A bacterial infection in which the third stage usually involves damage to the cardiovascular and nervous systems, resulting in confusion, dementia, and paralysis

b. Caused by the human immunodeficiency virus (HIV); can be transmitted in semen, vaginal secretions, or blood

c. Infection of the fallopian tubes and abdomen that can lead to infertility if untreated

d. The most commonly occurring STI; often causes no symptoms; can be treated with an antibiotic

e. In men, symptoms may include dysuria and a greenish discharge from the urethra

f. Caused by a virus. Known as HPV, may cause growths inside the urethra (in men) or around the vaginal opening, inside the vagina, or on the cervix (in women)

g. A viral infection that can cause painful blisters to form around the mouth, around the vaginal opening and perineum (in women), or around the external urinary opening (in men)

Activity T *Think About It! Briefly answer the following question in the space provided.*

Why is the prevention of sexually transmitted infections (STIs) important? List two ways to protect yourself from getting an STI.

_____

_____

_____

Many people are hesitant or embarrassed to discuss problems involving the reproductive organs. As a nursing assistant, you may be the first to notice a worrisome sign that could be a sign of a disorder affecting the reproductive system in a patient or resident. When you gently ask the person about the sign and then report your observations to the nurse, you are taking a very important first step toward making sure the person gets the treatment he or she needs.

SUMMARY

Activity U *Words shown in the picture have been jumbled. Use the clues below to form correct words using the letters given in the picture.*

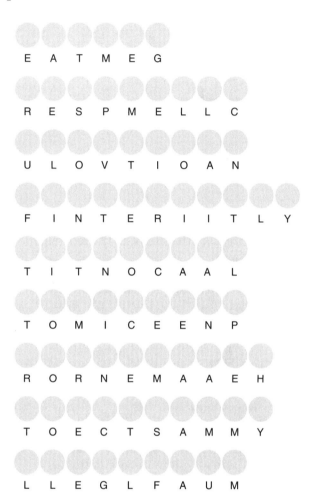

E A T M E G

R E S P M E L L C

U L O V T I O A N

F I N T E R I I T L Y

T I T N O C A A L

T O M I C E E N P

R O R N E M A A E H

T O E C T S A M M Y

L L E G L F A U M

1. Special cells contributed by each parent that contain half of the normal number of chromosomes
2. Male sex cell
3. The release of a ripe, mature egg from the female ovaries each month
4. The inability to become pregnant or to carry a pregnancy to full term
5. The process by which the glandular tissue of the female breast produces milk
6. The inability to achieve or maintain an erection long enough to engage in sexual activity
7. Absence of menstrual flow
8. Surgical removal of a breast
9. A sperm cell's "whip-like" tail, which allows it to move

CHAPTER 35

Caring for People With Rehabilitation Needs

Key Learning Points

- The terms *rehabilitation* and *restorative care*.
- Reasons why a person may require rehabilitation services, restorative care, or both.
- The major goals of rehabilitation and describe settings in which rehabilitation can take place.
- The three phases of the rehabilitation process.
- The responsibilities of key members of the rehabilitation team.

Activity A *Fill in the blanks using the words given in brackets.*

[disability, rehabilitation, OBRA, restorative care, independence]

1. One of the goals of the health care team is to help patients and residents learn to manage their disabilities and regain as much _____ as possible.

2. Many of the patients or residents that you will care for have some degree of _____, or impaired function.

3. The process of helping a person with a disability to return to his highest level of physical, emotional, or economic function is known as _____.

4. _____ requires long-term care facilities to provide rehabilitation services that meet the specific needs of the residents who live in the facility.

5. The care provided by all of the members of the health care team that supports the rehabilitation effort is called _____.

Activity B *Mark each statement as either "true" (T) or "false" (F). Correct the false statements.*

1. T F In most health care settings, the term "rehabilitation" usually refers to services provided by licensed therapists who specialize in various aspects of rehabilitation.

2. T F Traumatic injuries that involve the brain and the spinal cord are less likely to require long-term rehabilitation.

3. T F The rehabilitation effort focuses on the individual needs and capabilities of the health care facility.

4. T F In most health care settings, the term "restorative care" usually refers to the actions taken by the nursing team to support the rehabilitation effort.

Activity C *Think About It! Briefly answer the following question in the space provided.*

1. List some conditions that may require rehabilitation in a specialized rehabilitation center.

_____

Activity D *The following are descriptions of phases of rehabilitation. Place an "A" next to descriptions indicating the acute phase, an "S" next to descriptions indicating the subacute phase, and a "C" next to descriptions indicating the chronic phase.*

1. _____ Restores the person's mental health

2. _____ Focuses on stabilizing the person's medical condition

3. _____ Restores the person's ability to communicate

4. _____ Focuses on keeping the person alive

5. _____ Prevents complications associated with immobility

6. _____ Focuses on maintaining the person's ability to move independently

Activity E *Match the health care workers who specialize in rehabilitation given in Column A with their function given in Column B.*

Column A

____ 1. Rehabilitation nurse

____ 2. Occupational therapist

____ 3. Physical therapist

____ 4. Speech-language pathologist

____ 5. Orthotist

Column B

a. Helps the person regain or maintain the ability to perform ADLs

b. Helps the person regain or maintain strength, endurance, coordination, posture, and flexibility

c. Fits the person with supportive devices to correct deformity, aid movement, and relieve discomfort

d. Develops a nursing care plan to maximize the person's functioning and quality of life

e. Helps the person regain or maintain the ability to communicate with others, chew, and swallow

TYPES OF REHABILITATION

Key Learning Points

■ Types of rehabilitation that may be used in a rehabilitation program.

Activity F *Select the single best answer for the following questions.*

1. The rehabilitation process that is achieved through a program of exercise, often combined with the use of supportive devices, assistive devices, and/or prosthetic devices is called:
   a. Occupational therapy
   b. Physical therapy
   c. Vocational therapy
   d. ADL therapy

2. The health specialty that can help a person regain the skills needed for personal enjoyment, such as a craft or a hobby is known as:
   a. Physical therapy
   b. Vocational rehabilitation
   c. Emotional rehabilitation
   d. Occupational therapy

3. Speech-language pathology is a specialty that can help a person regain the ability to:
   a. Cope emotionally
   b. Engage in crafts and hobbies
   c. Speak, chew, and swallow
   d. Train for a new job

4. The goal of vocational rehabilitation is to return a person to:
   a. Gainful employment
   b. Medicare assistance
   c. Subacute care
   d. Emotional stability

5. Occupational therapy is a specialty listed under:
   a. Vocational rehabilitation
   b. Physical rehabilitation
   c. Emotional rehabilitation
   d. Speech-language pathology

FACTORS AFFECTING THE REHABILITATION EFFORT

Key Learning Points

- Factors that can affect the outcome of the rehabilitation effort.
- Why an elderly person might require rehabilitation.

Activity G *Think About It! Briefly answer the following question in the space provided.*

Give some examples of how a person's attitude and coping skills can affect the rehabilitation effort.

_____

_____

_____

Activity H *Place an "X" next to each correct answer for the following question.*

When family members treat a disabled person as a responsible, capable person, they have a positive effect on the person's rehabilitation by helping to:

a. _____ Build self-esteem

b. _____ Promote independence

c. _____ Perform all activities for the person

d. _____ Promote dependence on others

e. _____ Assist in rehabilitation

Activity I *Think About It! Briefly answer the following question in the space provided.*

What factors can affect the outcome of a rehabilitation effort?

_____

_____

_____

THE NURSING ASSISTANT'S ROLE IN REHABILITATION AND RESTORATIVE CARE

Key Learning Points

- The nursing assistant's role in rehabilitation and restorative care.
- How the concept of humanistic care applies to rehabilitation and restorative care.

Activity J *Place an "X" next to the practices that a nursing assistant is responsible for as part of the rehabilitation team.*

1. _____ You observe the patient or resident for any physical changes, positive or negative, that are related to the rehabilitation process.

2. _____ You make sure that the person is taken to the bathroom on schedule

3. _____ You assist your patient or resident with the use of new equipment or supportive devices, even though you may not be sure how to use them yourself.

4. _____ You will be the one who notices and reports that a splint or supportive device has caused redness or chafing of the skin.

5. _____ If a new rehabilitation measure does not seem to be working for the person, perhaps change is necessary. Your input is not an important part of this process.

Activity K *Think About It! Briefly answer the following questions in the space provided.*

1. Mrs. Rice has just had a stroke and this has affected her ability to care for herself physically, as well as her ability to function emotionally. As her nursing assistant, you should apply the concept of holistic care while caring for her. What is a holistic approach? Other than physical therapy, what should you focus on to help Mrs. Rice?

_____

_____

_____

2. Mr. Chin is an engineer by profession, and he works in the sales department in an engineering firm. One day, Mr. Chin lost both of his feet in a car accident. As a result of the accident, Mr. Chin will need to learn how to walk again with prosthetic feet, and he has grown very depressed. He is also worried about his ability to return to his job, since the accident shattered his physical, emotional, and economic functions. Presently, he is undergoing rehabilitation in one of the city's long-term care facilities. As his nursing assistant, what steps would you take to help Mr. Chin overcome his feelings of helplessness and anger?

_____

_____

_____

⬤ Rehabilitation is the process of helping a person with a disability to return to his highest level of physical, emotional, or economic function. Rehabilitation is achieved through restorative care, which includes treatment, education, and the prevention of further disability. As a nursing assistant, you will play a key role in the successful rehabilitation of a patient or resident.

SPECIFIC REHABILITATION MEASURES

Key Learning Points

■ Rehabilitation measures that are commonly used in the health care setting specific to different body systems.

Activity L *There are different types of rehabilitation that are specific for disorders of the body systems. Match the body system in Column A with the rehabilitation measures listed in Column B.*

Column A

___ **1.** Integumentary system

___ **2.** Musculoskeletal system

___ **3.** Cardiovascular system

___ **4.** Nervous system

___ **5.** Endocrine system

Column B

a. Dietary changes that help control obesity and blood cholesterol levels

b. Specialized care for people recovering from brain or spinal cord injuries

c. Diet management, weight loss, and exercise to control diabetes mellitus

d. Dressing changes, VAC therapy, and position changes

e. Range-of-motion exercises and heat and cold applications

SUMMARY

Activity M *Fill in the blanks.*

1. Disability is impaired function and can be physical, mental, or _____.

2. Restorative care is the care provided by the _____ that supports the rehabilitation effort.

3. During the chronic phase of rehabilitation, the health care team focuses on helping the person regain _____.

4. Rehabilitation involves a team of people working together to address the specific needs of the _____ or _____.

5. _____ therapy focuses on helping the person regain or maintain strength, endurance, coordination, balance, posture, and flexibility.

6. Emotional rehabilitation focuses on helping the person come to terms with the disability and cope with _____.

7. Because of the unique relationship that develops between the nursing assistant and the people he cares for, the nursing assistant becomes the _____ of the rehabilitation team.

8. Rehabilitation for disorders of the digestive, urinary, and reproductive systems involves measures such as _____ and _____.

Caring for People With Developmental Disabilities

WHAT IS A DEVELOPMENTAL DISABILITY?

Key Learning Points

■ The meaning of the term *developmental disability*
■ The various causes of developmental disabilities

Activity A *Fill in the blanks using the words given in brackets.*

[acquired, permanent, congenital]

1. A developmental disability is a _____ disability that interferes with the person's ability to achieve developmental milestones.

2. A developmental disability may be _____ (something a child is born with) or _____ (occurring after birth, as a result of trauma or illness).

Activity B *Developmental disabilities can be either congenital or acquired. Place a "C" next to causes that are congenital and an "A" next to causes that are acquired.*

1. ____ Genetic (inherited) disorders

2. ____ Consumption of alcohol, drugs, or other toxic substances during pregnancy

3. ____ Head injury

4. ____ Near-drowning

5. ____ Infections during pregnancy, such as German measles (rubella) or HIV

6. ____ Poisoning

7. ____ Poor nutrition during pregnancy

8. ____ Conditions that deprive the baby of oxygen during pregnancy or labor and delivery

SPECIAL NEEDS OF PEOPLE WITH DEVELOPMENTAL DISABILITIES

Key Learning Points

■ The special needs of people with developmental disabilities

Activity C *Match the terms, given in Column A, with their descriptions, given in Column B.*

Column A

___ **1.** Special educational programs focused on self-care skills

___ **2.** Special educational programs focused on life skills

___ **3.** Special educational programs focused on social skills

___ **4.** The Americans with Disabilities Act

___ **5.** The Arc of the United States

___ **6.** Special Olympics

Column B

a. Teach people with developmental disabilities skills such as how to count money

b. Teach people with developmental disabilities appropriate behavior and "limits" when interacting with people in society

c. Ensures that people who have disabilities are treated the same as those without disabilities, by guaranteeing people with disabilities access to public education, employment, and public places such as parks, restaurants, and transportation

d. One notable way in which people with developmental disabilities gain self-esteem; also promotes their physical health

e. An organization that promotes the rights of people with mental disabilities

f. Teach people with developmental disabilities skills such as how to eat or dress independently

Activity D *Think About It! Briefly answer the following question in the space provided.*

What is mainstreaming? Briefly describe the benefits mainstreaming offers to children with developmental disabilities, and to children without developmental disabilities.

_____

_____

_____

TYPES OF DEVELOPMENTAL DISABILITIES

Key Learning Points

- The characteristics of common developmental disabilities

Activity E *Fill in the blanks using the words given in brackets.*

[severe, intelligence quotient, mild, Down syndrome, moderate, below-average, intellectual functioning, profound, adaptive]

1. A person with mental retardation has _____ intellectual functioning and problems with adaptive skills.

2. _____ is the ability to reason, think, and understand.

3. _____ skills are skills needed to live and work, such as communication skills, social skills, and self-care skills.

4. A mentally retarded person has an _____ score of less than 70 points and limited adaptive skills in two or more areas.

5. With special education, a person with _____ mental retardation is usually able to achieve a third- to sixth-grade learning level and master the skills needed for socially appropriate behavior.

6. People with _____ mental retardation have delays in both motor (manual) skills and speech development.

7. With special education, people with
_____ mental retardation are able to
learn some communication and basic self-care
skills, such as how to feed themselves.

8. People with _____ mental retardation
have minimal function in all developmental
areas, physical and mental.

9. _____ is a developmental disability
that is the result of a genetic disorder.

Activity F *Think About It! Briefly answer
the following question in the space provided.*

Allison is a 15-year-old with moderate mental
retardation. Although Allison's intellectual
capacity is about the same as that of an 8-year-
old, physically she is developing like the teenager
that she is. What challenges might this present
for Allison? As a nursing assistant, what can you
do to help Allison meet these challenges and
protect her from harm?

_____

_____

_____

Activity G *Mark each statement as either
"true" (T) or "false" (F). Correct the false
statements.*

1. T F A person with Down syndrome has
45 chromosomes.

2. T F A person with Down syndrome has
certain characteristic physical features,
such as eyelid folds that give the eyes an
almond-shaped appearance; a large
tongue in a small mouth; square hands
with short, stubby fingers; a small, wide
nose and small ears; short stature; and a
wide, short neck.

3. T F A person with autism has extreme
difficulty walking.

4. T F Cerebral palsy is caused by damage to
the cerebellum, the part of the brain
involved with motor control.

5. T F Varying degrees of mental retardation
may accompany the physical disabilities
associated with cerebral palsy.

6. T F Fragile X syndrome is an inherited
type of mental retardation caused by
a decrease in the number of
chromosomes.

7. T F Fetal alcohol syndrome is a combination
of physical and mental problems that
affect a child whose mother consumed
alcohol during pregnancy.

8. T F Many people with autism have below-
average intelligence.

9. T F Some people with developmental
disabilities are able to enter the
workforce.

10. T F Spina bifida is a congenital defect of the
spinal column.

11. T F Hydrocephalus, sometimes called
"water on the brain," results from a
build-up of cerebrospinal fluid (CSF).

12. T F People who have fetal alcohol
syndrome are usually moderately to
severely mentally retarded and may
have physical characteristics such as
large, cupped ears; a slim build; wide-
set, somewhat squinting eyes; and
velvet-like skin.

Activity H *Chad has cerebral palsy. Place an
"X" on the part of his brain that is affected.
Then fill in the blanks in the sentences below
using the words given in brackets.*

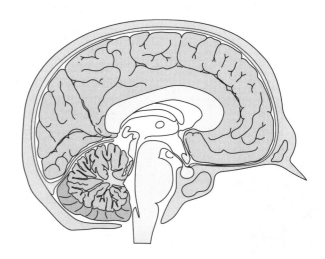

[contractures, involuntary movements, facial, tongue, spasms, shortening]

Cerebral palsy can affect body movements in two different ways. One type of cerebral palsy causes _____ and _____ of the muscles. The affected joints may develop _____. The second type of cerebral palsy causes _____ of the arms, legs, and upper body. _____ and _____ muscles may also be involved, making the person appear to be chewing constantly.

CARING FOR A PERSON WITH A DEVELOPMENTAL DISABILITY

Key Learning Points

- Techniques for communicating with a person with a developmental disability
- Physical problems that people with developmental disabilities may have
- Types of rehabilitation that may be used to help people with developmental disabilities

Activity I *Think About It! Briefly answer the following questions in the spaces provided.*

1. Good communication is especially important when working with people with developmental disabilities. List three reasons a person with developmental disabilities may have difficulty communicating. Then list three things a nursing assistant can do to improve his or her ability to communicate with a person with a developmental disability.

_____

_____

_____

_____

_____

_____

2. You are working in a group home that provides care for people with developmental disabilities. For each of the following residents, briefly describe the assistance you would need to provide in the given situation.

a. Joe has cerebral palsy that has caused contractures in the joints of his hands and arms. Joe also has mild mental retardation. Joe is getting ready to eat his lunch.

_____

_____

b. Brendan has profound mental retardation. It's time for Brendan to get ready for bed.

_____

_____

c. Susan has mild mental retardation accompanied by hearing loss. Susan is a member of the housekeeping staff at a local hotel. It's time for Susan to put on her uniform so that she can go to work.

_____

_____

When working with a person who has a developmental disability, the care that you provide must be specific to the person's abilities and disabilities. Learn as much as you can about each person in your care. Focusing on each person's abilities, whether developmentally disabled or not, will help you to provide the standard of care that each of your patients or residents needs from you.

SUMMARY

Activity J *Use the clues to complete the crossword puzzle.*

Across

5. Adjective used to describe a disorder that a person is born with
6. A developmental disability characterized by extreme difficulty communicating and relating to other people and surroundings

Down

1. A developmental disability that is the result of having 47 chromosomes instead of 46; people with this disorder have mental retardation and certain key physical features, such as almond-shaped eyes and square hands with short, stubby fingers
2. A congenital defect of the spinal column that occurs when the vertebrae do not close properly during development, leaving the spinal cord exposed
3. An inherited type of mental retardation caused by a defect in the X chromosome
4. Below-average intellectual functioning and problems with adaptive skills
5. A developmental disability caused by damage to the cerebrum, the part of the brain involved with motor control

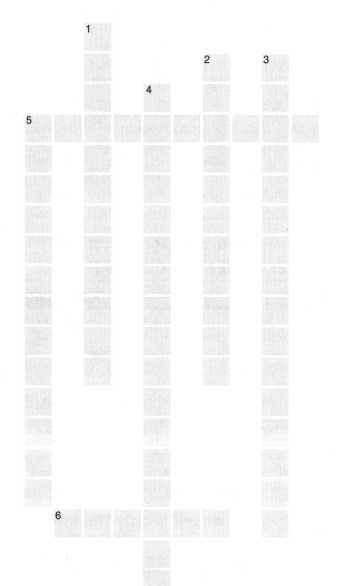

Caring for People With Mental Illness

MENTAL HEALTH

Key Learning Points

- The meaning of the term *mental illness*
- Some of the qualities that define good mental health
- Methods that people use to cope with stress effectively

Activity A *Think About It! Briefly answer the following question in the space provided.*

List at least eight sources of common mental stress.

_____

_____

_____

Activity B *Think About It! Briefly answer the following question in the space provided.*

What coping mechanism do you use when you start to feel overwhelmed or "stressed out"? Is this a positive or negative way of coping?

_____

_____

_____

Activity C *Place an "X" next to examples of positive coping mechanisms.*

1. ____ Thomas goes jogging

2. ____ Jane leaves her office and goes to the park to smoke a cigarette

3. ____ Neil bites his nails

4. ____ Sharon practices yoga

5. ____ Mr. Gagliardi does the crossword puzzle in the newspaper

6. ____ Josh takes his sports car out for a drive

7. ____ Lisa goes for a swim

8. ____ Peter goes to a bar to drink with his friends every night after work

9. ____ Amy calls her best friend on the telephone

Activity D *Match the common defense mechanisms, given in Column A, with their examples, given in Column B.*

Column A

____ **1.** Compensation

____ **2.** Conversion

____ **3.** Denial

____ **4.** Displacement

____ **5.** Projection

____ **6.** Rationalization

____ **7.** Regression

____ **8.** Repression

Column B

a. Mrs. Dellarosa accuses Joan, a nursing assistant, of being racist, when in fact it is Mrs. Dellarosa who made an unkind remark about her roommate, who is of another race.

b. Tony, a 6-year-old child hospitalized for acute illness, has taken up thumb sucking.

c. Mrs. Zorger feels lonely so she eats a large pizza all by herself.

d. Maria cannot remember her childhood between the ages of 8 and 10 when she lived with a stepfather who abused her.

e. Mr. Thomson refuses to believe the doctor when she tells him his test results show cancer.

f. Ronnie complains of a stomachache and refuses to attend school.

g. Mrs. Lombardi, who is angry with her daughter for moving her to long-term care facility, snaps at Rita, a nursing assistant.

h. Remy tells himself it is OK to smoke because if he quits smoking, he will gain weight.

CAUSES AND TREATMENT OF MENTAL ILLNESS

Key Learning Points

- Possible causes of mental illness
- The different treatments that are available for people with mental illness

Activity E *Place an "X" next to the sentences that describe people who are at risk for developing a mental illness.*

1. ____ Mrs. Alonzo's mother was clinically depressed.

2. ____ Tony has left his job and started his own business.

3. ____ Nita was sexually abused by her uncle when she was a child.

4. ____ Mr. Noh's brain does not produce the proper amount of some neurotransmitters.

5. ____ Sylvia is a poet.

TYPES OF MENTAL ILLNESSES

Key Learning Points

- Common mental illnesses that you may encounter in the health care setting

Activity F *Fill in the blanks using the words given in brackets.*

[phobia, anxiety, addiction, compulsion, panic, obsession]

1. _____ is a feeling of uneasiness, dread, apprehension, or worry.

2. _____ is a sudden, overpowering fright.

3. An _____ causes a person to suffer intensely from recurrent unwanted thoughts.

4. A _____ is a ritual that the person cannot control.

5. A _____ is an excessive, abnormal fear of an object or situation.

6. An _____ is a physical need that results in withdrawal signs and symptoms if the substance is withheld.

Activity G *Match the phobias, given in Column A, with their descriptions, given in Column B.*

Column A

____ **1.** Simple phobia

____ **2.** Social phobia

____ **3.** Agoraphobia

Column B

a. Mr. Carin has an intense fear of having a panic attack while traveling on a crowded bus.

b. Mona is abnormally afraid of cats.

c. Rob's fear of public humiliation has prevented him from being able to get and keep a job.

Activity H *Think About It! Briefly answer the following question in the space provided.*

List six signs of clinical depression.

_____

_____

_____

Activity I *Select the single best answer for the following question.*

1. Mrs. Walker, a resident at your facility, is 72 years old. You think she may be depressed because several of her friends have died recently, and you have noticed a change in her behavior. For example, she used to like to go to the activity room, but now whenever you try and get her to come to an activity, she gives you an excuse for not going. Based on your suspicions, what should you do?

a. Be supportive of Mrs. Walker and wait for her mood to improve. She is grieving for the loss of her friends.

b. Assume that Mrs. Walker is just getting older, and her behavior is a normal part of getting older.

c. Report your observations to the nurse. Mrs. Walker could be suffering needlessly.

d. Try to cheer Mrs. Walker up by bringing her special treats.

Activity J *Each of the following people is suffering from a mental illness. Use the words given in brackets to identify the type of mental illness each person has.*

[bulimia nervosa, panic attack, post-traumatic stress disorder, obsessive-compulsive disorder, anorexia nervosa]

1. Alexis, a 20-year-old college student, allows herself to eat one apple and 10 baby carrots each day. _____

2. Jack must wash each part of his body a specified number of times. If he makes a mistake, then he must start all over again from the beginning. As a result, Jack spends 2 hours every day in the shower.

_____

3. Julie will eat an entire box of doughnuts and a bag of potato chips in one sitting, and then go to the bathroom and make herself vomit. _____

4. Mrs. Schmidt has sudden feelings of overwhelming anxiety and intense fear, accompanied by a pounding heart, dizziness, and shortness of breath. _____

5. Mr. Jeffs has recurring nightmares and flashbacks about his military service in Vietnam. _____

Activity K *Place a "D" next to the phrases that describe delusions, and an "H" next to the phrases that describe hallucinations.*

1. ____ Mrs. Ainsley believes that she is the Queen Mother.

2. ____ Mr. Wohl hears voices in his head telling him to kill his neighbor.

3. ____ Mrs. Evans sees mice crawling all over her bed.

4. ____ Mrs. McMahon believes that aliens have planted a device for spying on her in her refrigerator.

5. ____ Mrs. Velker believes that her handiman has stolen her deceased husband's tools.

6. ____ Mrs. Martinez insists that there is a foul odor coming from her closet.

● Clinical depression is one of the most common mental illnesses. It affects more than 19 million Americans each year. Many of the people with clinical depression are elderly. If you will be working with elderly patients or residents, pay attention to changes in their behaviors or moods that could indicate clinical depression. Prompt treatment is needed to help a clinically depressed person return to an enjoyable, productive life.

CARING FOR A PERSON WITH MENTAL ILLNESS

Key Learning Points

■ Special concerns related to the health care setting and aging that may affect a person's mental health
■ The responsibilities of the nursing assistant when caring for mentally ill patients and residents

Activity L *Mark each statement as either "true" (T) or "false" (F). Correct the false statements.*

1. T F   A physical problem, such as a urinary tract infection, can sometimes cause an elderly person's behavior or mental status to change.

2. T F   Only young people are likely to abuse alcohol as a way of reducing stress.

3. T F   Serious mental health problems usually only affect young people.

4. T F   Many mental health problems cannot be treated, so recognizing that a person has a mental health problem is not important.

5. T F   Nearly 25% of people who commit suicide are 65 years of age or older.

6. T F   A nursing assistant is only likely to care for people with mental illnesses if he or she chooses to work in a facility that specializes in caring for mentally ill people.

SUMMARY

Activity M *Words shown in the picture have been jumbled. Use the clues below to form correct words using the letters given in the picture.*

1. Episodes when a person sees, feels, hears, or tastes something that does not really exist
2. A mental health disorder that affects how a person thinks, feels and acts; the person has difficulty determining what is real from what is imaginary.
3. A physical or emotional factor that changes the body's normal balance or equilibrium
4. An excessive, abnormal fear of an object or situation
5. A mental health disorder characterized by mood swings; people with this disorder experience excessively "high" or happy periods, followed by excessively "low" or depressed periods
6. A person with education and training that allows him to provide counseling services to people who are mentally ill
7. A doctor trained in diagnosing and treating mental illnesses
8. The intentional and voluntary taking of one's own life
9. An emotional and physical reaction that occurs when use of an addictive substance is discontinued

L L A H C I N S N O I T A U

A I N E R H P O I Z C H S

T S E S S R

I A O B H P

R E D R O S D I R O A L B I P

T S I C O L O H G Y P S

I R S T A I T Y S C H P

I E D S I C U

D I A W L R T W A H

CHAPTER 38

Caring for People With Dementia

WHAT IS DEMENTIA?

Key Learning Points

- The difference between dementia and delirium
- The three stages of dementia

Activity A *Fill in the blanks using the words given in brackets.*

[dementia, delirium]

1. _____ is the permanent and progressive loss of mental functions, caused by damage to the brain tissue.

2. _____ is a temporary state of confusion that can be a symptom of an underlying disorder, such as an infection.

Activity B *Mark each statement as either "true" (T) or "false" (F). Correct the false statements.*

1. **T F** Once the cause of dementia is identified and treated, the dementia will go away.

2. **T F** A person with dementia is likely to have problems with memory, especially short-term memory.

3. **T F** A person with dementia may act in socially inappropriate ways.

4. **T F** A person with dementia is able to make responsible decisions.

5. **T F** Dementia usually has a rapid onset.

Activity C *The following list includes symptoms of the different stages of dementia. Please place an "E" beside the one's that indicate Early stage, an "M" beside the one's that indicate Middle stage, and an "L" beside the one's that indicate Late stage.*

____ 1. The person's personality may change, and she may begin to behave differently, often in challenging ways.

____ 2. The person becomes totally incontinent of urine and feces.

____ 3. The person begins to experience memory loss and is aware of these memory changes.

____ 4. The person is no longer able to speak, swallow, or smile.

____ 5. The person begins to have difficulty remembering the steps that are necessary to complete familiar tasks, such as getting dressed.

____ 6. The person loses the ability to walk and sit independently.

____ 7. The person begins to have difficulty communicating.

____ 8. The person dies.

TYPES OF DEMENTIA

Key Learning Points

■ Four major causes of dementia

Activity D *Match the types of dementia, given in Column A, with their causes, given in Column B.*

Column A

____ **1.** Alzheimer's disease

____ **2.** Vascular dementia

____ **3.** Lewy body dementia

____ **4.** Frontotemporal dementia

Column B

a. is caused by the build-up of abnormal protein deposits in areas of the brain that are responsible for thinking and movement.

b. the person with this type of dementia may show changes in personality and have difficulty with language skills.

c. the person with this type of dementia may have abnormal plaques and tangles in the part of the brain that affects memory.

d. mental functions are lost because areas of brain tissue die due to a lack of adequate oxygen and nutrients.

Activity E *Fill in the blanks using the words given in brackets.*

[frontal lobe, vascular dementia, Alzheimer's disease, 14 million, 10%, Lewy body dementia]

1. Four of the most common causes of dementia are Alzheimer's disease, vascular dementia, _____, and frontotemporal dementia.

2. The _____ is the area of the brain that is responsible for personality and behavior.

3. _____ is the most common type of dementia, accounting for more than 50% of cases of dementia.

4. If no cure is found for Alzheimer's disease, it is estimated that around _____ people will have the disease by the year 2050.

5. Alzheimer's disease occurs in _____ of people older than 65 years.

Activity F *Think About It! Briefly answer the following question in the space provided.*

Barry's grandfather died of vascular (multi-infarct) dementia, and Barry is worried about his chances of developing the disease. List at least five risk factors for vascular (multi-infarct) dementia that Barry should be aware of.

_____

_____

_____

BEHAVIORS ASSOCIATED WITH DEMENTIA

Key Learning Points

■ Behaviors that are common in people with dementia
■ Strategies for managing difficult behaviors in people with dementia

Activity G *Match the behaviors shown by people with dementia, given in Column A, with their descriptions, given in Column B.*

Column A

____ **1.** Wandering

____ **2.** Pacing

____ **3.** Repetition (perseveration)

____ **4.** Rummaging

____ **5.** Delusions

____ **6.** Hallucinations

____ **7.** Agitation

Column B

a. False beliefs

b. Searching through drawers or closets

c. Walking back and forth

d. Doing the same thing over and over again

e. Straying away from home

___ **8.** Catastrophic reactions

___ **9.** Sundowning

___ **10.** Inappropriate sexual behaviors

f. Attempting to get into bed with another resident, or masturbating in a public area

g. Worsening of a person's behavioral symptoms in the late afternoon and evening, as the sun goes down

h. Becoming very upset and excited

i. Overreacting to something that would cause a healthy person minimal or no stress

j. Seeing, hearing, tasting, or smelling something that is not really there

Activity H *Mark each statement as either "true" (T) or "false" (F). Correct the false statements.*

1. T F A resident who tends to wander may wear a bracelet or an anklet that will set off an alarm if the resident tries to leave the facility through a doorway that leads to an unsafe area.

2. T F A person with dementia may do the same thing over and over again. This is called pacing.

3. T F If one of your residents is delusional, try to correct the person.

4. T F Reality orientation is useful for people with delirium. It is not an effective technique to use with a person who has dementia.

5. T F Reality therapy stresses the importance of acknowledging the person's reality, rather than correcting the person.

Activity I *Match the behaviors seen in people with dementia, given in Column A, with actions that can be taken to help the person, given in Column B.*

Column A

___ **1.** Wandering

___ **2.** Pacing

___ **3.** Repetition

___ **4.** Rummaging

___ **5.** Delusions

___ **6.** Hallucinations

___ **7.** Sundowning

___ **8.** Inappropriate sexual behaviors

Column B

a. Try to redirect the conversation. For example, you might say, "Tell me about your day" or "Would you like to take a walk now?"

b. Helping to ensure periods of quiet and rest during the day might help to reduce fatigue; turning on lights earlier in the evening may help too

c. Reassure the person and then gently redirect the person's attention

d. Gently, but firmly, lead the person back to her room and redirect the person's attention by introducing another activity

e. If the facility has a fenced-in garden area, suggest to the person that he or she walk with you outside

f. Show the person a special drawer or a box filled with small personal items

g. Distracting the person by offering to take her for a walk, or by getting her involved in an activity such as looking through a magazine, may help to break the cycle

h. Moving the person to a quieter area, offering a snack, or taking the person to the bathroom might help relieve this behavior

Activity J *Think About It! Briefly answer the following questions in the spaces provided.*

1. Mrs. Wyatt has dementia, and she shows many of the behaviors typical of people with dementia. In particular, she likes to wander and pace a lot. Lately, though, she has also been having more catastrophic reactions and showing more sundowning behavior as well. Why is it important to determine the cause of Mrs. Wyatt's behaviors, when everyone knows that these behaviors are "normal" for people who have dementia?

_____

_____

2. Mr. Murphy has Alzheimer's disease. He insists that his son is coming to visit him today. Unfortunately, you know that his son died in a plane crash when he was 24, more than 20 years ago. How would you respond to Mr. Murphy?

_____

_____

> Try to remember that a person with dementia does not want to act the way she is acting. She is not trying to be difficult or annoying. She simply cannot help it. Often, there is a physical or emotional reason for the person's behavior. When you make the effort to find the underlying cause of the behavior and address it, you provide relief to the person (and to yourself!)

CARING FOR A PERSON WITH DEMENTIA

Key Learning Points

- Special considerations that the nursing assistant must keep in mind while helping a person with dementia with activities of daily living (ADLs), such as bathing, eating, and toileting
- Special care measures that are taken to help maintain quality of life for a person with dementia

Activity K *Think About It! Briefly answer the following questions in the spaces provided.*

1. When you are helping a person with dementia with her activities of daily living (ADLs), there are five things you can do to make the task at hand go more smoothly. What are these five things?

_____

_____

_____

2. You work in a facility that cares exclusively for people with dementia. What special considerations would you have when you are assisting each of the following residents in the situations given?

a. It is time for Mr. Rodriguez's tub bath.

_____

_____

b. It is time for Mrs. Cheng to get dressed.

_____

_____

c. Miss Myrtle is having lunch in the dining room. _____

_____

d. Mr. Rider needs to go to the bathroom.

_____

_____

3. Four different types of therapy are used to help meet the emotional needs of people with dementia. List these therapies and give examples of each.

_____

_____

_____

_____

_____

_____

_____

Activity L *Mark each statement as either "true" (T) or "false" (F). Correct the false statements.*

1. **T F**   It is not necessary to assist a person with dementia with personal hygiene and grooming, since the person cannot appreciate being clean and well-groomed anyway.

2. **T F**   When assisting a person with dementia with a task, it is important to use short words and short sentences.

3. **T F**   A person with dementia cannot benefit from a kind word, a gentle touch, or a smile.

4. **T F**   It is not important to help the person to maintain his independence because eventually he will be dependent on you for everything anyway.

5. **T F**   People with dementia respond best to a calm, structured environment.

6. **T F**   People with dementia can benefit from visual cues, such as a large "STOP" sign on the door or a large calendar in the person's room.

EFFECTS OF CARING FOR THE PERSON WITH DEMENTIA ON THE CAREGIVER

Key Learning Points

- The effects of caring for a person with dementia on the caregiver, and strategies for coping

Activity M *Mark each statement as either "true" (T) or "false" (F). Correct the false statements.*

1. **T F**   It is acceptable to physically punish a resident with dementia who has cursed at you, spit on you, slapped you, scratched you, pulled your hair, pinched you, or called you something offensive.

2. **T F**   Many of the behaviors of people with dementia can be very annoying, because they are crazy.

3. **T F**   Caring for a person with dementia is emotionally, but not physically, demanding.

4. **T F**   A person with dementia will be punished by a court of law if he causes any harm to the caregiver.

5. **T F**   When you become tired and frustrated, take time out, be good to yourself, and share your feelings with the nurse.

Caring for people with dementia is very important work. The difference you make in the life of the person with dementia, as well as those of her family members, is significant.

SUMMARY

Use the clues to find words that are present in the grid of letters, either horizontally from left to right or vertically from top to bottom.

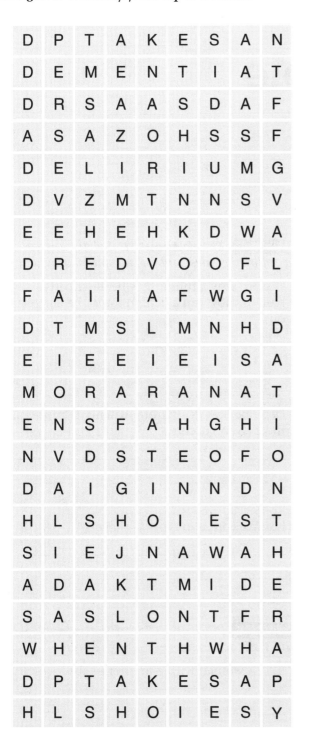

D	P	T	A	K	E	S	A	N
D	E	M	E	N	T	I	A	T
D	R	S	A	A	S	D	A	F
A	S	A	Z	O	H	S	S	F
D	E	L	I	R	I	U	M	G
D	V	Z	M	T	N	N	S	V
E	E	H	E	H	K	D	W	A
D	R	E	D	V	O	O	F	L
F	A	I	I	A	F	W	G	I
D	T	M	S	L	M	N	H	D
E	I	E	E	I	E	I	S	A
M	O	R	A	R	A	N	A	T
E	N	S	F	A	H	G	H	I
N	V	D	S	T	E	O	F	O
D	A	I	G	I	N	N	D	N
H	L	S	H	O	I	E	S	T
S	I	E	J	N	A	W	A	H
A	D	A	K	T	M	I	D	E
S	A	S	L	O	N	T	F	R
W	H	E	N	T	H	W	H	A
D	P	T	A	K	E	S	A	P
H	L	S	H	O	I	E	S	Y

Down

1. The inappropriate and constant repetition of a phrase or act
2. The most common type of dementia; characterized by the permanent and progressive loss of the ability to think and remember caused by damage to the brain
3. The worsening of a person with dementia's behavioral symptoms in the late afternoon and evening (as the sun goes down)
4. A technique used for interacting with people who have dementia, in which the caregiver acknowledges the person's reality; rather than correcting the person, the caregiver attempts to distract the person and redirect the conversation whenever possible

Across

5. The permanent and progressive loss of mental function
6. A temporary state of confusion

CHAPTER 39

Caring for People With Cancer

WHAT IS CANCER?

Key Learning Points

- The difference between benign and malignant tumors
- The common causes of cancer
- Some common types of cancer

Activity A *Fill in the blanks using the words given in brackets.*

[malignant, benign, crab, metastasis, kind, tumor, evil]

1. The word *cancer* comes from the Greek word karkinos, or _____.

2. A _____ is an abnormal growth of tissue.

3. Tumors that are not cancerous are called _____.

4. *Benign* means _____.

5. Cancerous tumors are called _____.

6. *Malignant* means _____.

7. The process by which cancer cells spread from their original location in the body to a new location is called _____.

Activity B *Think About It! Briefly answer the following questions in the spaces provided.*

1. Explain why a tumor may be described as benign. How can a benign tumor be dangerous?

_____

_____

_____

2. Describe how death from malignant tumors almost always occurs.

_____

_____

_____

3. List five common types of cancer.

_____

_____

_____

Activity C *Place an "X" next to the people who have risk factors for developing cancer.*

1. ___ A woman with a mother or sister who has breast cancer

2. ___ A person who smokes

3. ___ A person who exercises on a regular basis

4. ___ A person who spends a lot of time around people who smoke

5. ___ A person who works in a job that exposes him to radiation

6. ___ A person who lives in a damp, humid place

7. ___ A person who lives in a highly polluted town

8. ___ A person whose diet is high in fruit and vegetables

9. ___ A person whose diet is high in fat

DETECTION OF CANCER

Key Learning Points

- The seven warning signs of cancer
- How early detection and treatment affects the outcome of a cancer diagnosis

Activity D *Our bodies are very good at letting us know when something is not quite right. Using the words given in brackets, write the type of cancer associated with the "warning sign" given by the body.*

[cancers of the respiratory tract, skin cancer, cancers of the digestive system, bladder or kidney cancer, uterine cancer, oral cancer, colon cancer, breast cancer]

1. _____ Diarrhea or constipation, or stool that has become smaller in diameter

2. _____ A sore that does not heal or small, scaly patches on the skin that bleed or do not heal

3. _____ A sore in the mouth that does not heal

4. _____ Unusual bleeding or discharge from the vagina

5. _____ Blood in the urine

6. _____ Thickening or lumps in and around the breast

7. _____ Indigestion, heartburn, or difficulty swallowing

8. _____ A cough that does not go away or a hoarse (rough) voice

Activity E *Think About It! Briefly answer the following question in the space provided.*

List the eight warning signs of cancer. Remember the word CAUTIONS.

_____

_____

_____

_____

_____

_____

_____

Many people who are diagnosed with cancer survive it, especially when the cancer is diagnosed and treated early. As a nursing assistant, you will play an important role in making sure that changes in a patient or resident that may be early signs of cancer are reported to the nurse promptly.

Activity F *Fill in the blanks using the words given in brackets.*

[gastroscopy, biopsy, Pap smears, exploratory surgery, endoscopic, bronchoscopy, mammograms, colonoscopy, imaging studies]

1. Examples of screening tests include _____ (used to detect breast cancer) and _____ (used to detect cervical cancer).

2. _____ is performed when a person is thought to have a significant medical problem but the doctors do not know exactly how bad the problem is or exactly what is causing it.

3. _____, such as x-rays, computed tomography (CT) scans, and magnetic resonance imaging (MRI) scans, allow the doctor to see the tumor without actually entering the body.

4. _____ studies involve the use of a special lighted instrument to look inside the body and obtain tissue or fluids for analysis.

5. _____ involves using a scope that is passed into the lungs through the mouth.

6. _____ involves the use of a scope that is passed into the stomach through the mouth.

7. _____ involves passing a scope into the large intestine through the anus.

8. _____ is the surgical removal of cells or a small piece of tissue for microscopic examination.

TREATMENT OF CANCER

Key Learning Points

■ The types of treatment used for people with cancer

Activity G *Mark each statement as either "true" (T) or "false" (F). Correct the false statements.*

1. T F Palliative therapy involves cutting away the tumor and surrounding tissue to remove the cancer and stop the spread of the disease.

2. T F Chemotherapy is often used in combination with surgery to help destroy any malignant cells that the surgery may not have removed completely.

3. T F Radiation therapy involves the use of medications (chemical agents) to destroy the cancer cells.

4. T F Surgery involves the use of powerful x-ray beams to destroy the cancer.

5. T F Surgery is only performed with the goal of curing the person of cancer by completely removing the cancerous cells from the body.

6. T F When the cancer cannot be cured, the goal of treatment is to make the person as comfortable as possible until death occurs. This sort of treatment is referred to as *curative*.

7. T F Stomatitis means the loss of hair.

Activity H *Think About It! Briefly answer the following questions in the spaces provided.*

1. What are the three main approaches to treating cancer? What would make the doctor decide upon one type of treatment over another?

_____

_____

_____

2. Explain how radiation therapy works.

_____

_____

_____

3. Explain how chemotherapy works.

_____

_____

_____

4. List at least two ways that cancer treatment can change a person's physical appearance.

_____

_____

_____

CARING FOR A PERSON WITH CANCER

Key Learning Points

■ Some of the side effects of cancer treatment and how a nursing assistant can help a person who is experiencing these side effects feel more comfortable
■ How cancer affects a person emotionally and how a nursing assistant can provide holistic care

Activity I *Write down the measures a nursing assistant can take to help minimize the following side effects:*

1. Pain _____

2. Nausea and vomiting _____

3. Skin irritation _____

4. Stomatitis _____

5. Fatigue _____

6. Increased risk for infection _____

_____

Activity J *Think About It! Briefly answer the following questions in the spaces provided.*

1. List some of the fears a person who has been diagnosed with cancer might have.

_____

_____

_____

2. Each cancer patient has the right to choose his or her type of treatment, if any at all. Given this right to choose, how can a nursing assistant truly provide holistic care to a patient with cancer?

_____

_____

_____

> As a nursing assistant, you must take steps to prevent any discomfort you may have with the subject of cancer from compromising your ability to care for a patient or resident with the disease. Often, the best thing you can do is listen if the person wants to talk, or just spend quiet time with the person, if he does not want to talk.

SUMMARY

Activity K *Words shown in the picture have been jumbled. Use the clues to form correct words using the letters given in the picture.*

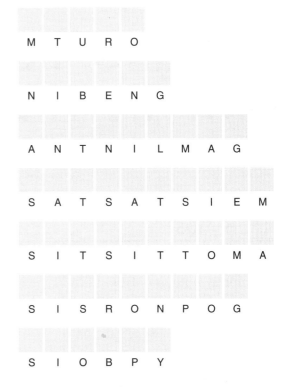

M	T	U	R	O			
N	I	B	E	N	G		
A	N	T	N	I	L	M	A	G
S	A	T	S	A	T	S	I	E	M
S	I	T	S	I	T	T	O	M	A
S	I	S	R	O	N	P	O	G
S	I	O	B	P	Y	

1. An abnormal growth of tissue; the cells may be benign or malignant

2. An adjective used to describe a non-cancerous tumor

3. An adjective used to describe a cancerous tumor

4. The process by which cancer cells spread from their original location in the body to a new location, which may be quite distant from the first

5. Inflammation of the mouth, often seen in people who are receiving chemotherapy

6. A doctor's prediction of the course of a person's disease, and his or her estimation of the person's chances for recovery

7. A diagnostic procedure that involves obtaining a tissue sample and examining it under a microscope for cancerous cells

CHAPTER 40

Caring for People With HIV/AIDS

WHAT IS AIDS?

Key Learning Points

- Common symptoms of HIV infection
- How AIDS affects a person physically
- People who are at risk for HIV infection and AIDS

Activity A *Fill in the blanks using the words given in brackets.*

[33.4, dysphagia, 40, HIV-positive, 1 million, Kaposi's sarcoma]

1. A person who is infected with HIV is said to be _____, because he or she has tested positive on the blood test for HIV antibodies.

2. Bruises or dark bumps on the skin that do not heal are called _____.

3. Pain or difficulty swallowing is called _____.

4. Currently, more than _____ people in the United States are infected with HIV.

5. The Centers for Disease Control and Prevention (CDC) reports that people _____ years and older make up approximately 10% of the total number of AIDS cases nationwide.

6. At the end of 2008, the World Health Organization reported that an estimated _____ million people worldwide were HIV-positive.

Activity B *Mark each statement as either "true" (T) or "false" (F). Correct the false statements.*

1. T F The test for HIV will always be positive if the person is tested for the virus within 3 to 6 months of acquiring it.

2. T F Although very expensive, medications have been developed that can cure AIDS in HIV-positive people.

3. T F Medications can kill the HIV virus, virtually without side effects.

4. T F HIV invades the white blood cells of the body and destroys them.

5. T F HIV is transmitted from one person to another through body fluids, such as blood, semen, and vaginal secretions.

6. T F A person can have HIV without ever developing AIDS.

7. T F Anyone can become infected with the HIV virus, although past the age of 50 years, it is a very rare occurrence.

8. T F In developing countries, such as those in Africa and Southeast Asia, the rate of HIV infection is declining.

Activity C *Place an "X" next to the symptoms a person who is infected with HIV may experience.*

1. ____ Loss of appetite, nausea, vomiting, or diarrhea

2. ____ Weight loss

3. ____ Loss of finger- and toenails

4. ____ Fever (with or without night sweats)

5. ____ Dysphagia

6. ____ Constipation

7. ____ Fatigue

8. ____ Swollen lymph nodes in the neck, armpits, and groin

9. ____ A cough or recurrent episodes of pneumonia

10. ____ Reduced eye sight, eventually leading to blindness

11. ____ Sores or white patches in the mouth

12. ____ Bruises or dark bumps on the skin, which do not heal

13. ____ Forgetfulness and confusion

14. ____ Reduced or complete hearing loss

15. ____ Delusions

Activity D *Think About It! Briefly answer the following questions in the spaces provided.*

1. Name the three most common behaviors and situations that increase a person's risk for becoming infected with HIV.

   _____

   _____

   _____

2. Explain why people with AIDS do not actually die from the virus that has infected their bodies.

   _____

   _____

   _____

3. Explain the point at which HIV is considered to be AIDS.

   _____

   _____

   _____

4. Why are more and more babies in developing nations are being born with HIV?

   _____

   _____

   _____

Today, AIDS is considered a global health crisis. Since it was first identified in the early 1980s, AIDS has spread rapidly, killing a large number of people throughout the world in a short period of time. Currently, the only "cure" for AIDS is to prevent infection with HIV from occurring in the first place!

PROTECTION OF RIGHTS

Key Learning Points

- Legal concerns related to caring for people with HIV/AIDS

Activity E *Think About It! Briefly answer the following question in the space provided.*

What are the factors that contribute to the negative attitude many people have toward those with HIV/AIDS?

_____

_____

_____

Activity F *Mark each statement as either "true" (T) or "false" (F). Correct the false statements.*

1. T F   To protect a person with HIV/AIDS from discrimination, many states have laws that ensure the person's right to employment, education, privacy, and health care.

2. T F   Since laws are in place to protect the person with HIV/AIDS from discrimination; this person is free from discrimination.

3. T F   As a nursing assistant, you are not held responsible for failing to maintain confidentiality about a person's HIV/AIDS status.

4. T F   It is mandatory that you inform every visitor coming to visit a patient or resident who has tested positive for the HIV virus of the patient's or resident's health status.

> As a nursing assistant, you are responsible for maintaining absolute confidentiality about a person's HIV status. You need to know the HIV status of a person to whom you are providing care. However— no one else needs to know.

CARING FOR A PERSON WITH AIDS

Key Learning Points

- How AIDS affects a person emotionally
- The importance of the nursing assistant's responsibility to provide for the physical and emotional needs of the person with HIV/AIDS

Activity G *Write down the measures a nursing assistant can take when caring for a person with the following physical changes that are the result of AIDS.*

1. Fatigue and disability _____

_____

2. Painful sores in the mouth _____

_____

3. Chronic diarrhea _____

_____

4. Weak immune system _____

_____

Activity H *Think About It! Briefly answer the following question in the space provided.*

What are the sources of emotional stress in a person with HIV/AIDS? As a nursing assistant, how can you help the person to cope with this stress?

_____

_____

_____

> A patient or resident with HIV/AIDS needs your care and support, perhaps more than anything else she has ever needed before. Your ability to provide supportive and compassionate care to your patients or residents with HIV/AIDS will make a significant difference in their quality of life.

Caring for Surgical Patients

INTRODUCTION TO CARING FOR SURGICAL PATIENTS

Key Learning Points

- The various reasons surgery is done
- Definition of the term *anesthesia*
- The three main types of anesthesia
- Changes in the health care field that affect the care of the surgical patient

Activity A *Fill in the blanks using the words given in brackets.*

[definitive, general, elective, urgent, exploratory, emergent, anesthesia, regional, local, surgery]

1. _____ is a branch of medicine that involves treating diseases and disorders by entering the body and physically removing or repairing damaged organs or tissues.

2. _____ surgery may be performed when a person has a significant medical problem but the doctors do not know exactly how bad the problem is or exactly what is causing it.

3. _____ surgery is performed when the person's medical problem is known and the best way to address it is through surgery.

4. Surgeries are performed on an _____ basis when the procedure is planned for and scheduled ahead of time.

5. _____ surgeries are planned and scheduled ahead of time, but usually an effort is made to schedule the procedure as soon as possible to prevent the person's condition from getting worse.

6. An _____ surgery is one that must be performed immediately to prevent the person from dying or becoming disabled.

7. _____ prevents the person from feeling pain during the surgery, and is accomplished through the use of medications.

8. _____ anesthesia causes a loss of consciousness.

9. To numb the body from the waist down during childbirth a woman is given _____ anesthesia.

10. Eye surgeries, breast biopsies, and hernia repairs are examples of surgeries that are often performed under _____ anesthesia.

Activity B *Select the single best answer for each of the following questions.*

1. Which of the following would be considered an elective surgical procedure?
   a. Mastectomy
   b. Cardiac bypass surgery
   c. A face lift
   d. Appendectomy

2. All of the following conditions can be treated with definitive surgery EXCEPT:

 a. Pneumonia

 b. Appendicitis

 c. Hernia

 d. Fracture

3. One of Mrs. Hernandez's heart valves is "leaky" and the doctor has recommended that she schedule heart valve replacement surgery within the next week or so. If she does not have the surgery, she will be at risk for all kinds of complications and possibly even death. What kind of surgery will Mrs. Hernandez be having?

 a. Emergent

 b. Urgent

 c. Elective

 d. Imperative

Activity C *Label the figure below using the words given in brackets. Then fill in the blanks in the sentences below, using the same words.*

[pre-operative phase, post-operative phase, intra-operative phase, peri-operative]

1. During the _____, the person is prepared physically and emotionally for the surgery.

2. During the _____, the surgery is performed.

3. During the _____, the person recovers under the watchful eye of the health care team.

4. These phases together are called the _____.

> Because many surgeries are now done on an outpatient basis, you may be responsible for helping a person to prepare for and recover from surgery, even if you do not work in a hospital or other acute care setting.

CARE OF THE PRE-OPERATIVE PATIENT

Key Learning Points

- The fears and concerns that a person who is about to have surgery may have, and the actions the nursing assistant can take to help relieve some of these worries
- What needs to be done to physically prepare a person for surgery
- The nursing assistant's role in preparing a person for surgery

Activity D *Think About It! Briefly answer the following question in the space provided.*

List some of the fears that a person facing surgery may have. What does the nursing staff do in pre-operative teaching to help the person overcome these fears?

_____

_____

_____

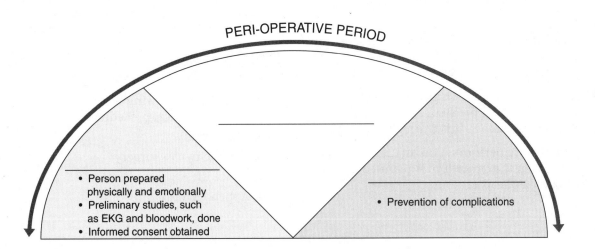

PERI-OPERATIVE PERIOD

- Person prepared physically and emotionally
- Preliminary studies, such as EKG and bloodwork, done
- Informed consent obtained

- Prevention of complications

Activity E *Place a "D" next to the pre-operative actions that are the responsibility of the doctor, an "NU" next to the pre-operative actions that are the responsibility of the nurse, and an "NA" next to the pre-operative actions that are the responsibility of the nursing assistant.*

1. _____ Explains the pre-operative procedures that are done to physically prepare the person for surgery

2. _____ Assists the person to bathe with an antimicrobial soap

3. _____ Informs the person about what complications can occur as a result of the procedure

4. _____ Explains the purpose of any medications or tests that are required during the pre-operative period

5. _____ Measures and records vital signs

6. _____ Reinforces what the nurse has told the person, and keeps the nurse informed of any questions the person may ask about the procedure

7. _____ Ensures that the person signs a form giving permission for the procedure to take place (in other words, ensures that informed consent has been obtained)

8. _____ Informs the person why he or she feels the procedure is the best treatment option for the person

9. _____ Brings the bedpan/urinal, or assists the person to the bathroom after sedative medication is administered

10. _____ Explains what will need to be done both before and after the surgery

11. _____ Informs the person what other treatment options, if any, are available

12. _____ or _____ Answers the person's questions regarding the surgical procedure

13. _____ Answers the person's questions regarding the reason for the NPO status prior to the procedure or the purpose of taking vital signs frequently after the procedure

14. _____ Explains what will happen during the post-operative period

15. _____ Teaches the person how to do any exercises that may be necessary to prevent complications following the surgery

16. _____ Informs the person about what will actually occur during the procedure

Activity F *Match the things done to physically prepare a person for surgery, given in Column A, with when they are done during the pre-operative period, given in Column B.*

Column A

____ 1. The patient may be given an anti-emetic drug and a sedative

____ 2. The patient may bathe with a special soap and have an enema or a vaginal douche administered

____ 3. The patient may undergo diagnostic testing such as blood work, urinalysis, and tests to assess the functioning of the cardio-vascular and respiratory systems

____ 4. The patient is placed on NPO status

Column B

a. In the days leading up to the surgery

b. The evening before the surgery

c. The morning of the surgery

d. Immediately before the surgery

Activity G *Think About It! Briefly answer the following questions in the spaces provided.*

1. Why is a person who is scheduled for surgery placed on NPO status for 6 to 8 hours before surgery? List two things a nursing assistant can do to help make being on NPO status easier for the patient.

_____

_____

2. List two precautions that are taken after a patient is given a sedative, and the reason why these precautions are taken.

_____

_____

> Although as a nursing assistant you will not participate directly in pre-operative teaching, you will still play a very important supporting role. By listening to your patients and promptly relaying any questions they may have to the nurse, you can make an important contribution to the pre-operative teaching process.

CARE OF THE POST-OPERATIVE PATIENT

Key Learning Points

- Potential complications of surgery, and the measures taken to prevent them
- Observations that would be important to report to the nurse, relevant to the care of a patient who is recovering from surgery
- The proper way to apply anti-embolism (TED) stockings

Activity H *Fill in the blanks using the words given in brackets.*

[sequential compression device, suctioning, deep breathing, surgical bed, coughing, supine, laterally, supplemental oxygen, blood clot, thrombophlebitis, Sims', pneumonia, atelectasis, incentive spirometry, thrombus, embolus, post-anesthesia care unit (PACU), nasogastric tube]

1. Immediately after surgery, the person is taken to the _____, also known as the recovery room.

2. While in the PACU, the person usually receives _____. _____ is also available, in case the person vomits or has secretions that interfere with respiration.

3. A _____ is prepared for a patient who is in surgery so that it is ready to receive the patient after surgery.

4. If the person is recovering from an anesthetic that was injected into the spinal canal, she may need to remain in the _____ position for a period of time.

5. Children may be positioned _____ or in _____ position to help prevent aspiration in the event of vomiting.

6. Common respiratory complications of surgery include _____ and _____.

7. Exercises commonly used to prevent respiratory complications include _____, and _____.

8. When blood flow slows and blood pools, a _____, or _____, may form.

9. A thrombus in one of the veins of the legs causes inflammation and pain, a condition known as _____.

10. A blood clot that breaks loose and moves through the bloodstream is known as an _____.

11. A _____ is a device that is applied to the calves to help prevent pooling of blood in the lower legs.

12. If the person has had surgery involving the digestive system, then she may have a _____ connected to suction to keep the stomach empty.

Activity I *Think About It! Briefly answer the following questions in the spaces provided.*

1. What are the duties of a nursing assistant while the person is in surgery, for preparing the person's room for his arrival post-operatively? What is the likely equipment that you should gather that may be needed at the time of arrival?

_____

_____

_____

2. Post-operatively, what is the schedule for taking the person's vital signs? Why is it important to report a change in a surgical patient's vital signs immediately?

_____

_____

Activity J *Think About It! Briefly answer the following questions in the spaces provided.*

1. Look at the figure below. What respiratory exercise is the patient doing? What complications does this exercise help to prevent?

_____

_____

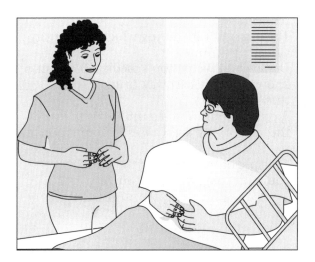

2. Look at the figure below. What respiratory exercise is the patient doing? What is the person supposed to do in this exercise?

_____

_____

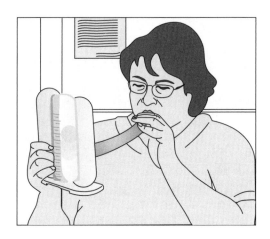

Activity K *Think About It! Briefly answer the following question in the space provided.*

Anesthetic agents, pain medications, and immobility after surgery can cause the body's circulation to slow down, putting the person at risk for thrombus formation. List three things that could happen if a person develops a thrombus. Then list three things that are done to help lower the person's risk of thrombus formation.

_____

_____

_____

Activity L *Anti-embolism (TED) stockings apply pressure to the legs, helping to return blood to the heart and prevent cardiovascular complications of surgery, such as thrombus formation. Some of the steps for applying anti-embolism stockings are given below. Write down the correct order of the steps in the boxes provided below.*

1. Turn the stocking inside out down to the heel.
2. Grasp the top of the stocking and pull it up the person's leg.
3. Help the person into a comfortable position, straighten the bottom linens, and draw the top linens over the person. Make sure that the bed is lowered to its lowest position and that the wheels are locked.
4. Help the person into the supine position.
5. Slip the foot of the stocking over the person's toes, foot, and heel.
6. Make sure that the bed is positioned at a comfortable working height and that the wheels are locked. Lower the side rail on the working side of the bed and keep the side rail on the opposite side of the bed up.
7. Fanfold the top linens to the foot of the bed and adjust the person's hospital gown or pajama bottoms as necessary to expose one leg at a time.
8. Check to make sure that the stocking is not twisted and that it fits snugly against the person's leg and over the heel and toe region.

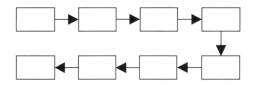

Activity M *Write down the nursing assistant's responsibilities with regard to each of the following during the post-operative period:*

1. Assisting with positioning

   _____

2. Assisting with nutrition

   _____

3. Assisting with elimination

   _____

4. Assisting with hygiene

   _____

5. Assisting with ambulation

   _____

> As a nursing assistant, you will play a large role in helping a person who has had surgery to make a good recovery! Many of your duties will involve helping to prevent complications of surgery. In addition, you may be the first to recognize a change in the patient that could indicate that he or she has developed a complication. Reporting your observations to the nurse promptly helps to prevent the person's condition from getting worse, and may actually save his or her life.

SUMMARY

Activity N *Words shown in the picture have been jumbled. Use the clues below to form correct words using the letters given in the picture.*

1. The term used to describe all three phases of the surgical process as a whole—the pre-operative, intra-operative, and post-operative phases
2. The phase of care during which the surgery is actually performed
3. Done when the person's medical problem is known and the best way to address it is through surgery
4. A condition in which a thrombus in one of the veins of the legs causes inflammation and pain
5. Collapse of the alveoli of the lungs; a common complication of surgery

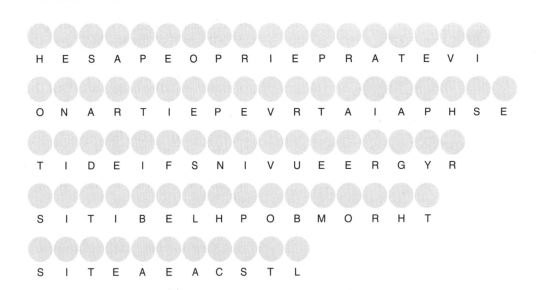

H E S A P E O P R I E P R A T E V I

O N A R T I E P E V R T A I A P H S E

T I D E I F S N I V U E E R G Y R

S I T I B E L H P O B M O R H T

S I T E A E A C S T L

CHAPTER 42

Caring for Mothers and Newborns

THE ANTEPARTUM (PRENATAL) PERIOD

Key Learning Points

- Physical changes that occur in the female reproductive system during pregnancy
- Reasons that an expectant mother may need home care or hospitalization during her pregnancy

Activity A *The body of a pregnant woman undergoes changes that allow for the growth and development of the new life she carries inside of her. Fill in the blanks using the words given in brackets.*

[morning sickness, uterus, placenta, prolactin, fetus, blood]

1. The _____ develops from the inside lining of the uterus during pregnancy.

2. The developing baby is called a _____.

3. _____, a hormone secreted by the pituitary gland, causes the woman's breasts to enlarge and prepare for the production of milk.

4. The _____ enlarges to make room for the growing baby.

5. More _____ is formed to meet the baby's need for oxygen and nutrients.

6. Changes in hormone levels may be responsible for the _____ that many women have early in their pregnancies.

Activity B *Select the single best answer for each of the following questions.*

1. Why is a pregnant woman advised to consume 3 to 4 servings of dairy foods each day (versus 2 to 3 servings for a woman who is not pregnant)?
   a. To lower her risk of miscarriage
   b. To meet the growing baby's need for calcium
   c. To prevent kidney stones
   d. To prevent morning sickness

2. Which of the following things should a pregnant woman do to provide the best care for herself and her developing baby?
   a. Avoid smoking and alcohol
   b. Engage in moderate exercise
   c. Eat a nutritious diet
   d. All of the above

3. How long is a trimester?
   a. 9 months
   b. 3 months
   c. 6 months
   d. 1 week

4. Which of the following is a normal change seen in pregnant women during the third trimester?

   a. Swollen ankles

   b. Morning sickness

   c. Hypertension

   d. All of the above

Activity C *Fill in the blanks using the words given in brackets.*

[preeclampsia, protein, eclampsia, glucose, pre-term labor]

1. _____ means that labor begins too early, before the fetus is capable of surviving on its own.

2. _____ or _____ is a complication that can develop during pregnancy that causes the woman to develop dangerously high blood pressure.

3. A pregnant woman may need to provide urine samples on a regular basis to be tested for _____ and _____.

Activity D *Think About It! Briefly answer the following question in the space provided.*

Mrs. Davis, who is 5 months' pregnant, has been admitted to the hospital because of pre-term labor. She will remain in the hospital on complete bed rest, so that the health care team can monitor her for signs that labor is starting again, and take measures to try and stop it if it does start again. The goal is to allow the baby to mature as much as possible so that it stands a better chance of surviving if it is born early. What responsibilities might the nursing assistant have in caring for Mrs. Davis and helping to meet both her physical and her emotional needs?

_____

_____

_____

Pregnancy can be a time of great joy and anticipation. It can also be a time of great stress, especially if complications develop that jeopardize the mother's health or that of the baby.

LABOR AND DELIVERY

Key Learning Points

■ The two ways of delivering a baby

Activity E *Fill in the blanks using the words given in brackets.*

[labor, cesarean section, vaginally, oxytocin, epidural block]

1. When it is time for a baby to be born, the mother's pituitary gland releases _____, a hormone that stimulates the uterus to contract.

2. The contractions of the uterus squeeze the baby downward, forcing his head against the cervix so that it opens, or dilates. This process is known as _____.

3. A woman may deliver (give birth to) the baby _____ or by _____.

4. Many women choose to have an _____, anesthesia given through a catheter that is placed in the spinal canal.

Activity F *Think About It! Briefly answer the following question in the space provided.*

How does the health care team care for the baby immediately after he or she is born?

_____

_____

_____

THE POSTPARTUM PERIOD

Key Learning Points

■ The responsibilities a nursing assistant would have when caring for a new mother
■ Observations a nursing assistant might make while caring for a new mother that should be reported to the nurse immediately
■ How to bottle-feed a baby
■ How to care for the umbilical cord stump
■ How to care for a baby boy who has been circumcised
■ How to bathe a baby
■ Important security and safety issues related to caring for a newborn

Activity G *Match the terms, given in Column A, with their definitions, given in Column B.*

Column A

___ **1.** Lochia alba

___ **2.** Lochia rubra

___ **3.** Lochia serosa

___ **4.** Colostrum

___ **5.** Vernix

___ **6.** Umbilical cord

___ **7.** Areola

Column B

a. Supplies the growing fetus with nutrients and oxygen, and removes waste

b. Thin, yellowish fluid produced by the breasts immediately following childbirth

c. The colored portion of the breast surrounding the nipple

d. Creamy white to yellow discharge from the vagina following child-birth

e. Bright red discharge from the vagina follow-ing childbirth

f. Pink- or brown-tinged discharge from the vagina following child-birth

g. White, cheese-like sub-stance covering the baby immediately following birth

Activity H *Think About It! Briefly answer the following question in the space provided.*

List four general responsibilities a nursing assistant has when caring for a woman who has just delivered a baby.

_____

_____

_____

Activity I *Many of the normal ranges for vital sign measurements are different in newborns than in adults. Next to each vital sign listed below, write the normal range for a newborn.*

1. Temperature _____

2. Pulse rate _____

3. Respiratory rate _____

4. Blood pressure _____

Activity J *Think About It! Briefly answer the following question in the space provided.*

Most health care facilities that care for newborns have many policies and procedures in place to ensure the security of the newborn. List three common security procedures designed to protect the newborn.

_____

_____

_____

Activity K *Select the single best answer for each of the following questions.*

1. How is the umbilical cord stump cared for?

  a. It is wrapped tightly

  b. It is wiped with an alcohol swab at each diaper change

  c. A petrolatum dressing is applied to it

  d. It is washed in hot, soapy water

2. Which of the following statements about circumcision is correct?

  a. Bleeding and a foul odor are normal until the circumcision heals

  b. The circumcision should heal in 10 to 14 days

  c. The baby cannot wear a diaper until the cir-cumcision has healed

  d. Circumcision is a mandatory procedure done for hygienic reasons

3. When can a baby have a complete bath (in a bath basin)?

   a. After the umbilical cord stump has dried up and fallen off

   b. When the baby is able to hold his own head up

   c. As soon as the baby's temperature stabilizes

   d. After the baby reaches the age of 29 days

Activity L *Think About It! Briefly answer the following question in the space provided. For each of the scenarios below, state the nursing assistant's role in assisting the new mother with feeding her infant.*

1. Mrs. Kleiss is breastfeeding her baby boy.

   _____

   _____

2. Mrs. Sanders is bottlefeeding her baby girl using a commercial formula.

   _____

   _____

Activity M *Mark each statement as either "true" (T) or "false" (F). Correct the false statements.*

1. T F   Microwaving the bottle ensures even heating of the contents.

2. T F   The baby should be laid down to take the bottle.

3. T F   A baby can be burped by holding the baby upright on your knee and gently rubbing or patting his back.

4. T F   Bottles need to be boiled for sterility.

5. T F   Infants younger than 1 year may be fed breast milk, a commercial formula, or cow's milk.

6. T F   Even very small infants can roll off a changing table or other surface, leading to serious injury.

7. T F   When bathing the baby, the bath basin should be filled with 5 to 6 inches of water.

8. T F   A baby should be placed on his back or side to sleep.

9. T F   A baby should be put to bed with a fluffy comforter and a stuffed animal.

10. T F   It is against the law to transport a baby in a car without first securing the baby properly in a car seat.

11. T F   An infant car seat is placed in the front seat, facing the front of the car.

Activity N *Write down the correct order of the steps for diapering a baby in the boxes provided below.*

1. Put on the gloves, and remove the soiled diaper.

2. Place the baby in an infant carrier or some other secure place.

3. Before placing a cloth diaper that is soiled with stool in the diaper pail, rinse it in cool water to prevent the stool from drying in the diaper.

4. Clean the perineal area using baby wipes, wiping from front to back if the baby is a girl.

5. Apply diaper rash ointment or a light dusting of cornstarch powder, if used.

6. Position the clean diaper, fastening it with the provided tabs.

7. Wash your hands and gather your supplies.

8. Remove your gloves and wash your hands.

9. Dispose of the soiled diaper in an appropriate waste container.

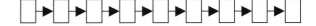

Activity O *Write down the correct order of the steps for bathing a baby in the boxes provided below.*

1. Dry the baby thoroughly and apply baby lotion as desired.
2. Place the baby in the bath basin and lather the baby's hair with a baby shampoo and rinse well.
3. Gather all of the supplies you will need before beginning the bath.
4. Wash the baby's face.
5. Move on to the rest of the body, making sure to rinse all soap from the skin.
6. Fill the bath basin with only 1 to 2 inches of warm water and check the water temperature with a bath thermometer.
7. Use a washcloth and soap formulated for infant skin.

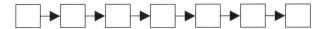

> Following the delivery of the baby, the nursing assistant cares for both the new mother and the baby. The immediate post-delivery period is a critical time physically for both the mother and the infant. You will play an important role during this time by reporting any unusual observations or vital sign measurements to the nurse promptly.

SUMMARY

Activity P *Use the clues to complete the crossword puzzle.*

Across

4. Dangerously high blood pressure in a pregnant woman

Down

1. The 6-week period of time following the birth of a baby
2. The first hour or two immediately following delivery of a baby, during which emotional and physical attachments between the parents and the infant develop
3. A newborn infant, 28 days or younger
5. The period of time from conception until the baby is born

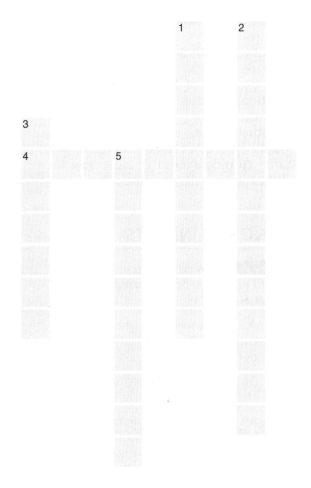

CHAPTER 43

Caring for Pediatric Patients

Key Learning Points

- The specific physical needs that children in health care settings have, according to their ages and abilities
- How the stages of development affect the emotional needs of children in health care settings
- Measures that the nursing assistant can use to assist a child in a health care setting
- Safety considerations that are specific for a child's age and developmental level

CARING FOR INFANTS

Activity A *Mark each statement as either "true" (T) or "false" (F). Correct the false statements.*

1. T F An infant who is ill or unable to drink or eat properly can quickly become dehydrated.

2. T F An infant's medical condition can change very quickly.

3. T F An infant will fail to grow and develop both physically and emotionally if he is not held and talked to.

4. T F Family members should avoid holding babies who are very sick.

Activity B *Safety precautions when caring for infants are given below. Under each precaution, write the reason why it is taken.*

1. Never leave an infant on a surface unattended, even for a moment.

_____

2. As the infant grows and is placed in an infant carrier, swing, or high chair, make sure that safety straps are securely fastened both across the infant's waist and between his legs.

_____

3. Always secure the infant in a car seat in the back seat of the car, facing the back of the car.

_____

4. Make sure that toys are appropriate for the age of the infant and that they have no small, removable parts.

_____

5. Keep plastic bags and balloons away from infants.

_____

6. Do not leave an infant unattended, even for a moment, in water of any depth.

_____

7. Make sure that electrical cords and window blind cords are out of the reach of the infant.

_____

CARING FOR TODDLERS

Activity C *Think About It! Briefly answer the following question in the space provided.*

1. Mary Jane is a 3-year-old who is receiving care in the hospital for an acute medical condition. Mary Jane's mother told you that Mary Jane was potty-trained, but as far as you can tell, she is not. What is going on here? How would you handle this situation?

_____

_____

_____

2. How can you promote a toddler's independence when assisting him to dress?

_____

_____

_____

Activity D *Select the single best answer for each of the following questions.*

1. It is time for lunch and you want Graham, a 2-year-old, to eat his lunch. What can you say to Graham that will increase your chance of success in getting him to eat?
   a. "Graham, honey, you have to eat to get well."
   b. "Graham, would you like a piece of apple or a piece of banana?"
   c. "Graham, sit down right this instant and eat!"
   d. "Graham, if you don't eat, I'm going to have to feed you."

2. Which of the following activities is most likely to be something a toddler would like to do?
   a. Completing an arts and craft project
   b. Playing a video game
   c. Singing along with a tape recording of children's songs
   d. Watching a mobile

3. Jimmy is almost 3 years old. You need to take Jimmy's blood pressure. What approach would work best?
   a. Say to Jimmy, "I'm going to take your blood pressure now."
   b. Restrain Jimmy for the duration of the procedure
   c. Explain to Jimmy what the blood pressure measurement means
   d. Let Jimmy play with your stethoscope and the blood pressure cuff before beginning the procedure

4. What characteristics of a toddler put him at risk for accidents?
   a. The toddler can easily roll off surfaces
   b. The toddler likes to run, jump, climb, and reach for things
   c. The toddler does not understand the meaning of the word "no"
   d. All of the above

CARING FOR PRESCHOOLERS

Activity E *Mark each statement as either "true" (T) or "false" (F). Correct the false statements.*

1. T F Preschoolers are children between the ages of 5 and 8 years.

2. T F Because the preschooler's attention span is a bit longer, she may enjoy activities that require her to sit still for a period of time, such as arts and crafts projects using paper, scissors, crayons, beads, and glue.

3. T F Most preschoolers enjoy eating many different types of foods.

4. T F Remember that during a procedure a frightened preschooler can be very strong if he feels cornered and may strike out to protect himself in any way possible.

5. T F "Magical thinking" is a thought process that is common among preschoolers.

Activity F *Think About It! Briefly answer the following question in the space provided.*

Janice is a 5-year-old who is about to have a very painful diagnostic procedure done. She asks you if the procedure is going to hurt. What will you tell her, and why?

_____

_____

_____

CARING FOR SCHOOL-AGE CHILDREN

Activity G *Fill in the blanks using the words given in brackets.*

[directions, 5 and 12, rewards, booster seat, praise, curiosity, active]

1. School-age children are children between the ages of _____ years.

2. School-age children like to be included as _____ participants in their own care and are very good at following _____.

3. _____ and _____ work very well for children of this age.

4. School-age children know not to drink poisonous liquids or stick objects into an electrical socket; however, their _____ and habit of pushing their physical abilities to the limit brings new dangers.

5. When transporting a school-age child in a car, a _____ is used until the car's lap and shoulder restraints fit the child properly.

Activity H *Think About It! Briefly answer the following question in the space provided.*

How can you help meet the emotional needs of the school-aged child in a health care facility?

_____

_____

_____

CARING FOR ADOLESCENTS

Activity I *Think About It! Briefly answer the following question in the space provided.*

Mandy is a 15-year-old who is receiving care following a skiing accident that resulted in several broken bones. She needs a great deal of assistance with her activities of daily living (ADLs), including bathing and elimination. Most of your interactions with Mandy have been fairly unpleasant—she's sarcastic and sullen. Why might Mandy be acting this way? What can you do to help make her time in the hospital easier for her?

_____

_____

_____

To provide holistic care for children, you must first understand that they are not just "little adults." An understanding of the basic stages of growth and development will better prepare you to provide the type of care that each child requires.

CHILD ABUSE

Key Learning Points

- The signs of abuse of a child and the nursing assistant's role in reporting suspected abuse

Activity J *Fill in the blanks using the words given in brackets.*

[Munchausen syndrome, psychological, shaken baby syndrome, neglect, 25%, sexual]

1. Violently shaking an infant or toddler can cause the child's brain to hit the inside of his skull repeatedly, leading to severe brain damage or death. This is called _____.

2. About _____ of children with shaken baby syndrome die, and the rest suffer from permanent disabilities.

3. In _____ by proxy the child's caregiver (usually the mother) deliberately does things to make the child appear ill.

4. Saying something like "I wish you had never been born!" to a child is a form of _____ abuse.

5. _____ abuse occurs when a caregiver touches or fondles a child's sexual organs.

6. _____ is a common form of physical abuse in children.

Activity K *Mark each statement as either "true" (T) or "false" (F). Correct the false statements.*

1. T F Caregivers who are very young, lack parenting skills, or lack knowledge about the normal behaviors and developmental stages of children are at risk for abusing children.

2. T F If a child tells you something that makes you think the child is being abused, you should ask the child questions designed to reveal the truth.

3. T F A child who is abused is likely to act withdrawn or fearful when in the presence of the abuser.

4. T F When a stranger sexually abuses a child, it is called sexual assault.

5. T F When reporting abuse, you should summarize what the child has told you for the nurse.

6. T F A child's play-acting may raise suspicions of abuse.

> It is very difficult to work with parents or caregivers if you suspect that their child has been abused. However, your top priority is to meet the child's physical and emotional needs as best you can while the child is in your care.

SUMMARY

Activity L *Words shown in the picture have been jumbled. Use the clues below to form correct words using the letters given in the picture.*

1. Placing oneself at the center of the world.
2. The child believes that if he wishes for something hard enough, it will happen.
3. To return to an earlier stage of development.
4. Occurs when an infant is not held and talked to.

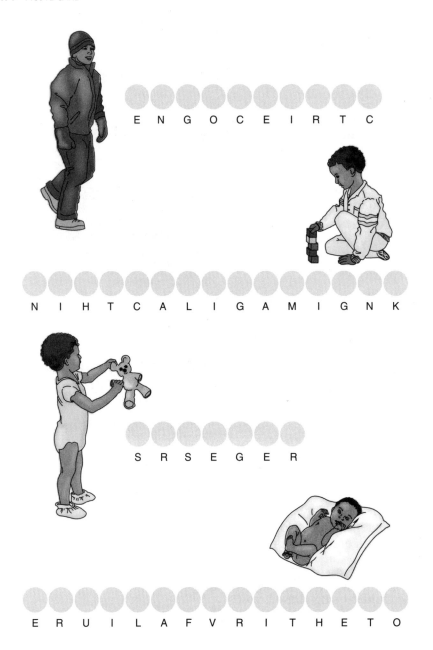

E N G O C E I R T C

N I H T C A L I G A M I G N K

S R S E G E R

E R U I L A F V R I T H E T O

CHAPTER 44

Introduction to Home Health Care

WHAT IS HOME HEALTH CARE?

Key Learning Points

- Why a person might need home health care
- How home health care is paid for
- How the home health care team works together to provide client care

Activity A *Fill in the blanks using the words given in brackets.*

[homebound, doctor, client *(used twice)*, case manager, Medicare, home health aide, Medicaid, documentation, hospice, client's family members, respite care, nurse, registered nurse, home care]

1. Home health care is also known as

   _____.

2. A person who is receiving the services of a home health care agency is called a

   _____

3. Care that allows the primary caregiver to rest or leave the house for a short period of time is called _____.

4. Insurance coverage for home health care is provided by insurance companies and by government agencies, such as _____ or state _____.

5. _____ means that that person is unable to leave the house without a lot of help from another person.

6. The health care team consists of the _____, the _____, the _____, a _____, a _____, a _____, and other specialists.

7. The case manager, usually a _____, is responsible for overseeing all of the client's care, from admission through discharge.

8. In the home health care setting, most communication among team members takes place through _____.

9. _____ care is often provided in the person's home if he or she is terminally ill.

Activity B *Think About It! Briefly answer the following questions in the spaces provided.*

1. List two reasons why it is important for a home health aide to properly document the care provided at each client visit.

   _____

   _____

   _____

2. List four reasons why a person might become a client of a home health care agency.

_____

_____

_____

3. What is the purpose of respite care? Why is it so important?

_____

_____

_____

RESPONSIBILITIES OF THE HOME HEALTH AIDE

Key Learning Points

■ Major duties of a home health aide

Activity C *Mark each statement as either "true" (T) or "false" (F). Correct the false statements.*

1. T F A home health aide's responsibilities are clearly outlined in the nursing care plan for the client.

2. T F The skills you use to assist with personal care in the home are no different from those you use in a hospital or long-term care setting.

3. T F Any changes to the client's care plan must first be approved by the case manager.

4. T F You are not required to keep a time and travel log for the day, since it's your responsibility to plan your activities for the day and execute them accordingly.

5. T F If you feel that something about a client's home environment puts the client at risk for injury, you must take care of it immediately.

6. T F You will document the homemaking duties that you perform on a homemaker flow sheet.

7. T F Some states require home health aides who will be preparing and serving food to have a food handler's permit.

8. T F As a home health aide, many of your light housekeeping duties will be related to helping your clients with activities such as bathing, eating, getting dressed, exercising, toileting, repositioning, and transferring.

Activity D *Think About It! Briefly answer the following question in the space provided.*

1. You have been assigned to care for a client, Mrs. Smith. She has an abusive relationship with her eldest son, who even threatens to slap and punch her at times. What should you do to protect Mrs. Smith from harm?

_____

_____

2. Mrs. Rader has no medical equipment in her home. She is confined to bed and frequently needs to be positioned in the semi-Fowler's position for different care procedures. How should you handle this situation?

_____

_____

3. One of your duties as a home health aide is to serve Mr. Salisbury his dinner. What are your responsibilities with regard to this task?

_____

_____

4. When providing housekeeping services, you should care for the client's home as if it were your own. Explain what must you do to ensure this.

_____

_____

5. Describe various housekeeping responsibilities that may be required of you as a home health aide.

_____

_____

QUALITIES OF THE SUCCESSFUL HOME HEALTH AIDE

Key Learning Points

- Personal qualities that a home health aide must have to be successful

Activity E *Look at the picture below and answer the questions.*

Identify the item shown in the picture. What is it used for? List five things you might find inside.

_____

_____

_____

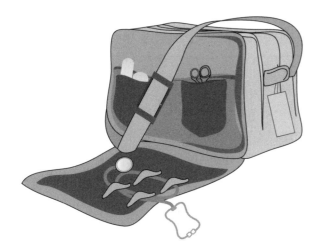

Activity F *Mark each statement as either "true" (T) or "false" (F). Correct the false statements.*

1. T F As a home health aide, you will be working in a client's home with direct supervision by the case manager most of the time.

2. T F Organization and planning are keys to working efficiently and safely.

3. T F A home health aide who leaves a client's home without completing the scheduled tasks is guilty of abandonment.

4. T F If you are not able to report to a client's home at the scheduled time, it is your responsibility both to call the client and to notify the home health care agency.

5. T F It is not appropriate to "drop in" on a client, or to go to the client's home after working hours to visit socially.

6. T F If a client offers you a tip, you should accept it.

Activity G *Think About It! Briefly answer the following questions in the spaces provided.*

1. List four qualities that characterize the most successful home health aides.

_____

_____

2. Why is it important that you complete your assigned duties as scheduled?

_____

_____

SUMMARY

Activity H *Use the clues to find words that are present in the grid of letters, either horizontally from left to right or vertically from top to bottom.*

Across

1. Adjective used to describe a person who cannot leave the house without a lot of help from another person

Down

1. A nursing assistant who provides skilled care in the home
2. In the home health care setting, the member of the health care team who is responsible for overseeing the client's total care
3. The act of withdrawing support or help from another person, in spite of duty or responsibility
4. A bag used by the home health aide to transport necessary supplies and equipment to each client's home

W	X	H	S	G	J	I	E	S
H	S	F	G	H	J	W	E	S
Y	S	W	E	R	T	H	J	K
H	G	C	F	D	T	Y	U	J
O	T	A	D	J	A	D	F	J
M	H	S	F	G	J	K	W	G
E	J	E	D	A	D	N	S	F
H	O	M	E	B	O	U	N	D
E	F	A	D	A	F	R	U	D
A	R	N	W	N	G	S	H	F
L	T	A	S	D	H	E	Q	R
T	H	G	I	O	N	S	W	E
H	N	E	J	N	J	B	S	S
A	J	R	H	M	U	A	R	C
I	K	E	T	E	W	G	R	V
D	I	D	F	N	S	P	F	B
E	A	C	C	T	D	D	C	V

CHAPTER 45

Safety and Infection Control in the Home Health Care Setting

WORKPLACE SAFETY

Key Learning Points

■ Safety concerns that are unique to the home health care environment

Activity A *Many factors in a person's home can put a person at risk for falling, or being injured due to a fire, especially if the person has limited mobility or poor eyesight. Place an "FA" next to the factors that can put a person at risk of falling and an "FI" next to the factors that can cause injury to a person due to a fire breakout. Place both an "FA" and an "FI" next to those factors that contribute to falling and are a fire hazard as well.*

1. ____ The wiring in the house may be old.

2. ____ Hallways, rooms, and staircases might be dimly lit, or not lit at all.

3. ____ Electrical cords may be covered by carpet.

4. ____ The home may be filled with a lifetime of collected objects and furniture, which can lead to crowding and clutter.

5. ____ Many homes are old, with worn carpets or uneven floors.

6. ____ Electrical outlets may be overloaded.

7. ____ Many people have pets, which can run underfoot.

8. ____ The family may rely on a space heater to provide heat and may not know how to use it properly.

9. ____ The bathroom may be small or not located in place that is easy for a person with poor mobility to reach.

10. ____ Many people do not have functioning smoke detectors in their homes.

Activity B *Match the actions taken to maintain a safe home environment, given in Column A, with their reasons, given in Column B.*

Column A	Column B
____ 1. Making sure that the furniture is arranged to allow for wide walkways	a. A house fire can have tragic consequences, especially when the people who live in the home are relatively unable to help themselves should a fire break out
____ 2. Providing adequate lighting	

_____ **3.** Installing night-lights as needed

_____ **4.** Cleaning up spills promptly

_____ **5.** Using a no-slip rubber bath mat on the floor of the bathtub

_____ **6.** Providing a bath bench or a shower chair for the person to use while showering

_____ **7.** Being aware of potential fire hazards and reporting these immediately

_____ **8.** Keeping chemicals, cleaning solutions, and other poisonous substances in a locked storage area

_____ **9.** Programming emergency telephone numbers into the telephone

b. This makes it easier for the person to summon help in the event of an emergency

c. An unsteady person will be more stable and at less risk for falling if he can sit down during the shower

d. This decreases a person's risk of tripping and falling

e. This enhances the person's ability to see, which helps to prevent falls

f. This increases the person's ability to see without turning on the lights in the room or hallway and helps to prevent falls

g. This decreases the person's risk of accidental poisoning

h. This reduces the person's chance of slipping on wet tile or linoleum floors

i. This helps to provide traction, reducing the person's risk of falling

Activity C *Mark each statement as either "true" (T) or "false" (F). Correct the false statements.*

1. T F It is the responsibility of the home health aide to make the changes necessary to ensure safe conditions in her client's home.

2. T F It is the responsibility of the home health aide in an emergency situation to call 911 or the emergency telephone number specified by the home health care agency and stay to provide appropriate care until help arrives.

3. T F It is the responsibility of the home health aide to investigate whether or not abuse has actually occurred before reporting it to the case manager.

INFECTION CONTROL

Key Learning Points

■ Ways that home health care aides can spread infection
■ Ways to reduce the spread of infection within the home
■ Ways to properly prepare and store food

Activity D *When working in a client's home, you will have responsibilities related to maintaining a sanitary environment and preventing the spread of infection. Fill in the blanks using the words given in brackets.*

[newspaper, "dirty," contamination, hands, clean, disinfect]

1. Bag technique is a procedure that is used to keep your nurse's bag free from _____ .

2. When you arrive at the client's home, place your nurse's bag on a clean surface, such as a piece of _____ on the kitchen table.

3. After washing your _____, remove the equipment you will need from the nurse's bag.

4. After you use your equipment, _____ it and _____ it, then return it to its proper location in your nurse's bag.

5. To transport specimens, such as urine or sputum samples, to the agency or laboratory, store them in the _____ area of the nurse's bag.

Activity E *Think About It! Briefly answer the following questions in the space provided.*

1. In order to maintain a sanitary environment and prevent the spread of infection, name three things that you should remember when cleaning floors and other household surfaces at a client's home.

_____

_____

_____

_____

2. When preparing foods for a client, you must first wash your hands and make sure that the surface where you will be preparing the food is clean. List at least five points that you need to remember when you are actually preparing the food.

_____

_____

_____

_____

3. What should you do with food left over from a client's meal?

_____

_____

_____

_____

4. Write some of the duties of a home health care aide related to assisting clients with personal hygiene.

_____

_____

_____

_____

5. Handwashing is the single most important method of preventing the spread of infection in any type of health care setting. List instances when handwashing is essential when working for a client in his home.

_____

_____

_____

6. Mrs. Sheen has diabetes and injects herself daily with insulin. When you start working for Mrs. Sheen, you find that she has been disposing of the syringes and needles simply by tossing them into the bathroom wastebasket. What should you do?

_____

_____

_____

_____

Infection control is a priority in the home, just as it is in any other health care setting. You will help to prevent the spread of infection by maintaining a sanitary environment and using standard precautions.

PERSONAL SAFETY

Key Learning Points

■ Measures that the home health aide can take to protect herself from personal harm while carrying out her duties

Activity F *Some aspects of the home health aide's job pose unique safety risks. Instead of working in one building, you will be required to travel from one client's home to another. What are the precautions that you should take in light of the following points?*

1. Your car's condition:

_____

_____

2. Your travel route:

_____

_____

3. Emergency car kit equipment:

_____

_____

4. Driving in ice and snow:

_____

_____

5. Personal cash and expensive personal items:

_____

_____

6. Visiting clients who live in unsafe neighborhoods:

_____

_____

7. Parking your car:

_____

_____

8. Choosing your walking route:

_____

_____

9. Self-defense in case of an attack:

_____

_____

10. Sharing your schedule:

_____

_____

11. Your cell phone:

_____

_____

> Working as a home health aide poses unique risks to your safety and well-being. Protecting yourself while traveling to and from your clients' homes is a top priority! Keeping your car in good repair, being prepared for roadside and weather emergencies, using common sense, and being aware of your surroundings are all ways that you can help to keep yourself safe.

Introduction to the Language of Health Care

MEDICAL TERMINOLOGY

Key Learning Points
- Roots, suffixes, prefixes, and combining vowels

Activity A *Break the following words into their roots, suffixes/prefixes, and combining vowels.*

1. Arthroscopy _____

_____

2. Blepharoplasty _____

_____

3. Cystitis _____

_____

4. Hepatomegaly _____

_____

5. Nocturia _____

_____

6. Stomatitis _____

_____

7. Bradycardia _____

_____

8. Hypogastric _____

_____

9. Pericarditis _____

_____

10. Intravascular _____

_____

11. Polydipsia _____

_____

12. Hyperemesis _____

_____

13. Leukocytopenia _____

_____

14. Electrocardiogram _____

Activity B *Match the common roots, given in Column A, with their meanings, given in Column B.*

Column A	Column B
___ **1.** Adip	**a.** Vessel
___ **2.** Erythr	**b.** Eyelid
___ **3.** Hepat	**c.** Fat
___ **4.** Proct	**d.** Gallbladder
___ **5.** Blephar	**e.** Red
___ **6.** Cholecyst	**f.** Bile, gall
___ **7.** Angi	**g.** Lower back
___ **8.** Lumb	**h.** Anus, rectum
___ **9.** Chol	**i.** Liver

Activity C *Mark each statement as either "true" (T) or "false" (F). Correct the false statements.*

1. T F   Retinopathy is a disease of the nose.

2. T F   Hepatomegaly means enlargement of the liver.

3. T F   Gastrectomy means removal of the colon.

4. T F   A glucometer is an instrument that is used to measure sugar (blood sugar.)

5. T F   Scleroderma is hardening of the skin.

6. T F   Hyperemesis means excessive vomiting.

Activity D *Fill in the blanks using the words given in brackets.*

[prefixes, roots, suffixes, combining vowels]

1. _____ contain the essential, basic meaning of the word.

2. _____ and _____ are attached to the root to make the root more specific.

3. _____ are often added in between the root and the suffix to make the new word easier to pronounce.

Activity E *Write the meaning of each of the following roots, suffixes, and prefixes.*

1. abdomin _____

_____

2. cephal _____

_____

3. –centesis _____

_____

4. –gram _____

_____

5. epi- _____

_____

6. inter- _____

_____

7. peri- _____

_____

8. pre- _____

_____

9. tachy- _____

_____

10. –rrhaphy _____

_____

11. –scope _____

_____

12. –tome _____

_____

13. blephar _____

_____

14. encephal _____

_____

15. hemangi _____

_____

> Make it a point to look up new words or abbreviations in a medical dictionary as soon as you hear or read them. Or, ask the nurse to explain the meaning of the word or the abbreviation to you. Before long, you will become very comfortable using and understanding the language of health care!

ANATOMICAL TERMS

Key Learning Points

- Anatomical planes
- Directional terms
- The terms used to describe body cavities
- The terms used to describe abdominal areas

Activity F *Mark each statement as either "true" (T) or "false" (F). Correct the false statements.*

1. T F Health care professionals use specific terms to describe the location of one body part in relation to another.

2. T F A person who is in normal anatomical position is standing upright and facing forward, with his feet close together.

3. T F The sagittal plane is a horizontal plane that divides the body into upper and lower segments.

4. T F Directional terms are used to describe the location of one body part in relation to the ground.

5. T F Changing a person's body position changes the directional reference.

Activity G *Label the figure using the words given in brackets.*

[frontal (coronal) plane, sagittal plane, transverse plane]

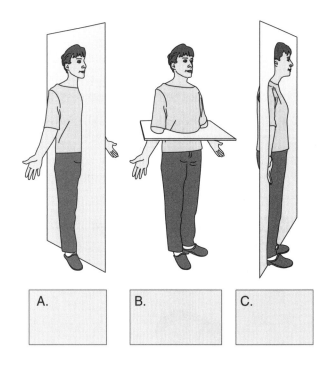

A. B. C.

Activity H *Fill in the blanks using the words given in brackets.*

[anterior, superior, medial, inferior, posterior, lateral, distal, proximal]

1. The nose is _____ to the eyes.

2. The ears are _____ to the nose.

3. The eyes are _____ to the breast.

4. The elbow is _____ to the wrist.

5. The chest is _____ to the throat.

6. The abdomen is _____ to the buttocks.

7. The buttocks are _____ to the abdomen.

8. The wrist is _____ to the elbow.

Activity I *Mark each statement as either "true" (T) or "false" (F). Correct the false statements.*

1. T F The dorsal cavity contains the brain and spinal cord.

2. T F The ventral cavity is toward the back of the body.

3. T F   The ventral cavity is divided by the pleura into the thoracic (chest) cavity and the abdominal (belly) cavity.

4. T F   The thoracic cavity contains the lungs, the heart, and the large blood vessels.

5. T F   The lower abdominal cavity contains the stomach, liver, and pancreas.

6. T F   The upper abdominal cavity contains the urinary bladder, the rectum, and female reproductive organs.

Activity J *Label the figure using the words given in brackets.*

[abdominal cavity, diaphragm, ventral cavity, dorsal cavity, thoracic cavity]

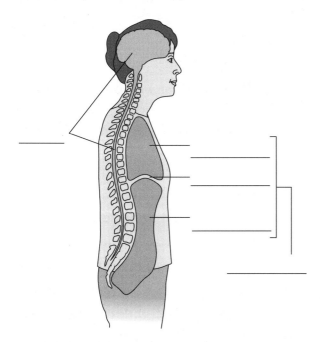

Activity K *Fill in the blanks using the words given in brackets.*

[umbilical, hypogastric, epigastric, regions, iliac, quadrants]

1. _____ are typically used to describe general information, such as where a person is experiencing pain.

2. _____ are used when it is necessary to be very specific (for example, when describing where an incision is located).

3. The _____ and _____ regions are named for their relation to the stomach.

4. The _____ region is named for the belly button.

5. The _____ regions are also sometimes called the inguinal (groin) regions.

Activity L *Label the figure using the words given in brackets.*

[left lower quadrant, left upper quadrant, right lower quadrant, right upper quadrant, umbilicus]

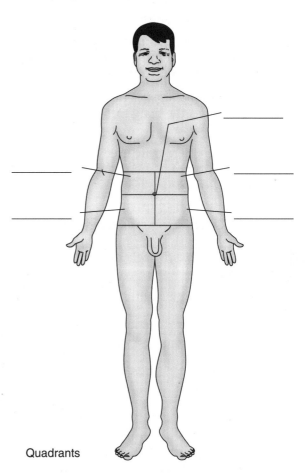

Quadrants

Activity M *Label the figure using the words given in brackets.*

[right iliac, left hypochondriac, left lumbar, left iliac, epigastric, hypogastric, right hypochondriac, umbilical, right lumbar]

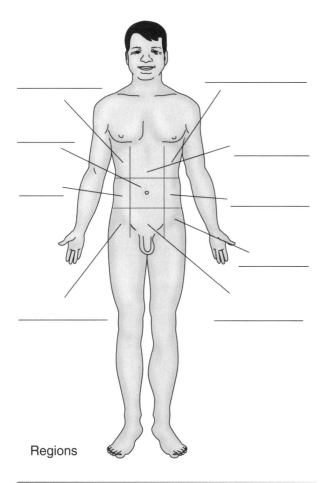

Regions

Understanding the terms and abbreviations that are unique to the health care profession is essential if you expect to be able to communicate effectively with other members of the health care team. Not knowing these terms and abbreviations will make it difficult for you to read and follow orders for patient or resident care. In addition, you will need to know these terms and abbreviations to accurately record and report.

ABBREVIATIONS

Key Learning Points

- Abbreviations commonly used in health care

Activity N *Let's play* Jeopardy! *The category is "Medical Abbreviations." We'll give you the answer. You must pick the correct question from the four choices below.*

1. These are proteins made by the body to protect itself from foreign substances such as bacteria or viruses.
   a. What is Au?
   b. What is Ab?
   c. What is ac?
   d. What is Adm?

2. It is a hospital unit specially staffed and equipped to treat patients with serious cardiac problems.
   a. What is a CCU?
   b. What is a CHD?
   c. What is a CHF?
   d. What is a CBR?

3. It is a colorless, odorless gas, necessary for combustion and life.
   a. What is OB?
   b. What is OJ?
   c. What is O_2?
   d. What is O?

4. It is designed, equipped, and staffed to meet the needs of people who are recovering from anesthesia, regional blocks, and intravenous sedation.
   a. What is an OR?
   b. What is a PAR?
   c. What is a PM?
   d. What is a PT?

Activity O *Write the meaning for each of the following abbreviations.*

1. AIDS _____

   _____

2. BKA _____

   _____

3. CCU _____

   _____

4. FBS _____

   _____

5. HBV _____

   _____

6. HIV _____

_____

7. LPN _____

_____

8. LVN _____

_____

9. NPO (npo) _____

_____

10. qt _____

_____

11. R _____

_____

12. STD _____

_____

13. Surg _____

_____

14. WNL _____

_____

15. wt _____

_____

Although abbreviations help save time and space when recording, it is very important to use abbreviations that are approved for use in your facility. Otherwise, other members of the health care team may be confused by the meaning. If unsure of the meaning of an abbreviation, please, either look the abbreviation up, or ask the nurse to explain it.

SUMMARY

Activity P *Use the clues to complete the crossword puzzle.*

Across

3. Closer to the mid-sagittal plane of the body (toward the inner side)
4. Toward the back, or *dorsal surface,* of the body
9. Toward the front, or *ventral surface*, of the body
12. The study of the structure of the body
13. The essential, basic meaning of the word
14. These are attached to the end of a root to make the root more specific
15. A vertical plane that divides the body into front and back segments

Down

1. Closer to the top of the body (closer to the head)
2. Further away from the mid-sagittal plane of the body (toward the outer side)
5. Further away from the top of the body (closer to the feet)
6. Cavity that contains the lungs, the heart, and the large blood vessels that enter and leave the heart
7. Directional term that is used to describe location of a body part further away from the point of origin in relation to something else
8. Directional term that is used to describe location of a body part closer to the point of origin in relation to something else
10. A horizontal plane that divides the body into upper and lower segments
11. The simplest way to describe the abdominal area
13. Smaller sections that the abdomen can be divided into

CHAPTER 7 PROCEDURE CHECKLISTS

PROCEDURE 7-1
Handwashing (Hand Hygiene)

	S	U	COMMENTS
1. Gather needed supplies, if not present at the handwashing area: *soap or the cleansing agent specified by your facility, hand lotion* (optional), *paper towels, a nailbrush* (optional), *an orange stick* (optional).	☐	☐	_____
2. Stand away from the sink, so that your uniform does not touch the sink. Push your sleeves up your arms 4 to 5 inches; if you are wearing a watch, push it up too.	☐	☐	_____
3. Use a clean paper towel to turn on the faucet, adjusting the water temperature until it is warm. Dispose of the paper towel in a facility-approved waste container.	☐	☐	_____
4. Wet your hands, keeping your fingers pointed down. This will cause the water to run off your fingertips and into the sink. Do not allow water to run up your forearms.	☐	☐	_____
5. Press the hand pump or step on the foot pedal to dispense the cleaning agent into one cupped hand.	☐	☐	_____
6. Lather well, keeping your fingers pointed down at all times. Make sure the lather extends at least 1 inch past your wrists.	☐	☐	_____
7. Rub your hands together in a circular motion, washing the palms and backs of your hands. Interlace your fingers to clean the spaces between your fingers. Continue for at least 15 seconds.	☐	☐	_____
8. Rub the fingernails of one hand against the palm of the opposite hand to force soap underneath the tips of the fingernails, *or* clean underneath the tips of the fingernails with the blunt edge of an orange stick or a nailbrush.	☐	☐	_____
9. Rinse your hands, keeping your fingers pointed down at all times.	☐	☐	_____
10. Dry your hands thoroughly with a clean paper towel. Dispose of the paper towel in a facility-approved waste container, being careful not to touch the container.	☐	☐	_____
11. With a new paper towel, turn off the faucet. Carefully dispose of the paper towel.	☐	☐	_____

12. As you leave the handwashing area, if there is a
    doorknob, open the door by covering the doorknob
    with a clean paper towel. If there is no doorknob,
    push the door open with your hip and shoulder to
    avoid contaminating your clean hands.   ☐ ☐ _____

13. After leaving the handwashing area, apply a small
    amount of hand lotion to keep your skin supple and
    moist.   ☐ ☐ _____

PROCEDURE 7-2
Removing Gloves

	S	U	COMMENTS

1. With one gloved hand, grasp the other glove at the palm and pull the glove off your hand. Keep the glove you have removed in your gloved hand. (Think, "glove to glove.") ☐ ☐ _____

2. Slip two fingers from the ungloved hand underneath the cuff of the remaining glove, at the wrist. Remove that glove from your hand, turning it inside-out as you pull it off. (Think, "skin to skin.") ☐ ☐ _____

3. Dispose of the soiled gloves in a facility-approved waste container. ☐ ☐ _____

4. Wash your hands. ☐ ☐ _____

PROCEDURE 7-3
Putting on a Gown

	S	U	COMMENTS
1. Gather needed supplies: *a gown, gloves.*	☐	☐	_____
2. Remove your watch and place it on a clean paper towel or in your pocket. (If you are wearing jewelry, remove that as well.) Roll up the sleeves of your uniform so that they are about 4-5 inches above your wrists.	☐	☐	
3. Wash your hands.	☐	☐	_____
4. Put on the gown by slipping your arms into the sleeves.	☐	☐	_____
5. Secure the gown around your neck by tying the ties in a simple bow or by fastening the Velcro™ strips.	☐	☐	_____
6. Reach behind yourself and overlap the edges of the gown so that your uniform is completely covered. Secure the gown at your waist by tying the ties in a simple bow or by fastening the Velcro™ strips.	☐	☐	_____
7. Put on the gloves. The cuffs of the gloves should extend over the cuffs of the gown.	☐	☐	_____

PROCEDURE 7-4
Removing a Gown

	S	U	COMMENTS
1. Remove and dispose of your gloves as described in Procedure 7-2.	☐	☐	_____
2. Untie the waist ties (or undo the Velcro™ strips at the waist).	☐	☐	_____
3. Untie the neck ties (or undo the Velcro™ strips at the neck). Be careful not to touch your neck or the outside of the gown.	☐	☐	_____
4. Grasping the gown at the neck ties, loosen it at the neck.	☐	☐	_____
5. Slip the fingers of your dominant hand under the cuff of the gown on the opposite sleeve, and pull the sleeve over your hand. Be careful not to touch the outside of the gown with either hand.	☐	☐	_____
6. Use your gown-covered hand to pull the sleeve over your other hand, and then pull the gown off both arms.	☐	☐	_____
7. Holding the gown away from your body, roll it downward, turning it inside out as you go. Take care to touch only the noncontaminated side of the gown.	☐	☐	_____
8. After the gown is rolled up, contaminated side inward, dispose of it in a facility-approved container.	☐	☐	_____
9. Wash your hands.	☐	☐	_____

PROCEDURE 7-5
Putting on and Removing a Mask

	S	U	COMMENTS

Putting on a Mask

1. Gather needed supplies: a mask.   ☐ ☐ _____

2. Wash your hands.   ☐ ☐ _____

3. Place the mask over your nose and mouth, being careful not to touch your face with your hands.   ☐ ☐ _____

4. Tie the top strings of the mask securely behind your head.   ☐ ☐ _____

5. Tie the bottom strings of the mask securely behind your neck. Make sure that the mask fits snugly around your face. You want to breathe through the mask, not around it.   ☐ ☐ _____

Removing a Mask

1. Wash your hands. (You do not want to touch your face with dirty hands.)   ☐ ☐ _____

2. Untie the bottom strings first, and then untie the top strings.   ☐ ☐ _____

3. Remove the mask by holding the top strings. Dispose of the mask, holding it by its ties only, in the facility-approved container located inside the patient's or resident's room.   ☐ ☐ _____

4. Wash your hands.   ☐ ☐ _____

PROCEDURE 7-6

Removing PPE at the Doorway Before Leaving the Patient Room

	S	U	COMMENTS
1. Remove and dispose of your gloves as described in Procedure 7-2.	☐	☐	_____
2. Remove your protective eyewear. Handle only by the "clean" headband or ear pieces.	☐	☐	_____
3. Untie the gown's waist ties (or undo the Velcro™ strips at the waist).	☐	☐	_____
4. Untie the gown's neck ties (or undo the Velcro™ strips at the neck), and loosen the gown at the neck. Remove and dispose of the gown as described in Procedure 7-4).	☐	☐	_____
5. Remove and dispose of the mask as described in Procedure 7-5.	☐	☐	_____
6. Wash your hands immediately after removing a PPE.	☐	☐	_____

PROCEDURE 7-7
Double-Bagging (Two Assistants)

	S	U	COMMENTS

1. The nursing assistant inside the person's room places the contaminated items into an isolation bag (usually a color-coded plastic bag) and secures the bag with a tie.
☐ ☐ _____

2. Another nursing assistant, referred to as the "clean" nursing assistant, stands outside of the person's room, holding a plastic bag cuffed over her hands. The cuff at the top of the bag protects the "clean" nursing assistant's hands.
☐ ☐ _____

3. The nursing assistant inside the isolation unit deposits the bag of contaminated items into the bag held by the "clean" nursing assistant.
☐ ☐ _____

4. The "clean" nursing assistant secures the top of the plastic bag tightly and disposes of the double-bagged items according to facility policy.
☐ ☐ _____

CHAPTER 10 PROCEDURE CHECKLISTS

PROCEDURE 10-1
Applying a Vest Restraint

	S	U	COMMENTS

Getting Ready

1. Complete the "Getting Ready" steps. ☐ ☐ _____

Procedure

2. Get help from a nurse or another personal support worker, if necessary. ☐ ☐ _____

3. Assist the person to a sitting position by locking arms with him or her. ☐ ☐ _____

4. Support the person's back and shoulders with one arm while slipping the person's arms through the armholes of the vest using your other hand. Apply the restraint according to the manufacturer's instructions. The vest should cross in the front, across the person's chest. ☐ ☐ _____

5. Make sure there are no wrinkles across the front or back of the restraint. ☐ ☐ _____

6. Bring the ties through the slots. ☐ ☐ _____

7. Help the person to lie or sit down. ☐ ☐ _____

8. Make sure the person is comfortable and in good body alignment. ☐ ☐ _____

9. If the person is in a chair, thread the straps *between* the seat and the armrest or *between* the back of the seat and the back of the chair, according to the manufacturer's directions. If the person is in bed, attach the straps to the bed frame, never the side rails. Always use the quick-release knot approved by your facility. ☐ ☐ _____

10. Make sure the restraint is not too tight. You should be able to slide a flat hand between the restraint and the person. Adjust the straps if necessary. ☐ ☐ _____

11. **a.** Raise the side rails if the person is in bed. ☐ ☐ _____
    b. Lock the wheels and make sure front wheels are facing forward if the person is in a wheelchair. ☐ ☐ _____

Finishing Up

12. Complete the "Finishing Up" steps. ☐ ☐ _____
13. Check on the restrained person every 15 minutes. ☐ ☐ _____

14. Release the restraint every 2 hours and:

    a. Reposition the person. □ □ _____

    b. Meet the person's needs for food, fluids, and elimination. □ □ _____

    c. Give skin care and perform range-of-motion exercises. □ □ _____

15. Reapply the restraint. □ □ _____

PROCEDURE 10-2
Applying Wrist or Ankle Restraints

	S	U	COMMENTS

Getting Ready

1. Complete the "Getting Ready" steps. ☐ ☐ _____

Procedure

2. Get help from a nurse or another personal support worker, if necessary. ☐ ☐ _____

3. Apply the wrist or ankle restraint following the manufacturer's instructions. Place the soft part of the restraint against the skin. ☐ ☐ _____

4. Secure the restraint so that it is snug, but not tight. You should be able to slide two fingers under the restraint. ☐ ☐ _____

5. Attach the straps to the bed frame. Always use the quick-release knot approved by your facility. ☐ ☐ _____

6. If applying more than one restraint, repeat steps 3 through 5. ☐ ☐ _____

7. Raise side rails if person is in bed. ☐ ☐ _____

Finishing Up

8. Complete the "Finishing Up" steps. ☐ ☐ _____
9. Check on the restrained person every 15 minutes. ☐ ☐ _____
10. Release the restraint every 2 hours and: ☐ ☐ _____
    a. Reposition the person. ☐ ☐ _____
    b. Meet the person's needs for food, fluids, and elimination. ☐ ☐ _____
    c. Give skin care and perform range-of-motion exercises. ☐ ☐ _____
11. Reapply the restraint. ☐ ☐ _____

PROCEDURE 10-3

Applying Lap or Waist (Belt) Restraints

	S	U	COMMENTS

Getting Ready

1. Complete the "Getting Ready" steps.   ☐ ☐ _____

Procedure

2. Get help from a nurse or another nursing assistant, if necessary. ☐ ☐ _____

3. If the person is in a chair, assist him or her to a proper sitting position, making sure that the person's hips are as far back against the back of the chair as possible. (If the person is in a wheelchair, make sure the brakes are locked first, and position the footrests to support the person's feet.) ☐ ☐

4. Wrap the restraint around the person's abdomen, crossing the straps behind the person's back. ☐ ☐ _____

5. Bring the ties through the loops at the sides of the restraint, according to the manufacturer's directions. ☐ ☐ _____

6. Make sure the person is comfortable and in good body alignment. ☐ ☐ _____

7. Thread the straps between the chair arm and the chair back before securing the straps out of the person's reach, at the back of the chair. Always use the quick-release knot approved by your facility. ☐ ☐ _____

8. Secure the restraint, making sure it is not too tight. You should be able to slide a flat hand between the restraint and the person. ☐ ☐ _____

9. Raise side rails if person is in bed. ☐ ☐ _____

Finishing Up

10. Complete the "Finishing Up" steps. ☐ ☐ _____
11. Check on the restrained person every 15 minutes. ☐ ☐ _____
12. Release the restraint every 2 hours and:
    a. Reposition the person, ☐ ☐ _____
    b. Meet the person's needs for food, fluids, and elimination. ☐ ☐ _____
    c. Give skin care and perform range-of-motion exercises. ☐ ☐ _____
13. Reapply the restraint. ☐ ☐ _____

CHAPTER 11 PROCEDURE CHECKLISTS

PROCEDURE 11-1
Moving a Person to the Side of the Bed (One Assistant)

	S	U	COMMENTS

Getting Ready

1. Complete the "Getting Ready" steps. ☐ ☐ _____

Procedure

2. Make sure that the bed is positioned at a comfortable working height (to promote good body mechanics) and that the wheels are locked. ☐ ☐ _____

3. Place the pillow at the head of the bed, on its edge against the headboard. This gets the pillow out of the way. ☐ ☐ _____

4. If the side rails are in use, lower the side rail on the working side of the bed. The side rail on the opposite side of the bed should remain up. Lower the head of the bed so that the bed is flat (as tolerated). Fanfold the top linens to the foot of the bed. ☐ ☐ _____

5. Stand at the side of the bed with your feet spread about 12 inches apart and with your knees slightly bent to protect your back. ☐ ☐ _____

6. Gently slide your hands under the person's head and shoulders and move the person's upper body toward you. ☐ ☐ _____

7. Gently slide your hands under the person's torso and move the person's torso toward you. ☐ ☐ _____

8. Gently slide your hands under the person's hips and legs and move the person's lower body toward you. ☐ ☐ _____

9. Now, position the person as planned (e.g., in the prone or lateral position). ☐ ☐ _____

10. Reposition the pillow under the person's head and straighten the bottom linens. Draw the top linens over the person. Raise the head of the bed as the person requests. ☐ ☐ _____

11. Make sure that the bed is lowered to its lowest position and that the wheels are locked. If the side rails are in use, return them to the raised position. ☐ ☐ _____

Finishing Up

12. Complete the "Finishing Up" steps. ☐ ☐ _____

PROCEDURE 11-2
Moving a Person to the Side of the Bed (Two Assistants)

	S	U	COMMENTS

Getting Ready

1. Complete the "Getting Ready" steps. ☐ ☐ _____

Procedure

2. Make sure that the bed is positioned at a comfortable working height (to promote good body mechanics) and that the wheels are locked. ☐ ☐ _____

3. Place the pillow at the head of the bed, on its edge against the headboard. This gets the pillow out of the way. ☐ ☐ _____

4. If the side rails are in use, lower the side rails. Lower the head of the bed so that the bed is flat (as tolerated). Fanfold the top linens to the foot of the bed. ☐ ☐ _____

5. If the lift sheet is already on the bed, make sure that it is positioned so that it is under the person's shoulders and hips. (If a lift sheet is not already on the bed, position one under the person's shoulders and hips.) ☐ ☐ _____

6. Stand at the side of the bed, opposite your coworker, with your feet spread about 12 inches apart and with your knees slightly bent to protect your back. ☐ ☐ _____

7. Grasp the edge of the lift sheet and roll it over as close to the person's body as possible. This will provide for a better grip. (Your coworker does the same.) ☐ ☐ _____

8. Grasp the rolled edge of the lift sheet with both hands, palms and fingers facing down. One hand should be level with the person's shoulders and the other should be level with his or her hips. ☐ ☐ _____

9. On the count of "three," slowly and carefully lift up on the lift sheet in unison and move the person to the side of the bed. ☐ ☐ _____

10. Now, position the person as planned (e.g., in the prone or lateral position). ☐ ☐ _____

11. Reposition the pillow under the person's head and straighten the bottom linens. Draw the top linens over the person. ☐ ☐ _____

12. Make sure that the bed is lowered to its lowest position and that the wheels are locked. If the side rails are in use, return them to the raised position. ☐ ☐ _____

Finishing Up

13. Complete the "Finishing Up" steps. ☐ ☐ _____

PROCEDURE 11-3
Moving a Person up in Bed (One Assistant)

	S	U	COMMENTS

Getting Ready

1. Complete the "Getting Ready" steps. ☐ ☐ _____

Procedure

2. Make sure that the bed is positioned at a comfortable working height (to promote good body mechanics) and that the wheels are locked. ☐ ☐ _____

3. If the side rails are in use, lower the side rail on the working side of the bed. The side rail on the opposite side of the bed should remain up. Fanfold the top linens to the foot of the bed. ☐ ☐ _____

4. Place the pillow at the head of the bed, on its edge against the headboard. This gets the pillow out of the way. It also pads the headboard in case you move the person up a little too much or too fast! ☐ ☐ _____

5. Method "A":

   a. Face the head of the bed. Position your outside foot (i.e., the foot that is farthest away from the edge of the bed) 12 inches in front of the other foot and bend your knees slightly to protect your back. ☐ ☐ _____

   b. Place your arm that is nearest the head of the bed under the person's head and shoulders. Lock your other arm with the person's arm that is closest to you. ☐ ☐ _____

   c. Have the person bend her knees. ☐ ☐ _____

   d. Tell the person that on the count of "three," she is to lift her buttocks and press her heels into the mattress as you lift her shoulders. On the count of "three," help the person to move smoothly toward the head of the bed. ☐ ☐ _____

6. Method "B":

   a. Have the person grasp the head of the bed or a trapeze, if there is one. ☐ ☐ _____

   b. Face the head of the bed. Position your outside foot (i.e., the foot that is farthest away from the edge of the bed) 12 inches in front of the other foot and bend your knees slightly to protect your back. ☐ ☐ _____

   c. Place your hands under the person's back and buttocks. ☐ ☐ _____

   d. Have the person bend his knees. ☐ ☐ _____

   e. Tell the person that on the count of "three," he is to lift his buttocks and press his heels into the mattress. On the count of "three," help the person to move smoothly toward the head of the bed. ☐ ☐ _____

7. Reposition the pillow under the person's head and straighten the bottom linens. Draw the top linens over the person. Raise the head of the bed as the person requests.

□ □ _____

8. Make sure that the bed is lowered to its lowest position and that the wheels are locked. If the side rails are in use, return them to the raised position.

□ □ _____

Finishing Up

9. Complete the "Finishing Up" steps.

□ □ _____

PROCEDURE 11-4
Moving a Person up in Bed (Two Assistants)

	S	U	COMMENTS

Getting Ready

1. Complete the "Getting Ready" steps.   ☐ ☐ _____

Procedure

2. Make sure that the bed is positioned at a comfortable working height (to promote good body mechanics) and that the wheels are locked.   ☐ ☐ _____

3. Place the pillow at the head of the bed, on its edge against the headboard. This gets the pillow out of the way. It also pads the headboard in case you move the person up a little too much or too fast!   ☐ ☐ _____

4. If the side rails are in use, lower the side rails. Lower the head of the bed so that the bed is flat (as tolerated). Fanfold the top linens to the foot of the bed.   ☐ ☐ _____

5. If the lift sheet is already on the bed, make sure that it is positioned so that it is under the person's shoulders and hips. (If a lift sheet is not already on the bed, position one under the person's shoulders and hips).   ☐ ☐ _____

6. Stand at the side of the bed, opposite your co-worker, with your feet spread about 12 inches apart and with your knees slightly bent to protect your back.   ☐ ☐ _____

7. Grasp the edge of the lift sheet and roll it over as close to the person's body as possible. This will provide for a better grip. (Your coworker does the same.)   ☐ ☐ _____

8. Grasp the rolled edge of the lift sheet with both hands, palms and fingers facing down. One hand should be level with the person's shoulders and the other should be level with his or her hips.   ☐ ☐ _____

9. On the count of "three," slowly and carefully lift up on the lift sheet in unison and move the person toward the head of the bed. Avoid dragging the person across the bottom linens.   ☐ ☐ _____

10. Reposition the pillow under the person's head and straighten the bottom linens. Draw the top linens over the person. Raise the head of the bed as the person requests.   ☐ ☐ _____

11. Make sure that the bed is lowered to its lowest position and that the wheels are locked. If the side rails are in use, return them to the raised position.   ☐ ☐ _____

Finishing Up

12. Complete the "Finishing Up" steps.   ☐ ☐ _____

PROCEDURE 11-5

Raising a Person's Head and Shoulders

	S	U	COMMENTS

Getting Ready

1. Complete the "Getting Ready" steps.   ☐ ☐ _____

Procedure

2. Make sure that the bed is positioned at a comfortable working height (to promote good body mechanics) and that the wheels are locked.   ☐ ☐ _____

3. Place the pillow at the head of the bed, on its edge against the headboard. This gets the pillow out of the way.   ☐ ☐ _____

4. If the side rails are in use, lower the side rail on the working side of the bed. The side rail on the opposite side of the bed should remain up. Fanfold the top linens to the foot of the bed.   ☐ ☐ _____

5. Face the head of the bed. Position your outside foot (i.e., the foot that is farthest away from the edge of the bed) 12 inches in front of the other foot, and bend your knees slightly to protect your back.   ☐ ☐ _____

6. Slide one hand under the person's shoulder that is nearest to you.   ☐ ☐ _____

7. Slide the other hand under the person's upper back.   ☐ ☐ _____

8. On the count of "three," slowly and carefully lift the person's head and shoulders.   ☐ ☐ _____

9. Reposition the pillow under the person's head and straighten the bottom linens. Draw the top linens over the person. Raise the head of the bed as the person requests.   ☐ ☐ _____

10. Make sure that the bed is lowered to its lowest position and that the wheels are locked. If the side rails are in use, return them to the raised position.   ☐ ☐ _____

Finishing Up

11. Complete the "Finishing Up" steps.   ☐ ☐ _____

PROCEDURE 11-6
Turning a Person Onto His or Her Side

	S	U	COMMENTS

Getting Ready

1. Complete the "Getting Ready" steps. ☐ ☐ _____

Procedure

2. Make sure that the bed is positioned at a comfortable working height (to promote good body mechanics) and that the wheels are locked. ☐ ☐ _____

3. Place the pillow at the head of the bed, on its edge against the headboard. This gets the pillow out of the way. ☐ ☐ _____

4. If the side rails are in use, lower the side rail on the working side of the bed. The side rail on the opposite side of the bed should remain up. Lower the head of the bed so that the bed is flat (as tolerated). Fanfold the top linens to the foot of the bed. ☐ ☐ _____

5. Stand at the side of the bed with your feet spread about 12 inches apart and with your knees slightly bent to protect your back. ☐ ☐ _____

6. Move the person to the side of the bed nearest you. ☐ ☐ _____

7. Cross the person's arm that is nearest you over the person's chest. ☐ ☐ _____

8. Bend the person's leg that is nearest you, placing the foot on the bed. (Or, cross the person's leg that is nearest to you over his or her other leg.) ☐ ☐ _____

9. Roll the person onto his or her side:

   a. **To roll the person away from you:** Place one of your hands on the person's shoulder that is nearest you, and place your other hand on the person's hip that is nearest you. Gently roll the person away from you, toward the opposite side of the bed. ☐ ☐ _____

   b. **To roll the person toward you:** Raise the side rail and move to the other side of the bed. Lower that side rail. Place one hand on the person's shoulder that is farthest away from you, and place your other hand on the person's hip that is farthest away from you. Gently roll the person toward you. ☐ ☐ _____

10. Reposition the pillow under the person's head and straighten the bottom linens. Support the person by placing a pillow lengthwise between the person's legs. The person's lower leg should be straight, and the upper leg should be slightly bent at the knee. Place additional pillows under the person's upper arm, and behind his or her back. Draw the top linens over the person. ☐ ☐ _____

11. Make sure that the bed is lowered to its lowest position and that the wheels are locked. If the side rails are in use, return them to the raised position. ☐ ☐ _____

Finishing Up

12. Complete the "Finishing Up" steps. ☐ ☐ _____

PROCEDURE 11-7
Logrolling a Person (Two Assistants)

	S	U	COMMENTS

Getting Ready

1. Complete the "Getting Ready" steps. ☐ ☐ _____

Procedure

2. Make sure that the bed is positioned at a comfortable working height (to promote good body mechanics) and that the wheels are locked. ☐ ☐ _____

3. Place the pillow at the head of the bed, on its edge against the headboard. This gets the pillow out of the way. ☐ ☐ _____

4. If the side rails are in use, lower the side rail on the working side of the bed. The side rail on the opposite side of the bed should remain up. Lower the head of the bed so that the bed is flat (as tolerated). Fanfold the top linens to the foot of the bed. ☐ ☐ _____

5. Stand with the other assistant on the side of the bed with the lowered side rail. Stand facing the bed with your feet spread about 12 inches apart and with your knees slightly bent to protect your back. One assistant is aligned with the person's head and shoulders; the other is aligned with the person's hips. ☐ ☐ _____

6. Place your hands under the person's head and shoulders while your coworker places his or her hands under the person's hips and legs (or vice versa). Lifting in unison, gently move the person toward the side of the bed closest to you. ☐ ☐ _____

7. Place a pillow lengthwise between the person's legs and fold the person's arm so that it will be on top of his chest when he is turned. ☐ ☐ _____

8. Raise the side rail and make sure that it is secure. ☐ ☐ _____

9. Go to the opposite side of the bed and lower the side rail. ☐ ☐ _____

10. Working with the other assistant, turn the person onto his side.

   a. If a lift sheet is being used, turn the person by reaching over him and grasping the lift sheet. One assistant should place one hand on the lift sheet at the level of the person's shoulder and the other hand at the level of the person's hip; the other assistant should place one hand on the liftsheet at the level of the person's hip and the other at the level of the person's calves. ☐ ☐ _____

b. If a lift sheet is not being used, one assistant should position his or her hands on the person's shoulders and hips and the other assistant should place his or her hands on the person's thigh and calves.

☐ ☐ _____

11. On the count of "three," roll the person toward the side on which you are standing in a single movement, being sure to keep the person's head, spine, and legs aligned.

☐ ☐ _____

12. Reposition the pillow under the person's head and straighten the bottom linens. Support the person by bolstering his back with pillows. The pillow between the person's legs should remain in place, and additional pillows or folded towels should be used to support the person's arms. Draw the top linens over the person.

☐ ☐ _____

13. Make sure that the bed is lowered to its lowest position and that the wheels are locked. If the side rails are in use, return them to the raised position.

☐ ☐ _____

Finishing Up

14. Complete the "Finishing Up" steps.

☐ ☐ _____

PROCEDURE 11-8
Applying a Transfer (Gait) Belt

	S	U	COMMENTS

Getting Ready

1. Complete the "Getting Ready" steps. ☐ ☐ _____

Procedure

2. If the person is in bed, make sure that the bed is lowered to its lowest position and that the wheels are locked. If the side rails are in use, lower the side rail on the working side of the bed. The side rail on the opposite side of the bed should remain up. Fanfold the top linens to the foot of the bed. Assist the person to sit on the edge of the bed. ☐ ☐ _____

3. Apply the belt around the person's waist, over his or her clothing. Buckle the belt in the front by threading the tongue of the belt through the side of the buckle that has "teeth" first, and then placing the tongue of the belt through the other side of the buckle. ☐ ☐ _____

4. Before tightening the belt, turn it so that the buckle is off-center in the front or to the side. ☐ ☐ _____

5. Tighten the belt and check for fit. The belt should be snug, but you should be able to slip your fingers between the belt and the person's waist. When applying a transfer belt to a woman, make sure that her breasts are not trapped underneath the belt. ☐ ☐ _____

6. Use an underhand grasp when holding the belt to provide greater safety. ☐ ☐ _____

Finishing Up

7. When the person has finished transferring and is ready to return to bed, reverse the procedure. ☐ ☐ _____

8. Complete the "Finishing Up" steps. ☐ ☐ _____

PROCEDURE 11-9

Transferring a Person From a Bed to a Wheelchair (One Assistant)

	S	U	COMMENTS

Getting Ready

1. Complete the "Getting Ready" steps. ☐ ☐ _____

Procedure

2. Determine the person's strongest side, and then place the wheelchair alongside the bed. Position the wheelchair so that the person will move toward the chair "strong side first." Whenever possible, position the wheelchair so that it is against a wall or a solid piece of furniture so that it will not slide backward during the transfer. ☐ ☐ _____

3. Lock the wheelchair wheels, and either remove the footrests or swing them to the side. ☐ ☐ _____

4. Fanfold the top linens to the foot of the bed. ☐ ☐ _____

5. Make sure that the bed is lowered to its lowest position and that the wheels are locked. Raise the head of the bed as tolerated. ☐ ☐ _____

6. Help the person to move toward the side of the bed where the wheelchair is located. ☐ ☐ _____

7. Assist the person to dangle. ☐ ☐ _____

8. Allow the person to rest on the edge of the bed. The person should be sitting squarely on both buttocks, with her knees apart and both feet flat on the floor (to offer a broad base of support). The person's arms should rest alongside her thighs. Watch for signs of dizziness or fainting. Position yourself in front of the person so that you can offer assistance in case she loses balance. ☐ ☐ _____

9. Help the person to put her shoes or slippers on and help her to get into a robe. Apply a transfer belt. ☐ ☐ _____

10. Help the person to stand.

   a. Stand facing the person. ☐ ☐ _____

   b. Have the person put her hands on the edge of the bed, alongside each thigh. ☐ ☐ _____

   c. Make sure the person's feet are flat on the floor. ☐ ☐ _____

   d. Have the person lean forward. ☐ ☐ _____

   e. Grasp the transfer belt at each side, using an underhand grasp. (If you are not using a transfer belt, pass your arms under the person's arms and rest your hands on her upper back.) ☐ ☐ _____

f. Position your feet alongside the person's feet, flexing your knees. Place your shins against the person's shins to block the person's feet and keep her knees from buckling as she stands up. ☐ ☐ _____

g. Have the person push down on the bed with her hands and stand on the count of "three." Assist the person into a standing position by pulling on the transfer belt as you straighten your knees. (If you are not using a transfer belt, assist the person into a standing position by gently pulling her up and forward as you straighten your knees.) Remember to keep your back straight. ☐ ☐ _____

11. Support the person in the standing position by holding the transfer belt or by keeping your hands on her upper back. Continue to block the person's feet and knees with your feet and knees. ☐ ☐ _____

12. Help the person to turn by pivoting on the stronger leg toward the chair. This will allow the person to grasp the far arm of the wheelchair. ☐ ☐ _____

13. Continue to assist the person with turning until she is able to grasp the other armrest. The backs of the person's legs should touch the edge of the chair. ☐ ☐ _____

14. Lower the person into the wheelchair by bending your hips and knees. ☐ ☐ _____

15. Make sure the person's buttocks are at the back of the chair. Make sure the person is comfortable and in good body alignment. ☐ ☐ _____

16. Remove the transfer belt. ☐ ☐ _____

17. Position the person's feet on the footrests of the wheelchair. Buckle the wheelchair safety belt (if ordered) and cover the person's lap and legs with a lap blanket, if desired. Make sure that the lap blanket does not drag on the floor. ☐ ☐ _____

Finishing Up

18. Position the wheelchair according to the person's preference. ☐ ☐ _____

19. Complete the "Finishing Up" steps. ☐ ☐ _____

PROCEDURE 11-10
Transferring a Person From a Bed to a Wheelchair (Two Assistants)

	S	U	COMMENTS
Getting Ready			
1. Complete the "Getting Ready" steps.	☐	☐	_____
Procedure			
2. Place the wheelchair alongside the bed, facing the foot of the bed.	☐	☐	_____
3. Lock the wheelchair wheels and either remove the footrests or swing them to the side.	☐	☐	_____
4. Fanfold the top linens to the foot of the bed.	☐	☐	_____
5. Make sure that the bed is positioned at a comfortable working height (to promote good body mechanics) and that the wheels are locked. Raise the head of the bed as tolerated.	☐	☐	_____
6. Help the person to move toward the side of the bed where the wheelchair is located.	☐	☐	_____
7. Help the person to put his shoes or slippers on, and help him get into a robe.	☐	☐	_____
8. Stand by the side of the bed, behind the wheelchair. Standing behind the person, pass your arms under the person's arms and grasp his forearms. The other assistant grasps the person's thighs and calves.	☐	☐	_____
9. Working in unison with the other assistant, lift the person from the bed and bring him toward the wheelchair on the count of "three." Lower the person into the wheelchair.	☐	☐	_____
10. Make sure the person's buttocks are at the back of the chair. Make sure the person is comfortable and in good body alignment.	☐	☐	_____
11. Position the person's feet on the footrests of the wheelchair. Buckle the wheelchair safety belt (if ordered) and cover the person's lap and legs with a lap blanket, if desired. Make sure that the lap blanket does not drag on the floor.	☐	☐	_____
Finishing Up			
12. Position the wheelchair according to the person's preference.	☐	☐	_____
13. Complete the "Finishing Up" steps.	☐	☐	_____

PROCEDURE 11-11

Transferring a Person From a Wheelchair to a Bed

	S	U	COMMENTS

Getting Ready

1. Complete the "Getting Ready" steps. ☐ ☐ _____

Procedure

2. Make sure that the bed is lowered to its lowest position and that the wheels are locked. Raise the head of the bed, fanfold the top linens to the foot of the bed, and raise the opposite side rail. ☐ ☐ _____

3. Position the wheelchair close to the side of the bed so that the person's strong side is next to the bed. Lock the wheelchair wheels and either remove the footrests or swing them to the side. ☐ ☐ _____

4. Remove the person's lap blanket (if one was used) and release the wheelchair safety belt, if in use. Apply a transfer belt. ☐ ☐ _____

5. Stand facing the person with your feet spread about 12 inches apart and with your knees slightly bent to protect your back. With your back straight, slide the person to the front of the wheelchair seat. ☐ ☐ _____

6. Grasp the transfer belt (or pass your arms under the person's arms, placing your hands on her upper back). Position your feet alongside the person's feet, flexing your knees. Place your shins against the person's shins to block the person's feet and keep her knees from buckling as she stands up. ☐ ☐ _____

7. Have the person rest her hands on your arms and assist her to stand by pulling on the transfer belt as you straighten your knees. (If you are not using a transfer belt, assist the person into a standing position by gently pulling her up and forward as you straighten your knees.) Remember to keep your back straight. Alternatively, a person who requires less assistance can place her hands on the wheelchair arms for support and "push off" while you offer support. ☐ ☐ _____

8. Slowly help the person to turn toward the bed by pivoting on her strong leg. Help the person to sit on the edge of the bed. ☐ ☐ _____

9. Remove the person's robe and slippers, if appropriate. ☐ ☐ _____

10. Move the wheelchair out of the way. ☐ ☐ _____

11. Place one of your arms around the person's shoulders and one arm under her legs. Swing the person's legs onto the bed. ☐ ☐ _____

12. Help the person to move to the center of the bed and position her comfortably. ☐ ☐ _____

13. Straighten the bottom linens and make sure the person is comfortable and in good body alignment. Draw the top linens over the person.   ☐ ☐ _____

14. If the side rails are in use, return them to the raised position.   ☐ ☐ _____

Finishing Up

15. Complete the "Finishing Up" steps.   ☐ ☐ _____

PROCEDURE 11-12

Transferring a Person From a Bed to a Stretcher (Four Assistants)

	S	U	COMMENTS
Getting Ready			
1. Complete the "Getting Ready" steps.	☐	☐	_____
Procedure			
2. Raise the bed to its highest level. (The stretcher should be slightly lower than the bed.) Lower the head of the bed so that the bed is flat. Make sure that the bed wheels are locked. Lower the side rails. Fanfold the top linens to the side of the bed opposite the stretcher.	☐	☐	_____
3. If the lift sheet is already on the bed, make sure that it is positioned so that it is under the person's shoulders and hips. (If a lift sheet is not already on the bed, position one under the person's shoulders and hips.)	☐	☐	_____
4. Position the stretcher alongside the bed. Lock the stretcher wheels and move the stretcher safety belts out of the way.	☐	☐	_____
5. Two assistants stand at the side of the bed facing their coworkers, who are positioned along the outside edge of the stretcher.	☐	☐	_____
6. Grasp the edge of the lift sheet and roll it over as close to the person's body as possible. This will provide for a better grip. (Your coworkers do the same.)	☐	☐	_____
7. On the count of "three," all four assistants slowly and carefully lift up on the lift sheet in unison and move the person to the side of the bed.	☐	☐	_____
8. On the count of "three," all four assistants slowly and carefully lift up on the transfer sheet in unison and move the person to the side of the stretcher.	☐	☐	_____
9. Position the person on the stretcher and make sure he or she is in good body alignment. Reposition the pillow under the person's head and cover the person with a blanket for modesty and warmth. Buckle the stretcher safety belts across the person and raise the side rails on the stretcher. Raise the head of the stretcher as the person requests.	☐	☐	_____
Finishing Up			
10. Transport the person to the appropriate site. A person on a stretcher should always be transported "feet first." Remain with the person; never leave someone alone on a stretcher.	☐	☐	_____
11. Complete the "Finishing Up" steps.	☐	☐	_____

PROCEDURE 11-13

Transferring a Person From a Stretcher to a Bed (Four Assistants)

	S	U	COMMENTS

Getting Ready

1. Complete the "Getting Ready" steps.   ☐ ☐ _____

Procedure

2. Raise or lower the bed so that it is slightly lower than the stretcher. Lower the head of the bed so that the bed is flat. Make sure that the bed wheels are locked. Lower the side rails. Fanfold the top linens to the side of the bed opposite the stretcher.   ☐ ☐ _____

3. If the lift sheet is already on the stretcher, make sure that it is positioned so that it is under the person's shoulders and hips. (If a lift sheet is not already on the stretcher, position one under the person's shoulders and hips.)   ☐ ☐ _____

4. Unbuckle the stretcher safety belts and lower the side rails on the stretcher.   ☐ ☐ _____

5. Position the stretcher against the bed and lock the stretcher wheels.   ☐ ☐ _____

6. Two assistants stand at the far side of the bed facing their coworkers, who are positioned along the outside edge of the stretcher. (Some facilities allow the assistants on the far side of the bed to kneel on the bed to complete the transfer; follow your facility's policy.)   ☐ ☐ _____

7. Grasp the edge of the lift sheet and roll it over as close to the person's body as possible. This will provide for a better grip. (Your coworkers do the same.)   ☐ ☐ _____

8. On the count of "three," all four assistants slowly and carefully lift up on the lift sheet in unison and move the person to the bed. Move the stretcher away from the bed.   ☐ ☐ _____

9. Help the person to move to the center of the bed and, if desired, remove the lift sheet by turning the person first to one side, then the other. Position the person comfortably.   ☐ ☐ _____

10. Straighten the bottom linens and make sure the person is comfortable and in good body alignment. Draw the top linens over the person.   ☐ ☐ _____

11. Make sure the bed is lowered to its lowest position and that the wheels are locked. If the side rails are in use, return them to the raised position.   ☐ ☐ _____

Finishing Up

12. Complete the "Finishing Up" steps.   ☐ ☐ _____

PROCEDURE 11-14
Transferring a Person Using a Mechanical Lift (Two Assistants)

	S	U	COMMENTS

Getting Ready

1. Complete the "Getting Ready" steps. ☐ ☐ _____

Procedure

2. Make sure that the bed is positioned at a comfortable working height (to promote good body mechanics) and that the wheels are locked. ☐ ☐ _____

3. If the side rails are in use, lower the side rails. ☐ ☐ _____

4. Fanfold the top linens to the foot of the bed. ☐ ☐ _____

5. Center the sling under the person. (To get the sling under the person, move the person as if you were making an occupied bed.) The lower edge of the sling should be positioned underneath the person's knees. ☐ ☐ _____

6. Raise the head of the bed as tolerated. ☐ ☐ _____

7. Move the release valve on the lift to the closed position. ☐ ☐ _____

8. Raise the lift so that it can be positioned over the person. ☐ ☐ _____

9. Spread the legs of the lift to provide a solid base of support. The legs must be locked in this position, or the lift could tip over, injuring you, the person you are trying to transfer, or both. ☐ ☐ _____

10. Move the lift into position over the person. ☐ ☐ _____

11. Fasten the sling to the straps or chains of the lift. Make sure the hooks face away from the person. ☐ ☐ _____

12. Attach the sling to the swivel bar with the short side attached to the top of the sling and the long side attached to the bottom of the sling. ☐ ☐ _____

13. Cross the person's arms across her chest. The person may hold onto the straps, but do not let her hold onto the swivel bar. ☐ ☐ _____

14. Raise the lift until the person and the sling are clear of the bed. ☐ ☐ _____

15. Place the wheelchair alongside the bed, facing the foot of the bed. Lock the wheelchair wheels. ☐ ☐ _____

16. Have your coworker support the person's legs as you move the lift into position over the wheelchair. ☐ ☐ _____

17. Turn the person so that she is facing the mast of the lift and is centered over the base. (The person's back should be facing the wheelchair.) ☐ ☐ _____

18. Move the lift so that the person is over the seat of the wheelchair. ☐ ☐ _____

19. Slowly open the release valve on the lift. Gently lower the person into the wheelchair. Make sure the person's buttocks are at the back of the chair.   ☐ ☐ _____

20. Lower the swivel bar so that you can unhook the sling. Leave the sling under the person.   ☐ ☐ _____

21. Make sure the person's buttocks are at the back of the chair. Make sure the person is comfortable and in good body alignment.   ☐ ☐ _____

22. Position the person's feet on the footrests of the wheelchair. Buckle the wheelchair safety belt (or place a lap restraint, if ordered). Cover the person's lap and legs with a lap blanket, if desired. Make sure that the lap blanket does not drag on the floor.   ☐ ☐ _____

Finishing Up

23. Position the wheelchair according to the person's preference.   ☐ ☐ _____

24. Follow the "Finishing Up" steps.   ☐ ☐ _____

25. When the person is ready to return to bed, reverse the procedure.   ☐ ☐ _____

PROCEDURE 11-15

Assisting a Person With Sitting on the Edge of the Bed ("Dangling")

	S	U	COMMENTS

Getting Ready

1. Complete the "Getting Ready" steps.   ☐ ☐ _____

Procedure

2. Make sure that the bed is lowered to its lowest position and that the wheels are locked.   ☐ ☐ _____

3. If the side rails are in use, lower the side rail on the working side of the bed. The side rail on the opposite side of the bed should remain up. Raise the head of the bed as tolerated. Fanfold the top linens to the foot of the bed.   ☐ ☐ _____

4. Method "A":

   a. Stand at the side of the bed with your feet spread about 12 inches apart and with your knees slightly bent to protect your back.   ☐ ☐ _____

   b. Have the person bend her knees and plant her feet on the bed.   ☐ ☐ _____

   c. Gently slide one arm behind the person's upper back. Slide the other arm under her knees and rest your hand on the side of her thigh.   ☐ ☐ _____

   d. With a single smooth movement, slide the person's legs over the side of the bed while moving her head and shoulders upward so that she is sitting on the edge of the bed.   ☐ ☐ _____

5. Method "B":

   a. Help the person to move toward the side of the bed.   ☐ ☐ _____

   b. Have the person roll over onto her side, facing the side of the bed. Have the person flex her knees and bend the arm she is lying on in preparation for using it to prop her upper body up. Have the person bend her top arm so that her hand is in a position that will enable her to push off the bed.   ☐ ☐ _____

   c. Instruct the person to rise to a sitting position by using the elbow of her bottom arm to raise her upper body while pushing against the mattress with her other hand. Advise the person to allow her legs to swing over the edge of the bed while you help to guide her into an upright position.   ☐ ☐ _____

6. Have the person put her hands on the edge of the bed, alongside each thigh, for support. Watch for signs of dizziness or fainting. If the person feels faint, help her to lie down and call for the nurse.   ☐ ☐ _____

7. Allow the person to "dangle" her legs over the side of the bed for the specified period of time, and then either take her vital signs (if indicated), help her to lie back down, or assist her to a standing position. Stay with her during the entire time.

□ □ _____

Finishing Up

8. Complete the "Finishing Up" steps.

□ □ _____

PROCEDURE 11-16
Assisting a Person With Walking (Ambulating)

	S	U	COMMENTS

Getting Ready

1. Complete the "Getting Ready" steps.   ☐ ☐ _____

Procedure

2. If the person is in bed, make sure that the bed is lowered to its lowest position and that the wheels are locked.   ☐ ☐ _____

3. Assist the person to "dangle." Check the person's pulse; a weak pulse could lead to lightheadedness. If the person's pulse is weak, stay with her and alert the nurse before attempting ambulation.   ☐ ☐ _____

4. Help the person put her shoes or slippers on and help her into a robe. Apply a transfer belt.   ☐ ☐ _____

5. Help the person to stand.

   a. Stand facing the person.   ☐ ☐ _____

   b. Have the person put her hands on the edge of the bed, alongside each thigh.   ☐ ☐ _____

   c. Make sure the person's feet are flat on the floor.   ☐ ☐ _____

   d. Have the person lean forward.   ☐ ☐ _____

   e. Grasp the transfer belt at each side, using an underhand grasp. (If you are not using a transfer belt, pass your arms under the person's arms and rest your hands on her upper back.)   ☐ ☐ _____

   f. Position your feet alongside the person's feet, flexing your knees. Place your shins against the person's shins to block the person's feet and keep her knees from buckling as she stands up.   ☐ ☐ _____

   g. Have the person push down on the bed with her hands and stand on the count of "three." Assist the person into a standing position by pulling on the transfer belt as you straighten your knees. (If you are not using a transfer belt, assist the person into a standing position by gently pulling her up and forward as you straighten your knees.) Remember to keep your back straight.   ☐ ☐ _____

6. Have the person grasp the cane or walker, if she is using one, in order to maintain balance. The person should hold the cane on her strong side.   ☐ ☐ _____

7. Help the person to walk. Stand slightly behind the person on her weaker side. Grasp the transfer belt with an underhand grip from the back. If the person is using an ambulation device, make sure she is using it correctly.   ☐ ☐ _____

8. After returning to the person's room, help her back into bed or a chair. ☐ ☐ _____

Finishing Up

9. Complete the "Finishing Up" steps. ☐ ☐ _____

CHAPTER 12 PROCEDURE CHECKLISTS

Performing Abdominal Thrusts in Conscious Adults and Children Older Than 1 Year

	S	U	COMMENTS

1. Check the person's ability to breathe and speak by tapping him or her on the shoulder and saying, "Are you okay? Can you talk? I can help you." A person who cannot breathe or speak needs immediate help. ☐ ☐ _____

2. If the person starts to cough, wait and see whether the coughing will dislodge the object. If the person's cough is weak and ineffective, or if the person is in obvious distress, continue with step 3. ☐ ☐ _____

3. Stay with the person and call for help. Have the person who is helping you activate the facility's emergency response system. ☐ ☐ _____

4. Stand behind the person with the obstructed airway and wrap your arms around his or her waist. ☐ ☐ _____

5. Make a fist with one hand and place the thumb of the fist against the person's abdomen, just above the navel and below the sternum (breastbone). Grasp your fist with the other hand. (Do not tuck your thumb inside your fist.) ☐ ☐ _____

6. Being careful not to put pressure on the person's ribs or sternum with your forearms, press your fist inward and pull upward, using quick thrusting motions, until the object is expelled, the person begins to cough forcefully, or the person loses consciousness.

   a. If the object is expelled, stay with the person, and follow the nurse's directions. ☐ ☐ _____

   b. If the person begins to cough, wait and see whether the coughing results in expulsion of the object. If it does not, continue giving abdominal thrusts. ☐ ☐ _____

   c. If the person loses consciousness, lower the person to the floor and begin Procedure 12-2, beginning with step 3. ☐ ☐ _____

7. The person should be evaluated by a doctor following the choking incident. ☐ ☐ _____

8. Record your observations and actions according to your facility's policy. ☐ ☐ _____

PROCEDURE 12-2

Relieving an Obstructed Airway in Unconscious Adults and Children Older than 1 Year

Why you do it: If breathing and circulation are not restored, the person will die.

	S	U	COMMENTS
1. **Responsiveness:** Check the person's state of consciousness by gently shaking or tapping her. Quickly check to see if the person is breathing (at least 5 seconds, but no more than 10 seconds).	☐	☐	_____
2. Stay with the person and call for help. Have the person who is helping you activate the facility's emergency response system.	☐	☐	_____
3. Check for a pulse (no more than 10 seconds). If there is no pulse, go on to step 6.	☐	☐	_____
4. **Rescue breathing:** If you feel a definite pulse, open the airway, using a head tilt-chin lift, and deliver one breath into the person's mouth through a ventilation barrier device. Deliver enough air into the person to make the person's chest rise. (figure from procedure for step 4)	☐	☐	_____
5. If the chest does not rise, repeat the head tilt-chin lift and give a second breath. If you are unable to ventilate the person after 2 attempts, promptly begin chest compressions.	☐	☐	_____
6. **Chest compressions.** If the person does not have a pulse, or if you are unable to ventilate the person after 2 attempts, begin chest compressions. To give chest compressions:	☐	☐	_____
a. Kneel beside the person.	☐	☐	_____
b. Place the heel of your hand closest to the person's head on his sternum (breastbone) and place your other hand on top and interlock your fingers.	☐	☐	_____
c. Position your body forward so that your shoulders are over the center of the person's chest and your arms are straight. You will want to compress straight down and up. Do not rock back and forth.	☐	☐	_____
d. **Push hard, push fast:** Compress the chest at a rate of at least 100 compressions per minute with a depth of at least 2 inches for adults and approximately 2 inches for children. Allow the chest to recoil completely after each compression.	☐	☐	_____
7. After you have given 30 chest compressions, quickly open the person's mouth wide and look for the object. If you see an object that can easily be removed, remove it with your fingers.	☐	☐	_____
8. Perform the head tilt-chin lift maneuver. Blow one breath into the person's mouth through a ventilation barrier device. If the air does not go in, repeat the head tilt-chin lift maneuver and attempt one breath again.	☐	☐	_____

9. Repeat the chest compression – object check – rescue breathing sequence until the object is expelled, rescue breathing is successful, or other trained personnel arrive and take over.   ☐ ☐   _____

10. The person should be evaluated by a doctor following the chocking incident.   ☐ ☐   _____

11. Record your observations and actions according to facility policy.   ☐ ☐   _____

PROCEDURE 12-3
Performing Chest Thrusts in Conscious Adults and Children Older Than 1 Year

If the Person Is Conscious

	S	U	COMMENTS
1. Stand behind the person and place your arms under the person's armpits and around his or her chest.	☐	☐	_____
2. Make a fist with one hand and place the thumb of the fist against the center of the person's sternum. Be sure that your thumb is centered on the sternum, not on the lower tip of the sternum (the xiphoid process) and not on the ribs.	☐	☐	_____
3. Give up to five quick chest thrusts by grasping your fist with your other hand and pressing inward five times. Each thrust should compress the chest 1½ to 2 inches.	☐	☐	_____
4. Continue to give chest thrusts until the object is expelled, the person begins to cough forcefully, or the person loses consciousness.			
a. If the object is expelled, stay with the person, and follow the nurse's directions.	☐	☐	_____
b. If the person begins to cough, wait and see whether the coughing results in expulsion of the object. If it does not, continue giving chest thrusts in groups of five.	☐	☐	_____
c. If the person loses consciousness, lower the person to the floor and initiate procedure 12-2.	☐	☐	_____
5. The person should be evaluated by a doctor following the choking incident.	☐	☐	_____
6. Record your observations and actions according to facility policy.	☐	☐	_____

PROCEDURE 12-4
Clearing the Airway in a Conscious Infant

	S	U	COMMENTS

1. Check the infant's ability to breathe and cry. An infant who cannot breathe or cry needs immediate help.

2. Stay with the infant. Call for help and have the person who is helping you activate the emergency medical services (EMS) system.

3. Position the infant on his or her back on your forearm. Place your other arm on top of the infant, using your thumb and forefinger to hold the infant's jaw while sandwiching the infant between your forearms.

4. Rotate your arms, so that the infant is facing downward, still sandwiched between your forearms. Lower your arm onto your thigh so that the infant's head is lower than his or her chest.

5. Give five firm blows to the back (between the infant's shoulder blades), using the heel of your hand. Be sure that you continue to support the infant's head and neck by firmly holding the baby's jaw between your thumb and forefinger.

6. If the back blows do not dislodge the foreign body, you must turn the infant over in preparation for administering chest thrusts. Turn the infant over by placing your free hand and forearm along the infant's head and back so that the infant is sandwiched between your hands and forearms. Continue to support the infant's head between your thumb and forefinger from the front, while you cradle the back of the head with your other hand. Turn the infant onto his or her back. Lower your arm onto your thigh so that the infant's head is lower than his or her chest.

7. To locate the correct place to give chest thrusts, imagine a line running across the infant's chest between the nipples. Place the pads of your first three fingers on the infant's sternum (breastbone), even with this imaginary line. If you feel the notch at the end of the infant's sternum, move your fingers toward the infant's head so that your fingers are over the center of the sternum.

8. Lift your ring finger off the chest, and using the pads of the two remaining fingers, compress the sternum ½ to 1 inch, and then let the sternum return to its normal position. Give five chest thrusts.

9. Repeat the back blow-chest thrust sequence until the foreign body is expelled, the infant begins to cough forcefully, or the infant loses consciousness.   ☐ ☐ _____

   a. If the foreign body is expelled, stay with the infant, and follow the nurse's directions.   ☐ ☐ _____

   b. If the infant begins to cough, wait and see if the coughing results in expulsion of the object. If it does not, continue giving five back blows followed by five chest thrusts.   ☐ ☐ _____

   c. If the infant loses consciousness, initiate the procedure described in Procedure 12-5, beginning with step 4.   ☐ ☐ _____

10. The infant should be evaluated by a doctor following the choking incident.   ☐ ☐ _____

11. Record your observations and actions according to facility policy.   ☐ ☐ _____

PROCEDURE 12-5
Clearing the Airway in an Unconscious Infant

	S	U	COMMENTS

1. Check the infant's responsiveness by gently shaking the infant and speaking to him. An unresponsive infant needs immediate help.   ☐ ☐ _____

2. Stay with the infant and call for help. Have the person who is helping you activate the emergency medical services (EMS) system.   ☐ ☐ _____

3. **Head tilt/chin lift maneuver.** Position the infant on his or her back on a hard, flat surface. Open the infant's airway by tilting the head back slightly and lifting the chin until the infant's nose points toward the ceiling. Look, feel, and listen for signs of breathing.   ☐ ☐ _____

4. **Rescue breathing.** If the infant is not breathing, keep his or her head tilted back and the chin lifted. Cover the infant's nose and mouth with your mouth or an airway device and blow two slow breaths into the infant's mouth, removing your mouth from the infant's nose and mouth and inhaling between each breath. If the air does not go in, repeat the head tilt/chin lift maneuver and attempt rescue breathing once again.   ☐ ☐ _____

5. If no air enters the infant's lungs after the second attempt, assume that the infant's airway is blocked.   ☐ ☐ _____

6. **Chest compressions**

   a. Place the infant on a flat surface.   ☐ ☐ _____

   b. Open his airway and look for a foreign object in his throat. If an object is visible, remove it using a "pincer"-type motion with your fingers.   ☐ ☐ _____

   c. Begin quick downward chest compressions by placing two fingers in the center of the infant's chest, just below the nipple line. Compress ½ inch deep with each compressions at a rate of 100 per minute for 30 compressions.   ☐ ☐ _____

7. **Foreign body check**

   a. After completing a cycle of 30 chest compressions, open the infant's airway and look for a foreign object.   ☐ ☐ _____

   b. If you see an object, remove it.   ☐ ☐ _____

8. Blow two slow breaths into the infant's nose and mouth, removing your nose and mouth from the infant's mouth and inhaling between each breath. If the air does not go in, repeat the head tilt/chin lift maneuver and attempt rescue breathing once again.   ☐ ☐ _____

9. Repeat steps 6 through 8 until the foreign body is expelled, rescue breathing is successful, or other trained personnel arrive and take over. ☐ ☐ _____

10. The infant should be evaluated by a doctor following the choking incident. ☐ ☐ _____

11. Record your observations and actions according to facility policy. ☐ ☐ _____

CHAPTER 15 PROCEDURE CHECKLISTS

PROCEDURE 15-1
Making an Unoccupied (Closed) Bed

	S	U	COMMENTS

Getting Ready

1. Complete the "Getting Ready" steps. ☐ ☐ _____

Procedure

2. Place the linens on a clean surface close to the bed (e.g., the over-bed table). ☐ ☐ _____

3. Make sure that the bed is positioned at a comfortable working height (to promote good body mechanics) and that the wheels are locked. ☐ ☐ _____

4. Lower the side rails and move the mattress to the head of the bed (it may have shifted toward the foot of the bed if the occupant of the bed had the head of the bed elevated). ☐ ☐ _____

   Note: The mattress pad, bottom sheet, and draw sheet are positioned and tucked in on one side of the bed before moving to the other side to complete these actions. This is most efficient in terms of energy and time. ☐ ☐ _____

5. Place the mattress pad on the bed and unfold it so that only one vertical crease remains. Make sure that this crease is centered on the mattress. If the mattress pad is fitted, carefully pull the corners of the near side over the corners of the mattress and smooth down the sides. If the mattress pad is flat, make sure the top of the pad is even with the head of the mattress. Open the mattress pad across the bed, taking care to keep it centered. ☐ ☐ _____

6. Place the bottom sheet on the bed. If the bottom sheet is fitted, carefully pull the corners of the near side over the corners of the mattress and smooth down the sides. If the bottom sheet is flat:

   a. Place the sheet so that when you unfold it, the wide hem will be at the head of the bed and the hem stitching will be against the mattress, away from the person who will be occupying the bed. ☐ ☐ _____

   b. Unfold the sheet so that only one vertical crease remains. Make sure that this crease is vertically centered on the mattress. ☐ ☐ _____

   c. Open the sheet across the bed, taking care to keep it centered. The same length of sheet (approximately 12 to 18 inches) should hang over each side of the bed. Make sure that the lower edge of the sheet is even with the foot of the mattress. ☐ ☐ _____

d. Tuck the sheet under the mattress at the head of the bed and miter the corner. ☐ ☐ _____

e. Tuck the near side of the sheet underneath the mattress, working from the head of the bed toward the foot. As you tuck, make sure there are no wrinkles in the sheet and that the mattress pad remains smooth and in place. ☐ ☐ _____

7. Place the lift sheet on the bed so that the top of the sheet is approximately 12 inches from the head of the mattress. If you are using a plastic or rubberized lift sheet, place a cotton lift sheet on top of it. Smooth the lift sheet across the bed and tuck the near side under the mattress. ☐ ☐ _____

8. Now, move to the other side of the bed and repeat the process of aligning the mattress pad, mitering the corner, and tucking in the bottom sheet and lift sheet. ☐ ☐ _____

9. Place the top sheet on the bed so that when you unfold it, the wide hem will be at the head of the bed and the hem stitching will be facing upward, away from the person who will be occupying the bed.

a. Unfold the sheet so that only one vertical crease remains. Make sure that this crease is centered vertically on the mattress. ☐ ☐ _____

b. Open the sheet across the bed, taking care to keep it centered. The same length of sheet (approximately 12 to 18 inches) should hang over each side of the bed. Make sure that the top edge of the sheet is even with the head of the mattress. Pull the bottom of the sheet over the foot of the bed, but do not tuck it in yet (it will be tucked in with the blanket and bedspread). ☐ ☐ _____

10. Place the blanket on the bed and unfold it in the same manner as the sheet, keeping the center crease in the center of the bed. The same length of blanket (approximately 12 to 18 inches) should hang over each side of the bed. Make sure that the top edge of the blanket is approximately 6 to 8 inches from the head of the mattress. Fold the top edge of the sheet back over the top edge of the blanket, creating a cuff. Pull the bottom edge of the blanket over the sheet at the foot of the bed, but do not tuck anything in yet. ☐ ☐ _____

11. Place the bedspread on the bed and unfold it in the same manner as the sheet, keeping the center crease in the center of the bed. The sides of the bedspread should be even and cover all of the other bed linens. Make sure that the top of the bedspread is even with the head of the mattress, unless the pillow is to be tucked under the bedspread (in which case you will need to allow more length at the top). Pull the bottom of the bedspread over the blanket and sheet at the foot of the bed. ☐ ☐ _____

12. Together, tuck the bedspread, the blanket, and the top sheet under the foot of the mattress. Make a mitered corner at the foot of the bed on both sides. ☐ ☐ _____

13. Fold the top of the bedspread back over the blanket to make a cuff. ☐ ☐ _____

14. Rest the pillow on the bed. Grasping the closed end of the pillowcase, turn the pillowcase inside out over your hand and arm. Grasp the pillow through the pillowcase and pull the pillowcase down over the pillow. Make sure any tags or zippers are on the inside of the pillowcase. ☐ ☐ _____

15. Place the pillow on the bed with the open end of the pillowcase facing away from the door. ☐ ☐ _____

Finishing Up

16. Complete the "Finishing Up" steps. ☐ ☐ _____

PROCEDURE 15-2
Making an Occupied Bed

	S	U	COMMENTS

Getting Ready

1. Complete the "Getting Ready" steps. ☐ ☐ _____

Procedure

2. Place the linens on a clean surface close to the bed (e.g., the over-bed table). ☐ ☐ _____

3. Make sure that the bed is positioned at a comfortable working height (to promote good body mechanics) and that the wheels are locked. Make sure to position the table holding the linens close enough to the bed that you do not have to step away from the bedside to reach it. ☐ ☐ _____

4. Remove the call-light control and check the bed for dentures or any other personal items. ☐ ☐ _____

5. Lower the head of the bed so that the bed is flat (as tolerated). ☐ ☐ _____

6. Put on the gloves (the linens may be wet or soiled). ☐ ☐ _____

7. Remove the bedspread and blanket from the bed. If they are to be reused, fold them and place them on a clean surface, such as a chair. ☐ ☐ _____

8. Loosen the top sheet at the foot of the bed and spread a bath blanket over the top sheet (and the person). ☐ ☐ _____

9. If the person is able, have her hold the bath blanket. If not, tuck the corners under the person's shoulders. Remove the top sheet by pulling it out from underneath the bath blanket, being careful not to expose the person. ☐ ☐ _____

10. Place the top sheet in the linen hamper or linen bag. ☐ ☐ _____

11. If the side rails are in use, lower the side rail on the working side of the bed. The side rail on the opposite side of the bed should remain up. Turn the person onto her side so that she is facing away from you. Reposition the pillow under the person's head, and adjust the bath blanket to keep the person covered. ☐ ☐ _____

12. Loosen the lift sheet, bottom sheet, and (if necessary) the mattress pad. ☐ ☐ _____

13. Fanfold the bottom linens toward the person's back, tucking them slightly underneath her. ☐ ☐ _____

14. Straighten the mattress pad (if it is not being changed). If the mattress pad is being changed, place the clean mattress pad on the bed and unfold it so that only one vertical crease remains. Make sure that this crease is centered vertically on the mattress. If the mattress pad is fitted, carefully pull the corners of the near side over the corners of the mattress and smooth down the sides. If the mattress pad is flat, make sure the top of the pad is even with the head of the mattress. Fanfold the opposite side of the mattress pad close to the patient or resident.   ☐ ☐ _____

15. Place the clean bottom sheet on the bed. If the bottom sheet is fitted, carefully pull the corners over the corners of the mattress and smooth down the sides. If the bottom sheet is flat:

   a. Place the sheet so that when you unfold it, the wide hem will be at the head of the bed and the hem stitching will be against the mattress, away from the person who will be occupying the bed.   ☐ ☐ _____

   b. Unfold the sheet so that only one vertical crease remains. Make sure that this crease is centered vertically on the mattress.   ☐ ☐ _____

   c. Open the sheet across the bed, taking care to keep it centered. The same length of sheet (approximately 12 to 18 inches) should hang over each side of the bed. Make sure that the lower edge of the sheet is even with the foot of the mattress. Fanfold the opposite side of the sheet close to the patient or resident.   ☐ ☐ _____

   d. Tuck the sheet under the mattress at the head of the bed and miter the corner.   ☐ ☐ _____

   e. Tuck the near side of the sheet underneath the mattress, working from the head of the bed toward the foot. As you tuck, make sure there are no wrinkles in the sheet and that the mattress pad remains smooth and in place.   ☐ ☐ _____

16. Place the lift sheet on the bed so that the top of the sheet is approximately 12 inches from the head of the mattress. If you are using a plastic or rubberized lift sheet, place a cotton lift sheet on top of it. Fanfold the opposite side of the lift sheet close to the patient or resident. Smooth the lift sheet across the bed and tuck the near side under the mattress.   ☐ ☐ _____

17. Raise the side rail on the working side of the bed. Help the person to roll toward you, over the folded linens. Reposition the pillow under the person's head and adjust the bath blanket to keep the person covered.   ☐ ☐ _____

18. Move to the other side of the bed and lower the side rail.   ☐ ☐ _____

19. Loosen and remove the soiled bottom linens and place them in the linen hamper or linen bag. Change your gloves if they become soiled.   ☐ ☐ _____

20. Now, repeat the process of aligning the mattress pad, mitering the corner, and tucking in the bottom sheet and lift sheet.

□ □ _____

21. Help the person to move to the center of the bed and position her comfortably. Raise the side rail on the working side of the bed.

□ □ _____

22. Change the pillowcase and place the pillow under the person's head.

□ □ _____

23. Place the clean top sheet over the person (who is still covered with the bath blanket), being careful not to cover her face. The sheet should be placed so that when you unfold it, the wide hem will be at the head of the bed and the hem stitching will be facing upward, away from the person who will be occupying the bed.

   a. Unfold the sheet so that only one vertical crease remains. Make sure that this crease is centered vertically on the mattress.

□ □ _____

   b. Open the sheet across the bed, taking care to keep it centered. The same length of sheet (approximately 12 to 18 inches) should hang over each side of the bed.

□ □ _____

   c. If the person is able, have her hold the top sheet. If not, tuck the corners under her shoulders. Remove the bath blanket by pulling it out from underneath the top sheet, being careful not to expose the person. Place the bath blanket in the linen hamper or linen bag.

□ □ _____

24. Place the blanket and then the bedspread over the top sheet. Together, tuck the bedspread, the blanket, and the top sheet under the foot of the mattress. Make a mitered corner at the foot of the bed on both sides.

□ □ _____

25. Make a toe pleat by grasping the top sheet, the blanket, and the bedspread over the person's feet and pulling the linens straight up. The toe pleat allows the person to move her feet and helps to relieve pressure on the feet from tightly tucked linens.

□ □ _____

26. Lower the bed to its lowest position and make sure that the wheels are locked. Raise the head of the bed as the person requests.

□ □ _____

27. Remove your gloves and dispose of them in a facility-approved waste container.

□ □ _____

Finishing Up

28. Complete the "Finishing Up" steps.

□ □ _____

CHAPTER 16 PROCEDURE CHECKLISTS

PROCEDURE 16-1
Measuring an Oral Temperature (Glass or Electronic Thermometer)

	S	U	COMMENTS

Getting Ready

1. Complete the "Getting Ready" steps. ☐ ☐ _____

Procedure

2. Ask the person if he or she has eaten, consumed a beverage, chewed gum, or smoked within the last 15 minutes. If so, wait 15 to 30 minutes before proceeding (or follow facility policy). ☐ ☐ _____

3. Prepare the thermometer.

   a. **Glass thermometer:** Run cool water over the thermometer to rinse away the disinfectant. Dry the thermometer with a paper towel and inspect it for cracks or chips. Carefully shake down the glass thermometer so that the indicator material is below the 94° mark (if using a Fahrenheit thermometer) or the 34° mark (if using a Celsius thermometer). Cover the end of the glass thermometer with the thermometer sheath. ☐ ☐ _____

   b. **Electronic thermometer:** Cover the electronic probe with the probe sheath. Turn the thermometer on and wait until the "ready" sign appears on the display screen. ☐ ☐ _____

4. Ask the person to open his or her mouth. Slowly and carefully insert the thermometer, placing the tip under the person's tongue and to one side. ☐ ☐ _____

5. Ask the person to gently close his or her mouth around the thermometer without biting down. If necessary, hold the thermometer in place. Ask the person to breathe through his or her nose. ☐ ☐ _____

6. Leave the thermometer in place for the specified amount of time:

   a. **Glass thermometer:** 3 to 5 minutes (or follow facility policy) ☐ ☐ _____

   b. **Electronic thermometer:** until the instrument blinks or beeps (usually just a few seconds) ☐ ☐ _____

7. Ask the person to open his or her mouth. Remove the thermometer from the person's mouth. ☐ ☐ _____

8. Read the temperature measurement.

   a. **Glass thermometer:** Using a tissue, remove the thermometer sheath from the glass thermometer, being careful not to touch the bulb end of the thermometer. Dispose of the tissue and the thermometer sheath in a facility-approved waste container. Hold the thermometer horizontally by the stem at eye level while facing a light source. Rotate the thermometer until you can see the level of the indicator material. Read the temperature.

   b. **Electronic thermometer:** Read the temperature on the electronic thermometer's display screen. Remove the probe sheath from the probe by pushing the button on the top of the probe. Direct the probe sheath into a facility-approved waste container.

9. Prepare the thermometer for its next use.

   a. **Glass thermometer:** Shake down the glass thermometer, clean it according to facility policy, and return it to its disinfectant-filled case.

   b. **Electronic thermometer:** Replace the probe into the electronic thermometer. (Always read the temperature before placing the probe in the instrument because this action clears the display screen.) Turn the instrument off if it does not automatically turn itself off. Place the thermometer in its charger.

Finishing Up

10. Complete the "Finishing Up" steps.

PROCEDURE 16-2

Measuring a Rectal Temperature
(Glass or Electronic Thermometer)

	S	U	COMMENTS

Getting Ready

1. Complete the "Getting Ready" steps. ☐ ☐ _____

Procedure

2. Make sure that the bed is positioned at a comfortable working height (to promote good body mechanics) and that the wheels are locked. ☐ ☐ _____

3. Prepare the thermometer.

   a. **Glass thermometer:** Run cool water over the thermometer to rinse away the disinfectant. Dry the thermometer with a paper towel and inspect it for cracks or chips. Carefully shake down the glass thermometer so that the indicator material is below the 94° mark (if using a Fahrenheit thermometer) or the 34° mark (if using a Celsius thermometer). Cover the end of the glass thermometer with the thermometer sheath. ☐ ☐ _____

   b. **Electronic thermometer:** Cover the electronic probe with the probe sheath. Turn the thermometer on and wait until the "ready" sign appears on the display screen. ☐ ☐ _____

4. Place the thermometer on a clean paper towel on the over-bed table. Open the lubricant package and squeeze a small amount of lubricant onto the paper towel. Lubricate the tip of the thermometer to ease insertion. ☐ ☐ _____

5. If the side rails are in use, lower the side rail on the working side of the bed. The side rail on the opposite side of the bed should remain up. Lower the head of the bed so that the bed is flat (as tolerated). ☐ ☐ _____

6. Ask the person to lie on his or her side, facing away from you, in Sims' position. Help the person into this position, if necessary. ☐ ☐ _____

7. Fanfold the top linens to below the person's buttocks. Adjust the person's hospital gown or pajama bottoms as necessary to expose the person's buttocks. ☐ ☐ _____

8. Put on the gloves. ☐ ☐ _____

9. With one hand, raise the person's upper buttock to expose the anus. Suggest that the person take a deep breath and slowly exhale as the thermometer is inserted. Using your other hand, gently and carefully insert the lubricated end of the thermometer into the person's rectum (not more than 1 inch for adults, or ½ inch for children). Never force the thermometer into the rectum. If you are unable to insert the thermometer, stop and call the nurse.   ☐ ☐ _____

10. Hold the thermometer in place for the specified amount of time:

    a. **Glass thermometer:** 3 to 5 minutes (or follow facility policy)   ☐ ☐ _____

    b. **Electronic thermometer:** until the instrument blinks or beeps (usually just a few seconds)   ☐ ☐ _____

11. Remove the thermometer from the person's rectum. Wipe the person's anal area with a tissue to remove the lubricant, and adjust the person's hospital gown or pajama bottoms as necessary to cover the buttocks.   ☐ ☐ _____

12. Read the temperature measurement.

    a. **Glass thermometer:** Using a tissue, remove the thermometer sheath from the glass thermometer, being careful not to touch the bulb end of the thermometer. Dispose of the tissue and the thermometer sheath in a facility-approved waste container. Hold the thermometer horizontally by the stem at eye level while facing a light source. Rotate the thermometer until you can see the level of the indicator material. Read the temperature.   ☐ ☐ _____

    b. **Electronic thermometer:** Read the temperature on the electronic thermometer's display screen. Remove the probe sheath from the probe by pushing the button on the top of the probe. Direct the probe sheath into a facility-approved waste container.   ☐ ☐ _____

13. Remove your gloves and dispose of them according to facility policy. Wash your hands.   ☐ ☐ _____

14. Help the person back into a comfortable position, straighten the bottom linens, and draw the top linens over the person. Raise the head of the bed, as the person requests.   ☐ ☐ _____

15. Make sure that the bed is lowered to its lowest position and that the wheels are locked. If the side rails are in use, return the side rails to the raised position.   ☐ ☐ _____

16. Prepare the thermometer for its next use.

   a. **Glass thermometer:** Shake down the glass thermometer, clean it according to facility policy, and return it to its disinfectant-filled case. ☐ ☐ _____

   b. **Electronic thermometer:** Replace the probe into the electronic thermometer. (Always read the temperature before placing the probe in the instrument because this action clears the display screen.) Turn the instrument off if it does not automatically turn itself off. Place the thermometer in its charger. ☐ ☐ _____

Finishing Up

17. Complete the "Finishing Up" steps. ☐ ☐ _____

PROCEDURE 16-3
Measuring an Axillary Temperature (Glass or Electronic Thermometer)

	S	U	COMMENTS

Getting Ready

1. Complete the "Getting Ready" steps.   ☐ ☐ _____

Procedure

2. Ask the person if he or she has bathed or applied deodorant or antiperspirant within the last 15 minutes. If so, wait 15 to 30 minutes before proceeding (or follow facility policy).   ☐ ☐ _____

3. Prepare the thermometer.
   a. **Glass thermometer:** Run cool water over the thermometer to rinse away the disinfectant. Dry the thermometer with a paper towel and inspect it for cracks or chips. Carefully shake down the glass thermometer so that the indicator material is below the 94° mark (if using a Fahrenheit thermometer) or the 34° mark (if using a Celsius thermometer). Cover the end of the glass thermometer with the thermometer sheath.   ☐ ☐ _____

   b. **Electronic thermometer:** Cover the electronic probe with the probe sheath. Turn the thermometer on and wait until the "ready" sign appears on the display screen.   ☐ ☐ _____

4. Assist the person with removing his or her arm from the sleeve of his or her hospital gown or pajama top.   ☐ ☐ _____

5. Pat the axilla (underarm area) gently with a paper towel.   ☐ ☐ _____

6. Ask the person to lift his or her arm slightly. Position the tip of the thermometer in the center of the axilla and ask the person to hold the thermometer in place by holding his or her arm close to the body (or by grasping the arm with the opposite hand).   ☐ ☐ _____

7. Leave the thermometer in place for the specified amount of time:
   a. **Glass thermometer:** 10 minutes (or follow facility policy)   ☐ ☐ _____

   b. **Electronic thermometer:** until the instrument blinks or beeps (usually just a few seconds)   ☐ ☐ _____

8. Ask the person to lift his or her arm slightly. Remove the thermometer.   ☐ ☐ _____

9. Read the temperature measurement.

   a. **Glass thermometer:** Using a tissue, remove the thermometer sheath from the glass thermometer, being careful not to touch the bulb end of the thermometer. Dispose of the tissue and the thermometer sheath in a facility-approved waste container. Hold the thermometer horizontally by the stem at eye level while facing a light source. Rotate the thermometer until you can see the level of the indicator material. Read the temperature. ☐ ☐ _____

   b. **Electronic thermometer:** Read the temperature on the electronic thermometer's display screen. Remove the probe sheath from the probe by pushing the button on the top of the probe. Direct the probe sheath into a facility-approved waste container. ☐ ☐ _____

10. Help the person back into his or her hospital gown or pajama top. ☐ ☐ _____

11. Prepare the thermometer for its next use:

    a. **Glass thermometer:** Shake down the glass thermometer, clean it according to facility policy, and return it to its disinfectant-filled case. ☐ ☐ _____

    b. **Electronic thermometer:** Replace the probe into the electronic thermometer. (Always read the temperature before placing the probe in the instrument because this action clears the display screen.) Turn the instrument off, if it does not automatically turn itself off. Place the thermometer in its charger. ☐ ☐ _____

Finishing Up

12. Complete the "Finishing Up" steps. ☐ ☐ _____

PROCEDURE 16-4

Measuring a Tympanic Temperature (Tympanic Thermometer)

	S	U	COMMENTS

Getting Ready

1. Complete the "Getting Ready" steps. ☐ ☐ _____

Procedure

2. If the person wears a hearing aid, remove it carefully and wait 2 minutes before taking the person's temperature. ☐ ☐ _____

3. Inspect the ear canal for excessive cerumen (ear wax). If you see excessive wax build-up in the ear canal, gently wipe the ear canal with a warm, moist washcloth. ☐ ☐ _____

4. Cover the cone-shaped end of the thermometer with the probe sheath. Turn the thermometer on and wait until the "ready" sign appears on the display screen. ☐ ☐ _____

5. Stand slightly to the front of, and facing, the person. To straighten the ear canal (which will ease insertion of the thermometer), grasp the top portion of the person's ear and gently pull:

   a. Up and back (in an adult) ☐ ☐ _____

   b. Straight back (in a child) ☐ ☐ _____

6. Insert the covered probe into the person's ear canal, pointing the probe down and toward the front of the ear canal (pretend that you are aiming for the person's nose). This will seal off the ear canal by seating the probe properly, leading to a more accurate temperature reading. ☐ ☐ _____

7. To take the temperature, press the button on the instrument. Keep the button depressed and the probe in place until the instrument blinks or beeps (usually 1 second). ☐ ☐ _____

8. Remove the probe and read the temperature on the display screen. ☐ ☐ _____

9. Remove the probe sheath from the probe by pushing the button on the side of the instrument. Direct the probe sheath into a facility-approved waste container. ☐ ☐ _____

10. If your facility requires a tympanic temperature to be taken in both ears, repeat the procedure, using a clean probe cover for the other ear. ☐ ☐ _____

11. Turn the instrument off if it does not automatically turn itself off. Place the thermometer in its charger. ☐ ☐ _____

Finishing Up

12. Complete the "Finishing Up" steps. ☐ ☐ _____

PROCEDURE 16-5
Taking a Radial Pulse

	S	U	COMMENTS

Getting Ready

1. Complete the "Getting Ready" steps. ☐ ☐ _____

Procedure

2. Rest the person's arm on the over-bed table or on the bed. Locate the radial pulse in the person's wrist using your middle two or three fingers. (TIP: The radial pulse will be on the person's "thumb" side.) ☐ ☐ _____

3. Note the strength and regularity of the pulse. Look at your watch and wait until the second hand gets to the "12" or "6." When the second hand reaches the "12" or the "6," begin counting the pulse.

   a. If the pulse rhythm is regular, count the number of pulses that occur in 30 seconds and multiply the result by 2 to arrive at the pulse rate. ☐ ☐ _____

   b. If the pulse rhythm is irregular, count the number of pulses that occur in 60 seconds. Counting each pulse that occurs over the course of 1 full minute is the only way to obtain a truly accurate pulse rate when the pulse is irregular. ☐ ☐ _____

Finishing Up

4. Complete the "Finishing Up" steps. ☐ ☐ _____

PROCEDURE 16-6
Taking an Apical Pulse

	S	U	COMMENTS

Getting Ready

1. Complete the "Getting Ready" steps. ☐ ☐ _____

Procedure

2. Help the person to a sitting position by raising the head of the bed. ☐ ☐ _____

3. Using alcohol wipes, clean the earpieces, the diaphragm, and the bell of the stethoscope. Place the earpieces in your ears. ☐ ☐ _____

4. Place the diaphragm (or the bell, if the person is a child or infant) of the stethoscope under the person's clothing, on the apical pulse site (located approximately 2 inches below the person's left nipple). The diaphragm or bell must be placed directly on the person's skin because clothing will distort the sound. ☐ ☐ _____

5. Using two fingers, hold the diaphragm or bell firmly against the person's chest. Look at your watch and wait until the second hand gets to the "12" or "6." When the second hand reaches the "12" or the "6," begin counting the heartbeat. ☐ ☐ _____

6. Count the number of heartbeats that occur in 60 seconds. Each time the heart beats, you will hear two sounds, best described as a "lubb" and a "dupp." Both sounds make up one beat of the heart and should be counted as such. ☐ ☐ _____

7. After 60 seconds, remove the diaphragm of the stethoscope from the person's chest. Adjust the person's clothing as necessary and help the person back into a comfortable position. Lower the head of the bed, as the person requests. ☐ ☐ _____

8. Using alcohol wipes, clean the earpieces, the diaphragm, and the bell of the stethoscope. ☐ ☐ _____

Finishing Up

9. Complete the "Finishing Up" steps. ☐ ☐ _____

PROCEDURE 16-7
Counting Respirations

	S	U	COMMENTS

Getting Ready

1. Complete the "Getting Ready" steps.   ☐ ☐ _____

Procedure

2. Look at your watch and wait until the second hand
   gets to the "12" or "6." When the second hand
   reaches the "12" or the "6," look at the person's
   chest (or place your hand near the person's
   collarbone or on his or her side) and begin counting
   each rise and fall of the chest as one breath.

   a. If the respiratory rhythm is regular, count the   ☐ ☐ _____
      number of breaths that occur in 30 seconds and
      multiply the result by 2 to arrive at the respiratory
      rate.

   b. If the respiratory rhythm is irregular, count the   ☐ ☐ _____
      number of breaths that occur in 60 seconds.
      Counting each respiration that occurs over the
      course of 1 full minute is the only way to obtain a
      truly accurate respiratory rate when the person's
      breathing is irregular.

Finishing Up

3. Complete the "Finishing Up" steps.   ☐ ☐ _____

PROCEDURE 16-8
Measuring Blood Pressure

	S	U	COMMENTS

Getting Ready

1. Complete the "Getting Ready" steps.

Procedure

2. Assist the person into a sitting or lying position. Position the person's arm so that the forearm is level with the heart and the palm of the hand is facing upward. Assist the person with rolling up his or her sleeve so that the upper arm is exposed.

3. Using alcohol wipes, clean the earpieces, the diaphragm, and the bell of the stethoscope.

4. Stand no more than 3 feet away from the manometer. If it is not mounted on the wall, stand a mercury manometer upright on a flat surface, at eye level. Lay an aneroid manometer on a flat surface directly in front of you or leave it attached to the blood pressure cuff.

5. Squeeze the cuff to empty it of any remaining air. Turn the valve on the bulb clockwise to close it; this will cause the cuff to inflate when you pump the bulb.

6. Locate the person's brachial artery in the antecubital space by placing your fingers at the inner aspect of the elbow.

7. Place the arrow mark on the cuff over the brachial artery. Wrap the cuff around the person's upper arm so that the bottom of the cuff is at least 1 inch above the person's elbow. The cuff must be even and snug.

8. Place the stethoscope earpieces in your ears.

9. Pump the bulb until the pressure in the cuff is 30 mm Hg higher than the systolic pressure. There are two ways to do this:

   Method "A." Hold the bulb in one hand and position the diaphragm of the stethoscope over the brachial artery with the other hand. Inflate the cuff until you hear the pulse stop and then inflate the cuff 30 mm Hg more.

   Method "B." Hold the bulb in one hand and feel for the person's radial pulse (in his or her wrist) with the other hand. Inflate the cuff until you are no longer able to feel the radial pulse and then inflate the cuff 30 mm Hg more.

10. Position the diaphragm of the stethoscope over the brachial artery (or continue to hold it there if you used method "A" to inflate the cuff).

11. Turn the valve on the bulb slightly counterclockwise to allow air to escape from the cuff slowly. ☐ ☐ _____

12. Note the reading on the manometer where the first Korotkoff sound is heard. This is the systolic reading. ☐ ☐ _____

13. Continue to deflate the cuff. Note the reading on the manometer where the last Korotkoff sound is heard. This is the diastolic reading. ☐ ☐ _____

14. Deflate the cuff completely and remove it from the person's arm. Remove the stethoscope from your ears. ☐ ☐ _____

15. Return the sphygmomanometer to its case or wall holder. ☐ ☐ _____

16. Using alcohol wipes, clean the earpieces, the diaphragm, and the bell of the stethoscope. ☐ ☐ _____

Finishing Up

17. Complete the "Finishing Up" steps. ☐ ☐ _____

PROCEDURE 16-9
Measuring Height and Weight Using an Upright Scale

	S	U	COMMENTS

Getting Ready

1. Complete the "Getting Ready" steps. ☐ ☐ _____

Procedure

2. Ask the person to urinate. If necessary, assist the person to the bathroom or offer the bedpan or urinal. ☐ ☐ _____

3. Move the weights all the way to the left of the balance bar. ☐ ☐ _____

4. Help the person onto the scale platform so that she is facing the balance bar. Once the person is on the scale platform, do not allow her to hold on to you or to the scale. ☐ ☐ _____

5. Move the large weight on the lower scale bar to the right to the weight closest to the person's prior weight. For example, if the person weighed 155 pounds the last time you weighed her, you would move the large weight to the "150" mark. ☐ ☐ _____

6. Move the small weight on the upper scale bar to the right until the balance pointer is centered between the two scale bars. ☐ ☐ _____

7. Read the numbers on the upper and the lower scale bars where each weight has settled and add these two numbers together. This is the person's weight. ☐ ☐ _____

8. Have the person carefully turn around to face away from the scale bar. Slide the height scale up so that you can pull out the height rod, which extends from the top of the height scale. Be careful not to hit the person in the head with the height rod. ☐ ☐ _____

9. Slide the height rod down so that it lightly touches the top of the person's head. Read the number at the point where the height rod meets the height scale. This is the person's height. ☐ ☐ _____

10. Hold the height rod in your hand, and help the person step down from the scale. ☐ ☐ _____

11. Assist the person back to her room. ☐ ☐ _____

Finishing Up

12. Complete the "Finishing Up" steps. ☐ ☐ _____

PROCEDURE 16-10
Measuring Weight Using a Chair Scale

	S	U	COMMENTS

Getting Ready

1. Complete the "Getting Ready" steps. □ □ _____

Procedure

2. Ask the person to urinate. If necessary, assist the person to the bathroom or offer the bedpan or urinal. □ □ _____

3. Assist or wheel the person to the scale, using a transfer belt, a wheelchair, or both. □ □ _____

4. Reset the scale to "0" by turning it on. □ □ _____

5. Help the person onto the scale.

   a. If a regular chair scale is being used, help the person to sit in the chair on the scale. Make sure the person is seated properly, with his or her buttocks against the back of the chair and feet on the footrests. □ □ _____

   b. If a wheelchair scale is being used, roll the occupied wheelchair onto the platform and lock the wheels. □ □ _____

6. Read the weight on the display screen. If a wheelchair scale is being used, you must subtract the weight of the unoccupied wheelchair from this figure to determine the person's weight. □ □ _____

7. Help the person off of the scale.

   a. If a regular chair scale is being used, assist the person out of the chair and back into a wheelchair if one was used for the transfer. □ □ _____

   b. If a wheelchair scale is being used, unlock the wheels and roll the wheelchair off the platform. □ □ _____

8. Assist the person back to his or her room. □ □ _____

Finishing Up

9. Complete the "Finishing Up" steps. □ □ _____

PROCEDURE 16-11

Measuring Height and Weight Using a Tape Measure and a Sling Scale

	S	U	COMMENTS

Getting Ready

1. Complete the "Getting Ready" steps. ☐ ☐ _____

Procedure

2. Ask the person to urinate. If necessary, assist the person to the bathroom or offer the bedpan or urinal. ☐ ☐ _____

3. Position the sling scale next to the bed. Make sure that the bed is positioned at a comfortable working height (to promote good body mechanics) and that the wheels are locked. If the side rails are in use, lower the side rail on the working side of the bed. The side rail on the opposite side of the bed should remain up. ☐ ☐ _____

4. Fanfold the top linens to the foot of the bed. ☐ ☐ _____

5. Center the sling under the person. (To get the sling under the person, move the person as if you were making an occupied bed. see procedure 15-2) ☐ ☐ _____

6. Position the person in the supine position, or according to the manufacturer's instructions. ☐ ☐ _____

7. Move the release valve on the sling scale to the closed position. ☐ ☐ _____

8. Raise the sling scale so that it can be positioned over the person. ☐ ☐ _____

9. Spread the legs of the sling scale to provide a solid base of support. The legs must be locked in this position, or the scale could tip over, injuring you, the person you are trying to weigh, or both. ☐ ☐ _____

10. Move the scale into position over the person. ☐ ☐ _____

11. Fasten the sling to the straps or chains of the scale. Make sure the hooks face away from the person. ☐ ☐ _____

12. Cross the person's arms over her chest. ☐ ☐ _____

13. Slowly raise the sling until the person is clear of the bed. ☐ ☐ _____

14. Read the weight on the display screen. ☐ ☐ _____

15. Gently lower the person to the bed and remove the sling by gently rolling the person first to one side, then the other. ☐ ☐ _____

16. Position the person in the supine position, with her arms by her sides and her legs straight. ☐ ☐ _____

17. Using a pencil, make a small mark on the bottom sheet at the top of the person's head. Make another small mark at her heels. ☐ ☐ _____

18. Using the tape measure, measure the distance between the pencil marks. This is the person's height. ☐ ☐ _____

19. Make sure that the bed is lowered to its lowest position and that the wheels are locked. If the side rails are in use, return the side rails to the raised position. ☐ ☐ _____

Finishing Up

20. Complete the "Finishing Up" steps. ☐ ☐ _____

CHAPTER 17 PROCEDURE CHECKLISTS

PROCEDURE 17-1
Giving a Moist Cold Application

Getting Ready	S	U	COMMENTS
1. Complete the "Getting Ready" steps.	☐	☐	_____

Procedure

	S	U	COMMENTS
2. Check the pad for leaks. Make sure that the cord is not frayed and the plug is in good condition. Check the heating unit to be sure that it is filled with water. If you need to fill it, use distilled water. Tap water contains minerals that can corrode the unit.	☐	☐	_____
3. Place the heating unit so that the tubing and pad are level with the heating unit at all times. Make sure that the tubing is free of kinks. Plug the cord into an outlet.	☐	☐	_____
4. Allow the water to warm to the desired temperature, as specified by the nurse or the care plan. If the temperature is not preset, set the temperature with the key and then remove the key.	☐	☐	_____
5. Place the pad in its cover.	☐	☐	_____
6. Make sure that the bed is positioned at a comfortable working height (to promote good body mechanics) and that the wheels are locked.	☐	☐	_____
7. Help the person to a comfortable position and expose only the area to be treated.	☐	☐	_____
8. Apply the pad to the treatment site.	☐	☐	_____
9. Leave the pad in place for the designated amount of time, usually 15 to 20 minutes. The pad may be secured in place with ties or tape, or the resident may assist by holding the pad in place. (Do not use pins to secure the pad. Pins can puncture the pad, causing it to leak.)			
a. Check the skin beneath the pad every 5 minutes. If the skin appears red, swollen, or blistered or if the person complains of pain, numbness, or discomfort, discontinue treatment immediately and notify the nurse.	☐	☐	_____
b. Refill the heating unit if the water level drops below the fill line.	☐	☐	_____
c. If you must leave the room, place the call light control within easy reach and ask the person to signal if he or she experiences numbness or burning.	☐	☐	_____
10. When the treatment is complete, remove the pad.	☐	☐	_____

11. Straighten the bed linens and make sure the person is comfortable and in good body alignment. Draw the top linens over the person. ☐ ☐ _____

12. Make sure that the bed is lowered to its lowest position and that the wheels are locked. ☐ ☐ _____

13. Gather the soiled linens and place them in the linen hamper. Dispose of disposable items in a facility-approved waste container. Clean equipment and return it to the storage area. ☐ ☐ _____

Finishing Up

14. Complete the "Finishing Up" steps. ☐ ☐ _____

PROCEDURE 17-2
Giving a Dry Cold Application

	S	U	COMMENTS

Getting Ready

1. Complete the "Getting Ready" steps. ☐ ☐ _____

Procedure

2. Put the ice in the bath basin and fill the basin with cold water at the sink. ☐ ☐ _____

3. Make sure that the bed is positioned at a comfortable working height (to promote good body mechanics) and that the wheels are locked. ☐ ☐ _____

4. Help the person to a comfortable position and expose only the area to be treated. ☐ ☐ _____

5. Position the bed protector as necessary to keep the bed linens dry. ☐ ☐ _____

6. Moisten the compress with the ice water as ordered. Wring out the compress and apply it to the treatment site. ☐ ☐ _____

7. Leave the compress in place for the designated amount of time, usually 15 to 20 minutes. The compress may be secured in place with ties or rolled gauze, or the patient or resident may assist by holding the compress in place.

   a. Keep the compress moistened with ice water. ☐ ☐ _____

   b. Check the skin beneath the compress every 10 minutes. If the skin appears pale or blue or if the person complains of numbness or a burning sensation, discontinue treatment immediately and notify the nurse. ☐ ☐

   c. If you must leave the room, place the call light control within easy reach and ask the person to signal if he or she experiences numbness or burning. ☐ ☐ _____

8. When the treatment is complete, remove the compress and carefully dry the skin. ☐ ☐ _____

9. Remove the bed protector. Straighten the bed linens and make sure the person is comfortable and in good body alignment. Draw the top linens over the person. ☐ ☐ _____

10. Make sure that the bed is lowered to its lowest position and that the wheels are locked. ☐ ☐ _____

11. Gather the soiled linens and place them in the linen hamper. Dispose of disposable items in a facility-approved waste container. Clean equipment and return it to the storage area. ☐ ☐ _____

Finishing Up

12. Complete the "Finishing Up" steps. ☐ ☐ _____

PROCEDURE 17-3
Giving a Dry Heat Application With an Aquamatic Pad

	S	U	COMMENTS

Getting Ready

1. Complete the "Getting Ready" steps. ☐ ☐ _____

Procedure

2. Fill the ice bag with water, close it, and turn it upside down to check for leaks. Empty the bag. ☐ ☐ _____

3. Fill the bag one-half to two-thirds full with crushed ice. Do not overfill the ice bag. Squeeze the bag to force out excess air and close the bag. ☐ ☐ _____

4. Dry the outside of the bag with the paper towels and wrap it in the towel. ☐ ☐ _____

5. Make sure that the bed is positioned at a comfortable working height (to promote good body mechanics) and that the wheels are locked. ☐ ☐ _____

6. Help the person to a comfortable position and expose only the area to be treated. ☐ ☐ _____

7. Apply the ice bag to the treatment site. ☐ ☐ _____

8. Leave the compress in place for the designated amount of time, usually 15 to 20 minutes. The compress may be secured in place with ties or rolled gauze, or the resident may assist by holding the compress in place.

   a. Check the skin beneath the ice bag every 10 minutes. If the skin appears pale or blue or if the person complains of numbness or a burning sensation, discontinue treatment immediately and notify the nurse. ☐ ☐ _____

   b. Refill the bag with ice as necessary. ☐ ☐ _____

   c. If you must leave the room, place the call light control within easy reach and ask the person to signal if he or she experiences numbness or burning. ☐ ☐ _____

9. When the treatment is complete, remove the ice bag. ☐ ☐ _____

10. Straighten the bed linens and make sure the person is comfortable and in good body alignment. Draw the top linens over the person. ☐ ☐ _____

11. Make sure that the bed is lowered to its lowest position and that the wheels are locked. ☐ ☐ _____

12. Gather the soiled linens and place them in the linen hamper. Dispose of disposable items in a facility-approved waste container. Clean equipment and return it to the storage area. ☐ ☐ _____

Finishing Up

13. Complete the "Finishing Up" steps. ☐ ☐ _____

CHAPTER 18 PROCEDURE CHECKLISTS

PROCEDURE 18-1
Brushing and Flossing the Teeth

	S	U	COMMENTS

Getting Ready

1. Complete the "Getting Ready" steps. ☐ ☐ _____

Procedure

2. Cover the over-bed table with paper towels. Place the oral care supplies on the over-bed table. Fill a paper cup with water. ☐ ☐ _____

3. Make sure that the bed is positioned at a comfortable working height (to promote good body mechanics) and that the wheels are locked. ☐ ☐ _____

4. If the side rails are in use, lower the side rail on the working side of the bed. The side rail on the opposite side of the bed should remain up. ☐ ☐ _____

5. Raise the head of the bed as tolerated. Place a towel under the person's chin. ☐ ☐ _____

6. Put on the gloves. ☐ ☐ _____

7. Wet the toothbrush. Put a small amount of toothpaste on the toothbrush. ☐ ☐ _____

8. Brush the person's teeth as follows:

   a. Position the toothbrush at a 45° angle to the gums, against the outer surface of the top teeth. Starting at the back of the mouth, brush the outer surface of each tooth using a gentle circular motion. Repeat for the lower teeth. Allow the person to spit toothpaste into the emesis basin as necessary. ☐ ☐ _____

   b. Position the toothbrush at a 45° angle to the gums, against the inner surface of the top teeth. Starting at the back of the mouth, brush the inner surface of each tooth using a gentle circular motion. Repeat for the lower teeth. ☐ ☐ _____

   c. Brush the chewing surfaces of the upper and lower teeth using a gentle circular motion. ☐ ☐ _____

   d. Brush the tongue. ☐ ☐ _____

9. Offer the person the cup of water (and a straw, if desired) and ask her to rinse her mouth completely. Hold the emesis basin underneath the person's chin so that she can spit the water into the basin. ☐ ☐ _____

10. Place the emesis basin on the over-bed table and dry the person's mouth and chin thoroughly using a towel. ☐ ☐ _____

11. Cut a piece of dental floss measuring about 18 inches. Wrap the dental floss around the middle finger of each hand. Hold the dental floss between your thumb and index finger on each hand and stretch it tight. ☐ ☐ _____

12. Insert a segment of dental floss between two teeth, starting with the back upper teeth. Move the floss up and down gently, and then remove the dental floss from the person's mouth. Advance the floss a bit by releasing it from one middle finger and wrapping it around the other, and move on to the next two teeth. Use a new strand of dental floss as necessary. Offer the person the glass of water (and the straw, if desired) to rinse as necessary. Floss all of the person's teeth. ☐ ☐ _____

13. Offer the person the cup of water (and the straw, if desired) and ask her to rinse her mouth completely. Hold the emesis basin underneath the person's chin so that she can spit the water into the basin. ☐ ☐ _____

14. Place the emesis basin on the over-bed table and dry the person's mouth and chin thoroughly using a towel. ☐ ☐ _____

15. Pour a small amount of mouthwash (approximately ¼ cup) into another paper cup and help the person to rinse, as the person requests. ☐ ☐ _____

16. Apply lip lubricant to the lips, as the person requests. ☐ ☐ _____

17. If the side rails are in use, return the side rails to the raised position. Lower the head of the bed as the person requests. Make sure that the bed is lowered to its lowest position and that the wheels are locked. ☐ ☐ _____

18. Gather the soiled linens and place them in the linen hamper or linen bag. Dispose of disposable items in a facility-approved waste container. Clean equipment and return it to the storage area. ☐ ☐ _____

19. Remove your gloves and dispose of them in a facility-approved waste container. ☐ ☐ _____

Finishing Up

20. Complete the "Finishing Up" steps. ☐ ☐ _____

PROCEDURE 18-2
Providing Oral Care for a Person With Dentures

	S	U	COMMENTS

Getting Ready

1. Complete the "Getting Ready" steps.   ☐ ☐ _____

Procedure

2. Cover the over-bed table with paper towels. Place the oral care supplies on the over-bed table. Fill a paper cup with water.   ☐ ☐ _____

3. Make sure that the bed is positioned at a comfortable working height (to promote good body mechanics) and that the wheels are locked. Raise the head of the bed as tolerated. Place a towel under the person's chin.   ☐ ☐ _____

4. Put on the gloves.   ☐ ☐ _____

5. Ask the person to remove his dentures and place them in the emesis basin. If the person needs assistance with removing his dentures:

   a. Ask the person to open his mouth.   ☐ ☐ _____

   b. Holding a gauze square between your thumb and index finger, grasp the upper denture, moving it up and down slightly to break the seal. Ease the denture down, forward, and out of the mouth. Place the denture in the emesis basin.   ☐ ☐ _____

   c. Holding a gauze square between your thumb and index finger, grasp the lower denture. Turn the denture slightly, lifting it out of the mouth. Place the denture in the emesis basin.   ☐ ☐ _____

6. Take the emesis basin, the washcloth, the denture cup, the denture brush or toothbrush, and the denture cleaner or toothpaste to the sink. Line the sink with the washcloth to provide extra cushioning. Fill the sink partially with lukewarm water. Do not place the dentures in the sink.   ☐ ☐ _____

7. Wet the denture brush or the toothbrush. Put a small amount of toothpaste or denture cleaner on the denture brush or toothbrush. Working with one denture at a time, hold the denture in the palm of your hand and brush it on all surfaces until it is clean. Rinse the denture thoroughly under lukewarm running water and place it in the denture cup. Repeat with the other denture.   ☐ ☐ _____

8. If the dentures are to be stored, fill the denture cup with lukewarm water, a mixture of one part mouthwash to one part lukewarm water, or a denture solution so that the dentures are covered. Put the lid on the denture cup. Return the denture cup to the person's bedside table, making sure that it is within easy reach.   ☐ ☐ _____

9. If the dentures are to be reinserted in the person's mouth, take the emesis basin, the denture cup, and the toothbrush to the over-bed table. If the side rails are in use, lower the side rail on the working side of the bed. The side rail on the opposite side of the bed should remain up.

   a. Offer the person the cup of water (and a straw, if desired) and ask him to rinse his mouth completely. Some people may wish to use mouthwash instead of water. Hold the emesis basin underneath the person's chin so that he can spit the water or mouthwash into the basin.

     ☐ ☐ _____

   b. Place the emesis basin on the over-bed table and dry the person's mouth and chin thoroughly using a face towel.

     ☐ ☐ _____

   c. Gently clean the person's gums and tongue and the insides of the cheeks with the toothbrush or a foam-tipped applicator moistened with water or mouthwash. Use fresh applicators as needed.

     ☐ ☐ _____

   d. Ask the person to insert his dentures. If the person needs assistance with inserting his dentures:

     ☐ ☐ _____

   - Ask the person to open his mouth.
   - Gently lift the person's upper lip up. Grasp the upper denture between your thumb and index finger and insert it in the person's mouth. Press gently on the denture to be sure that it is seated properly.
   - Gently pull the person's lower lip down. Grasp the lower denture between your thumb and index finger and insert it in the person's mouth.

   e. Return the denture cup to the person's bedside table, making sure that it is within easy reach.

     ☐ ☐ _____

10. Dry the person's mouth and chin thoroughly using a towel. Apply lip lubricant to the lips, as the person requests.

      ☐ ☐ _____

11. Reposition the person comfortably and lower the head of the bed if necessary. If the side rails are in use, return the side rails to the raised position. Make sure that the bed is lowered to its lowest position and that the wheels are locked.

      ☐ ☐ _____

12. Gather the soiled linens and place them in the linen hamper or linen bag. Dispose of disposable items in a facility-approved waste container. Clean equipment and return it to the storage area.

      ☐ ☐ _____

13. Remove your gloves and dispose of them in a facility-
approved waste container.
☐ ☐ _____

Finishing Up

14. Complete the "Finishing Up" steps.
☐ ☐ _____

PROCEDURE 18-3
Providing Oral Care for an Unconscious Person

	S	U	COMMENTS

Getting Ready

1. Complete the "Getting Ready" steps. ☐ ☐ _____

Procedure

2. Cover the over-bed table with paper towels. Place the oral care supplies on the over-bed table. Fill the paper cup with water. ☐ ☐ _____

3. Make sure that the bed is positioned at a comfortable working height (to promote good body mechanics) and that the wheels are locked. If the side rails are in use, lower the side rail on the working side of the bed. The side rail on the opposite side of the bed should remain up. ☐ ☐ _____

4. Raise the head of the bed as tolerated. Turn the person's head to the side facing you. If it is difficult to keep the person's head turned to the side, roll the person onto his or her side. ☐ ☐ _____

5. If the person's condition permits, gently lift the person's head and place a towel on the pillow. Place the emesis basin on the towel, level with the person's chin. ☐ ☐ _____

6. Put on the gloves. ☐ ☐ _____

7. Open the person's mouth using the padded tongue blade. Be gentle; do not force the mouth open. Insert the tongue blade between the upper and lower teeth at the back of the mouth to hold the person's mouth open. ☐ ☐ _____

8. Clean the inside of the mouth:

   a. If the person has natural teeth, they should be gently brushed as described in Procedure 18-1. ☐ ☐ _____

   b. If the person is edentulous, gently clean the person's gums and tongue and the insides of the cheeks with the toothbrush or a foam-tipped applicator moistened with water, saline, or mouthwash. Use fresh applicators as needed. ☐ ☐ _____

9. Dry the person's mouth and chin thoroughly using a towel. Apply lip lubricant to the lips. Reposition the person comfortably. ☐ ☐ _____

10. If the side rails are in use, return the side rails to the raised position. Lower the head of the bed. Make sure that the bed is lowered to its lowest position and that the wheels are locked. ☐ ☐ _____

11. Gather the soiled linens and place them in the linen hamper or linen bag. Dispose of disposable items in a facility-approved waste container. Clean equipment and return it to the storage area.

☐ ☐ _____

12. Remove your gloves and dispose of them in a facility-approved waste container.

☐ ☐ _____

Finishing Up

13. Complete the "Finishing Up" steps.

☐ ☐ _____

PROCEDURE 18-4
Providing Female Perineal Care

	S	U	COMMENTS

Getting Ready

1. Complete the "Getting Ready" steps. ☐ ☐ _____

Procedure

2. Cover the over-bed table with paper towels. Place the wash basin, toiletries, clean clothing, and clean linens on the over-bed table. ☐ ☐ _____

3. Make sure that the bed is positioned at a comfortable working height (to promote good body mechanics) and that the wheels are locked. ☐ ☐ _____

4. Put on the gloves. ☐ ☐ _____

5. Because bathing often stimulates the urge to urinate, offer the bedpan. If the person uses the bedpan, empty and clean it before proceeding with the perineal care. Remove your gloves and dispose of them in a facility-approved waste container. Wash your hands and put on a clean pair of gloves. ☐ ☐ _____

6. Lower the head of the bed to a flat position (as tolerated). ☐ ☐ _____

7. Fill the wash basin with warm water [110°F (43.3°C) to 115°F (46.1°C) on the bath thermometer]. Place the basin on the over-bed table. ☐ ☐ _____

8. If the side rails are in use, lower the side rail on the working side. The side rail on the opposite side of the bed should remain up. ☐ ☐ _____

9. Spread the bath blanket over the top linens (and the person). If the person is able, have her hold the bath blanket. If not, tuck the corners under the person's shoulders. Fanfold the top linens to the foot of the bed. ☐ ☐ _____

10. Assist the person with undressing. ☐ ☐ _____

11. Ask the person to open her legs and bend her knees, if possible. If she is not able to bend her knees, help her spread her legs as much as possible. ☐ ☐ _____

12. Position the bath blanket over the person so that one corner can be wrapped under and around each leg. ☐ ☐ _____

13. Position the bed protector under the person's buttocks to keep the bed linens dry. ☐ ☐ _____

14. Lift the corner of the bath blanket that is between the person's legs upward, exposing only the perineal area. ☐ ☐ _____

15. Form a mitt around your hand with one of the washcloths. Wet the mitt with warm, clean water and apply soap. ☐ ☐ _____

16. Using the other hand, separate the labia. Clean the vulva by placing your washcloth-covered hand at the top of the vulva and stroking downward to the anus. Use a different part of the washcloth for each stroke. Repeat until the area is clean. ☐ ☐ _____

17. Rinse the vulva and perineum thoroughly: ☐ ☐ _____

   Form a mitt around your hand with a clean, wet washcloth. Using the other hand, separate the labia. Rinse the vulva by placing your washcloth-covered hand at the top of the vulva and stroking downward to the anus. Use a different part of the washcloth for each stroke. Repeat until the area is free of soap.

18. Dry the perineal area thoroughly using a towel. ☐ ☐ _____

19. Turn the person onto her side so that she is facing away from you. Help the person toward the working side of the bed so that her buttocks are within easy reach. Adjust the bath blanket to keep the person covered. ☐ ☐ _____

20. Form a mitt around your hand with one of the washcloths. Wet the mitt with warm, clean water and apply soap. ☐ ☐ _____

21. Using the other hand, separate the buttocks. Place your washcloth-covered hand at the front of the body and stroke toward the back. First clean one side, then the other side, and finally the middle, using a different part of the washcloth each time, until the anal area is clean. ☐ ☐ _____

22. Rinse and dry the anal area thoroughly. Remove the bed protector from underneath the person. ☐ ☐ _____

23. Remove your gloves and dispose of them in a facility-approved waste container. Put on a clean pair of gloves. ☐ ☐ _____

24. Assist the person into the supine position. Reposition the pillow under her head. Remove the bath blanket and help the person into the clean clothing. ☐ ☐ _____

25. If the bedding is wet or soiled, change the bed linens. ☐ ☐ _____

26. If the side rails are in use, return the side rail to the raised position. Raise the head of the bed as the person requests. Make sure that the bed is lowered to its lowest position and that the wheels are locked. ☐ ☐ _____

27. Gather the soiled linens and place them in the linen hamper or linen bag. Dispose of disposable items in a facility-approved waste container. Clean equipment and return it to the storage area. ☐ ☐ _____

28. Remove your gloves and dispose of them in a facility-approved waste container. ☐ ☐ _____

Finishing Up

29. Complete the "Finishing Up" steps. ☐ ☐ _____

PROCEDURE 18-5
Providing Male Perineal Care

	S	U	COMMENTS

Getting Ready

1. Complete the "Getting Ready" steps. ☐ ☐ _____

Procedure

2. Cover the over-bed table with paper towels. Place the wash basin, toiletries, clean clothing, and clean linens on the over-bed table. ☐ ☐ _____

3. Make sure that the bed is positioned at a comfortable working height (to promote good body mechanics) and that the wheels are locked. ☐ ☐ _____

4. Put on the gloves. ☐ ☐ _____

5. Because bathing often stimulates the urge to urinate, offer the bedpan or urinal. If the person uses the bedpan or urinal, empty and clean it before proceeding with the perineal care. Remove your gloves and dispose of them in a facility-approved waste container. Wash your hands and put on a clean pair of gloves. ☐ ☐

6. Lower the head of the bed to a flat position (as tolerated). ☐ ☐ _____

7. Fill the wash basin with warm water [110°F (43.3°C) to 115°F (46.1°C) on the bath thermometer]. Place the basin on the over-bed table. ☐ ☐ _____

8. If the side rails are in use, lower the side rail on the working side. The side rail on the opposite side of the bed should remain up. ☐ ☐ _____

9. Spread the bath blanket over the top linens (and the person). If the person is able, have him hold the bath blanket. If not, tuck the corners under the person's shoulders. Fanfold the top linens to the foot of the bed. ☐ ☐ _____

10. Assist the person with undressing. ☐ ☐ _____

11. Ask the person to open his legs and bend his knees, if possible. If he is not able to bend his knees, help him spread his legs as much as possible. ☐ ☐ _____

12. Position the bath blanket over the person so that one corner can be wrapped under and around each leg. ☐ ☐ _____

13. Position the bed protector under the person's buttocks to keep the bed linens dry. ☐ ☐ _____

14. Lift the corner of the bath blanket that is between the person's legs upward, exposing only the perineal area. ☐ ☐ _____

15. Form a mitt around your hand with one of the washcloths. Wet the mitt with warm, clean water and apply soap. ☐ ☐ _____

16. Using the other hand, hold the penis slightly away from the body.

    a. If the person is circumcised: Place your washcloth-covered hand at the tip of the penis and wash in a circular motion, downward to the base of the penis. Repeat, using a different part of the washcloth each time, until the area is clean. Rinse and dry the tip and the shaft of the penis thoroughly: ☐ ☐ _____

       Form a mitt around your hand with a clean, wet washcloth. Using the other hand, hold the penis slightly away from the body. Place your washcloth-covered hand at the tip of the penis and wipe in a circular motion, downward to the base of the penis. Repeat, using a different part of the washcloth each time, until the area is rinsed. Dry the penis thoroughly.

    b. If the person is uncircumcised: Retract the foreskin by gently pushing the skin toward the base of the penis. Place your washcloth-covered hand at the tip of the penis and wash in a circular motion, downward to the base of the penis. Repeat using a different part of the washcloth each time until the area is clean. Rinse and dry the tip and shaft of the penis thoroughly before gently pulling the foreskin back into its normal position. ☐ ☐ _____

17. Form a mitt around your hand with one of the washcloths. Wet the mitt with warm, clean water and apply soap. Wash the scrotum and perineum. Rinse and dry the scrotum and perineum thoroughly. ☐ ☐ _____

18. Turn the person onto his side so that he is facing away from you. Help the person toward the working side of the bed so that his buttocks are within easy reach. Adjust the bath blanket to keep the person covered. ☐ ☐ _____

19. Form a mitt around your hand with one of the washcloths. Wet the mitt with warm, clean water and apply soap. ☐ ☐ _____

20. Using the other hand, separate the buttocks. Place your washcloth-covered hand at the front of the body and stroke toward the back. First clean one side, then the other side, and finally the middle, using a different part of the washcloth each time, until the anal area is clean. ☐ ☐ _____

21. Rinse and dry the anal area thoroughly. Remove the bed protector from underneath the person. ☐ ☐ _____

22. Remove your gloves and dispose of them in a facility-approved waste container. Put on a clean pair of gloves. ☐ ☐ _____

23. Assist the person into the supine position. Reposition the pillow under the person's head. Remove the bath blanket and help the person into the clean clothing. ☐ ☐ _____

24. If the bedding is wet or soiled, change the bed linens. ☐ ☐ _____

25. If the side rails are in use, return the side rail to the raised position. Make sure that the bed is lowered to its lowest position and that the wheels are locked. ☐ ☐ _____

26. Gather the soiled linens and place them in the linen hamper or linen bag. Dispose of disposable items in a facility-approved waste container. Clean equipment and return it to the storage area. ☐ ☐ _____

27. Remove your gloves and dispose of them in a facility-approved waste container. ☐ ☐ _____

Finishing Up

28. Complete the "Finishing Up" steps. ☐ ☐ _____

PROCEDURE 18-6
Assisting With a Tub Bath or Shower

Getting Ready

	S	U	COMMENTS

1. Prepare the tub room. Place a nonskid mat on the floor of the tub or shower. If the person will be taking a tub bath, fill the tub halfway with warm water (105°F [43.3°C] to 115°F [46.1°C] on the bath thermometer). Obtain a shower chair if necessary and place it in the shower. Place a towel on the chair in the tub room where the person will sit while drying off. ☐ ☐ _____

2. Complete the "Getting Ready" steps. ☐ ☐ _____

Procedure

3. Ask the person if she needs to use the bathroom before bathing. ☐ ☐ _____

4. Assist the person to the tub room. ☐ ☐ _____

5. If the person will be taking a tub bath, check the temperature of the water and make sure the nonskid mat is secure. If the person will be taking a shower, turn on the water and adjust the temperature until the water is comfortable. ☐ ☐ _____

6. Assist the person with undressing. Assist the person into the bathtub or shower. ☐ ☐ _____

7. If the person is able to bathe herself, either partially or completely:

   a. Place bathing supplies within easy reach. ☐ ☐ _____

   b. Many facilities require you to remain in the room while the person bathes or showers. If facility policy permits you to leave the room, explain how to use the call-light control and ask the person to signal when bathing is complete or when she has done as much as she can on her own and needs help completing the bath. Stay nearby and check on the person every 5 minutes. The person should not remain in the bathtub or shower for longer than 20 minutes. Return when the person signals. Remember to knock before entering. ☐ ☐ _____

8. If the person is unable to bathe herself or requires assistance:

   a. Put on the gloves and form a mitt around your hand with one of the washcloths. ☐ ☐ _____

   b. If necessary, ask the person what parts of the body were not washed. Assist the person as needed with completing the bath. Wash the cleanest areas first and the dirtiest areas last: ☐ ☐ _____

- **Eyes.** Wet the mitt with warm, clean water. Ask the person to close her eyes. Place your washcloth-covered hand at the inner corner of the eye and stroke gently outward, toward the outer corner. Use a different part of the washcloth for each eye.

- **Face, neck, and ears.** Ask the person if you should use soap on the face. Rinse the washcloth and apply soap, if requested. Wash the face, neck, and ears, moving from the top of the head to the bottom (so that the nose and mouth are washed last). Rinse thoroughly.

- **Arms and axillae (armpits).** Rinse the washcloth and apply soap. Place your washcloth-covered hand at the shoulder and stroke downward, toward the hand, using long, firm strokes. Wash the hand. If necessary, assist the person with raising her arm so that you can wash the axilla. Repeat for the other arm and axilla.

- **Chest and abdomen.** Using long, firm strokes, wash the person's chest and abdomen.

- **Legs and feet.** Place your washcloth-covered hand at the top of the thigh and stroke downward, toward the foot, using long, firm strokes. Wash the foot. Repeat for the other leg.

- **Back and buttocks:** Wash the person's back and buttocks, moving from top to bottom and using long, firm strokes.

- **Perineal area:** Complete perineal care.

9. Make sure that soap is thoroughly rinsed from all parts of the body.

10. Remove your gloves and dispose of them in a facility-approved waste container. Put on a clean pair of gloves.

11. If the person is taking a tub bath, drain the water and carefully assist the person out of the tub and into the towel-covered chair. If the person is taking a shower, turn the water off and assist the person into the towel-covered chair.

12. Wrap a towel around the person. Using another bath towel, help the person to dry off, patting the skin dry. Take care to ensure that areas where "skin meets skin" are dried thoroughly (for example, in between the toes and underneath the breasts).

13. Help the person to apply lotion, powder, deodorant, antiperspirant, or other personal care products as the person requests.

14. Help the person into the clean clothing. If the person is wearing nightwear, help her into a robe. Help the person into her slippers.

15. Remove your gloves and dispose of them in a facility-approved waste container. ☐ ☐ _____

16. Assist the person back to her room. ☐ ☐ _____

Finishing Up

17. Complete the "Finishing Up" steps. ☐ ☐ _____

18. Gather the soiled linens and place them in the linen hamper or linen bag. Dispose of disposable items in a facility-approved waste container. Clean equipment and return it to the storage area. ☐ ☐ _____

19. Clean the tub room and shower chair (if used), if housekeeping is not responsible for this task at your facility. ☐ ☐ _____

PROCEDURE 18-7
Giving a Complete Bed Bath

	S	U	COMMENTS

Getting Ready

1. Complete the "Getting Ready" steps.

☐ ☐ _____

Procedure

2. Cover the over-bed table with paper towels. Place the wash basin, toiletries, clean clothing, and clean linens on the over-bed table.

☐ ☐ _____

3. Make sure that the bed is positioned at a comfortable working height (to promote good body mechanics) and that the wheels are locked.

☐ ☐ _____

4. Put on the gloves.

☐ ☐ _____

5. Because bathing often stimulates the urge to urinate, offer the bedpan or urinal. If the person uses the bedpan or urinal, empty and clean it before proceeding with the bath. Remove your gloves and dispose of them in a facility-approved waste container. Wash your hands and put on a clean pair of gloves.

☐ ☐ _____

6. Assist the person with oral care.

☐ ☐ _____

7. Remove the bedspread and blanket from the bed. If they are to be reused, fold them and place them on a clean surface, such as the chair.

☐ ☐ _____

8. Spread the bath blanket over the top linens (and the person). If the person is able, have him hold the bath blanket. If not, tuck the corners under the person's shoulders. Fanfold the top linens to the foot of the bed.

☐ ☐ _____

9. Assist the person with undressing.

☐ ☐ _____

10. Lower the head of the bed so that the bed is flat (as tolerated). Position the pillow under the person's head.

☐ ☐ _____

11. Fill the wash basin with warm water [110°F (43.3°C) to 115°F (46.1°C) on the bath thermometer]. Place the basin on the over-bed table.

☐ ☐ _____

12. If the side rails are in use, lower the side rail on the working side of the bed. The side rail on the opposite side of the bed should remain up.

☐ ☐ _____

13. Place a towel over the person's chest to keep the bath blanket dry.

☐ ☐ _____

14. To keep the bath water from becoming soapy too quickly, you can use two washcloths—one with soap, for washing; and one without soap, for rinsing. Form a mitt around your hand with one of the washcloths. Wet the mitt with warm, clean water. Ask the person to close his eyes. Place your washcloth-covered hand at the inner corner of the eye and stroke gently outward, toward the outer corner. Use a different part of the washcloth for each eye. Using a towel, dry the person's eyes.

☐ ☐ _____

15. Ask the person if you should use soap on the face. Rinse the washcloth and apply soap, if requested. Wash the face, neck, and ears, moving from the top of the head to the bottom (so that the nose and mouth are washed last). Using the clean washcloth, rinse thoroughly, and pat the person's face, neck, and ears dry with a towel.   ☐ ☐ _____

16. Place a bed protector under the person's far arm, to keep the linens dry. Form a mitt around your hand with the washcloth. Wet the mitt and apply soap. Place your washcloth-covered hand at the shoulder and stroke downward, toward the hand, using long, firm strokes. Wash the hand. If necessary, assist the person with raising his arm so that you can wash the axilla. Rinse thoroughly, and pat the person's arm, hand, and axilla dry with a towel. Remove the bed protector from underneath the person's arm.   ☐ ☐ _____

17. Repeat for the other arm.   ☐ ☐ _____

18. Place a towel horizontally across the person's chest. (The person is now covered with both a bath blanket and a towel.) With the towel in place, fold the bath blanket down to the person's waist. Wet the mitt and apply soap. Reach under the towel and wash the person's chest, using long, firm strokes. Using the clean washcloth, rinse thoroughly, and pat the person's chest dry with a towel.   ☐ ☐ _____

19. With the towel still in place, fold the bath blanket down to the pubic area. Form a mitt around your hand with the washcloth. Wet the mitt and apply soap. Reach under the towel and wash the person's abdomen, using long, firm strokes. Rinse thoroughly and pat the person's abdomen dry with a towel.   ☐ ☐ _____

20. Replace the bath blanket by unfolding it back over the towel and the person's body. Slide the towel out from underneath the bath blanket.   ☐ ☐ _____

21. Change the water in the wash basin if it is cool or soapy. (If the side rails are in use, raise the side rails before leaving the bedside.)   ☐ ☐ _____

22. Fold the bath blanket so that the far leg is completely exposed. Place a bed protector under the person's far leg to keep the linens dry. Wet the mitt and apply soap. Place your washcloth-covered hand at the top of the thigh and stroke downward, toward the foot, using long, firm strokes. Rinse thoroughly and pat the person's leg dry with a bath towel.   ☐ ☐ _____

23. Put the wash basin on the bed protector and place the person's foot in the basin. Wash the entire foot, including between the toes, with the soapy washcloth. Rinse thoroughly and pat the person's foot dry with a towel. Be sure to dry between the toes. Remove the wash basin. Remove the bed protector from underneath the person's leg.   ☐ ☐ _____

24. Repeat for the other leg and foot. ☐ ☐ _____

25. Change the water in the wash basin. (If the side ☐ ☐ _____
rails are in use, raise the side rails before leaving the
bedside.)

26. Turn the person onto his or her side so that he or she ☐ ☐ _____
is facing away from you. Help the person toward the
working side of the bed so that his back is within
easy reach. Adjust the bath blanket to keep the front
of the person covered (exposing only the back and
buttocks). Place a bed protector on the bed alongside
the person's back to keep the linens dry.

27. Form a mitt around your hand with the washcloth. ☐ ☐ _____
Wet the mitt and apply soap. Wash the person's back
and buttocks, moving from top to bottom and using
long, firm strokes. Rinse thoroughly and pat the person's back and buttocks dry using a bath towel. At
this point, a back massage may be given.

28. If the person is able to perform perineal care, assist ☐ ☐ _____
the person into Fowler's position and adjust the over-
bed table so that the bathing supplies are within easy
reach. Place the call-light control within easy reach
and ask the person to signal when perineal care is
complete. If the person is unable to perform perineal
care, assist the person onto his back and complete
perineal care.

29. Remove your gloves and dispose of them in a facility- ☐ ☐ _____
approved waste container. Put on a clean pair of
gloves.

30. Help the person to apply lotion, powder, deodorant, ☐ ☐ _____
antiperspirant, or other personal care products as the
person requests.

31. Help the person into the clean clothing. ☐ ☐ _____

32. If the bedding is wet or soiled, change the bed linens. ☐ ☐ _____

33. Carry out range-of-motion exercises as ordered. ☐ ☐ _____

34. If the side rails are in use, return the side rails to the ☐ ☐ _____
raised position. Raise or lower the head of the bed as
the person requests. Make sure that the bed is
lowered to its lowest position and that the wheels are
locked.

35. Gather the soiled linens and place them in the linen ☐ ☐ _____
hamper or linen bag. Dispose of disposable items in a
facility-approved waste container. Clean equipment
and return it to the storage area.

36. Remove your gloves and dispose of them in a facility- ☐ ☐ _____
approved waste container.

Finishing Up

37. Complete the "Finishing Up" steps. ☐ ☐ _____

PROCEDURE 18-8
Giving a Partial Bed Bath

	S	U	COMMENTS

Getting Ready

1. Complete the "Getting Ready" steps. ☐ ☐ _____

Procedure

2. Cover the over-bed table with paper towels. Place the wash basin, toiletries, clean clothing, and clean linens on the over-bed table. Put on the gloves. ☐ ☐ _____

3. Because bathing often stimulates the urge to urinate, offer the bedpan or urinal. If the person uses the bedpan or urinal, empty and clean it before proceeding with the bath. Remove your gloves and dispose of them in a facility-approved waste container. Wash your hands and put on a clean pair of gloves. ☐ ☐ _____

4. Assist the person with oral hygiene. Remove your gloves and dispose of them in a facility-approved waste container. Wash your hands. ☐ ☐ _____

5. Fill the wash basin with warm water (110°F [43.3°C] to 115°F [46.1°C] on the bath thermometer). Place the basin on the over-bed table. ☐ ☐ _____

6. If the person will be bathing independently, make sure that the bed is lowered to its lowest position and that the wheels are locked. If you will be assisting the person with bathing, make sure that the bed is positioned at a comfortable working height (to promote good body mechanics) and that the wheels are locked. If the side rails are in use, lower the side rail on the working side. The side rails on the opposite side of the bed should remain up. ☐ ☐ _____

7. The bath may either be carried out with the person in Fowler's position, or the person can be assisted to sit on the edge of the bed. Help the person to undress as necessary. ☐ ☐ _____

8. If the person is able to bathe herself, either partially or completely:

    a. Place bathing supplies within easy reach. ☐ ☐ _____

    b. Many facilities require you to remain in the room while the person bathes. If facility policy permits you to leave the room, explain how to use the call light control and ask the person to signal when bathing is complete or when she has done as much as she can on her own and needs help completing the bath. Stay nearby and check on the person every 5 minutes. Return when the person signals. Remember to knock before entering. ☐ ☐ _____

9. If the person is unable to bathe herself, or requires assistance:

   a. Put on the gloves and form a mitt around your hand with one of the washcloths. ☐ ☐ _____

   b. If necessary, ask the person what parts of the body were not washed. Assist the person as needed with completing the bath. Wash the cleanest areas first and the dirtiest areas last: ☐ ☐ _____

      ● **Face, neck, and ears.** Ask the person if you should use soap on the face. Rinse the washcloth and apply soap, if requested. Wash the face, neck, and ears, moving from the top of the head to the bottom (so that the nose and mouth are washed last). Rinse thoroughly, and pat the person's face, neck, and ears dry with a towel.

      ● **Hands.** Wash the hand. Rinse thoroughly, and pat the hand dry with a towel. Repeat for the other hand.

      ● **Axillae (armpits).** If necessary, assist the person with raising her arm so that you can wash the axilla. Rinse thoroughly, and pat the axilla dry with a towel. Repeat for the other axilla.

      ● **Back and buttocks.** Rinse the washcloth and apply soap. Wash the person's back and buttocks, moving from top to bottom and using long, firm strokes. Rinse thoroughly, and pat the back and buttocks dry with a towel.

      ● **Perineal area.** Complete male or female perineal care.

10. Remove your gloves and dispose of them in a facility-approved waste container. Put on a clean pair of gloves. ☐ ☐ _____

11. Help the person to apply lotion, powder, deodorant, antiperspirant, or other personal care products as the person requests. ☐ ☐ _____

12. Help the person into the clean clothing. ☐ ☐ _____

13. If the bedding is wet or soiled, change the bed linens. ☐ ☐ _____

14. Carry out range-of-motion exercises as ordered. ☐ ☐ _____

15. If the side rails are in use, return the side rails to the raised position. Raise or lower the head of the bed as the person requests. Make sure that the bed is lowered to its lowest position and that the wheels are locked. ☐ ☐ _____

16. Gather the soiled linens and place them in the linen hamper or linen bag. Dispose of disposable items in a facility-approved waste container. Clean equipment and return it to the storage area. ☐ ☐ _____

17. Remove your gloves and dispose of them in a facility-approved waste container. ☐ ☐ _____

Finishing Up

18. Complete the "Finishing Up" steps. ☐ ☐ _____

PROCEDURE 18-9
Giving a Back Massage

	S	U	COMMENTS

Getting Ready

1. Complete the "Getting Ready" steps. ☐ ☐ _____

Procedure

2. Fill the wash basin with warm water. Place the bottle of lotion in the basin of warm water to warm it. ☐ ☐ _____

3. Make sure that the bed is positioned at a comfortable working height (to promote good body mechanics) and that the wheels are locked. ☐ ☐ _____

4. Lower the head of the bed so that the bed is flat (as tolerated). If the side rails are in use, lower the side rail on the working side of the bed. The side rail on the opposite side of the bed should remain up. ☐ ☐ _____

5. Help the person into the prone position, or turn the person onto his or her side so that he or she is facing away from you. ☐ ☐ _____

6. Reposition the pillow under the person's head and adjust the bath blanket to keep the person covered, exposing only the back and buttocks. ☐ ☐ _____

7. Put on the gloves if contact with broken skin is likely. ☐ ☐ _____

8. Pour some lotion into your cupped palm and rub your hands together to distribute the lotion onto both palms. ☐ ☐ _____

9. Apply the lotion to the person's back with the palms of your hands. Massage the lotion into the person's skin, using long, gliding strokes (*effleurage*), moving up the center of the back from the buttocks to the shoulders, and then back down along the outside of the back. Do not directly rub any reddened areas. Repeat four times. ☐ ☐ _____

10. For the next set of strokes, move up the center of the back from the buttocks to the shoulders and then back down along the outside of the back. On the downstroke, massage the person's shoulders and back using a small circular motion. Repeat four times. ☐ ☐ _____

11. For the next set of strokes, move up the center of the back from the buttocks to the shoulders, and then back down along the outside of the back. On the downstroke, massage the person's shoulders, back, and buttocks using a small circular motion, paying special attention to the area at the base of the spine. Repeat four times. ☐ ☐ _____

12. Finish with long, gliding strokes (*effleurage*), moving up the center of the back from the buttocks to the shoulders and then back down along the outside of the back. Repeat four times. ☐ ☐ _____

13. Remove your gloves and dispose of them in a facility-approved waste container.   ☐ ☐ _____

14. If the back massage is being given as part of a bath, assist the person onto his or her back and continue with the bath. If the back massage is being given before bed or at any other time, help the person back into his or her pajamas, nightgown, or hospital gown.   ☐ ☐ _____

15. If the side rails are in use, return the side rails to the raised position. Make sure that the bed is lowered to its lowest position and that the wheels are locked.   ☐ ☐ _____

16. Gather the soiled linens and place them in the linen hamper or linen bag. Dispose of disposable items in a facility-approved waste container. Clean equipment and return it to the storage area.   ☐ ☐ _____

Finishing Up

17. Complete the "Finishing Up" steps.   ☐ ☐ _____

CHAPTER 19 PROCEDURE CHECKLISTS

PROCEDURE 19-1
Assisting With Hand Care

	S	U	COMMENTS

Getting Ready

1. Complete the "Getting Ready" steps. ☐ ☐ _____

Procedure

2. Make sure that the bed is lowered to its lowest position and that the wheels are locked. ☐ ☐ _____

3. Cover the over-bed table with paper towels. Pour some liquid soap into the emesis basin and fill the basin with warm water (100°F [37.7°C] to 115°F [46.1°C] on the bath thermometer). Place the emesis basin on the over-bed table, along with the nail care supplies and clean linens. ☐ ☐ _____

4. If the side rails are in use, lower the side rail on the working side of the bed. The side rail on the opposite side of the bed should remain up. ☐ ☐ _____

5. Help the person to transfer from the bed to a bedside chair, assist the person to sit on the edge of the bed, or raise the head of the bed as tolerated. ☐ ☐ _____

6. Put on the gloves if contact with broken skin is likely. ☐ ☐ _____

7. If the person is wearing nail polish and wants it removed, remove the nail polish by putting a small amount of nail polish remover on a cotton ball and gently rubbing each nail. ☐ ☐ _____

8. Help the person to position the tips of his or her fingers in the basin to soak. Let the person soak his or her fingers for about 5 minutes. ☐ ☐ _____

9. Working with one hand at a time, lift the person's hand out of the basin and wash the entire hand, including between the fingers, with the soapy washcloth. Use the orange stick to gently clean underneath the person's fingernails. Rinse thoroughly and pat the person's hand dry with a towel. Be sure to dry between the fingers. Repeat with the other hand. ☐ ☐ _____

10. Remove the emesis basin and dry the person's hands thoroughly. If facility policy allows it, gently push the cuticles back with the orange stick. ☐ ☐ _____

11. If facility policy allows it, use the nail clippers to cut the person's fingernails. If the person's nails need to be trimmed but this task is outside of your scope of practice, report this need to the nurse. ☐ ☐ _____

12. Use the emery board to file the fingernails into an oval shape and smooth the rough edges. ☐ ☐ _____

13. Apply lotion to the person's hands and gently massage it into the skin. ☐ ☐ _____

14. Apply nail polish as the person requests. ☐ ☐ _____

15. If necessary, help the person return to bed. If the side rails are in use, return the side rails to the raised position. Lower the head of the bed as the person requests. ☐ ☐ _____

16. Gather the soiled linens and place them in the linen hamper or linen bag. Dispose of disposable items in a facility-approved waste container. Clean equipment and return it to the storage area. ☐ ☐ _____

17. Remove your gloves and dispose of them in a facility-approved waste container. ☐ ☐ _____

Finishing Up

18. Complete the "Finishing Up" steps. ☐ ☐ _____

PROCEDURE 19-2
Assisting With Foot Care

	S	U	COMMENTS

Getting Ready

1. Complete the "Getting Ready" steps. ☐ ☐ _____

Procedure

2. Make sure that the bed is lowered to its lowest position and that the wheels are locked. ☐ ☐ _____

3. Cover the over-bed table with paper towels. Pour some liquid soap into the wash basin and fill the basin with warm water (100°F [37.7°C] to 115°F [46.1°C] on the bath thermometer). Place the wash basin on the over-bed table, along with the nail care supplies and clean linens. ☐ ☐ _____

4. If the side rails are in use, lower the side rail on the working side of the bed. The side rail on the opposite side of the bed should remain up. ☐ ☐ _____

5. If the person is able to get out of bed, help the person to transfer from the bed to a bedside chair. If the person is not able to get out of bed, raise the head of the bed as tolerated. Fanfold the top linens to the foot of the bed. ☐ ☐ _____

6. Put on the gloves if contact with broken skin is likely. ☐ ☐ _____

7. If the person is wearing nail polish and wants it removed, remove the nail polish by putting a small amount of nail polish remover on a cotton ball and gently rubbing each nail. ☐ ☐ _____

8. Place a bed protector on the floor in front of the chair (if the person is out of bed) or on the bottom sheet (if the person is in bed). Place the wash basin on the bed protector. ☐ ☐ _____

9. Help the person to position his or her feet in the basin to soak. Let the person soak his or her feet for about 5 minutes. ☐ ☐ _____

10. Working with one foot at a time, lift the person's foot out of the basin and wash the entire foot, including between the toes, with the soapy washcloth. Apply soap to the nailbrush and gently scrub any rough areas. Use the orange stick to gently clean underneath the person's toenails. Rinse thoroughly and pat the person's foot dry with a towel. Be sure to dry between the toes. Repeat with the other foot. ☐ ☐ _____

11. If facility policy allows it, use the nail clippers to cut the person's toenails. If the person's nails need to be trimmed but this task is outside of your scope of practice, report this need to the nurse. ☐ ☐ _____

12. Use the emery board to smooth the rough edges of the toenails. ☐ ☐ _____

13. Apply lotion to the person's feet and gently massage it into the skin.   ☐ ☐ _____

14. Apply nail polish as the person requests.   ☐ ☐ _____

15. If necessary, help the person return to bed. If the side rails are in use, return the side rails to the raised position. Lower the head of the bed as the person requests.   ☐ ☐ _____

16. Gather the soiled linens and place them in the linen hamper or linen bag. Dispose of disposable items in a facility-approved waste container. Clean equipment and return it to the storage area.   ☐ ☐ _____

Finishing Up

17. Complete the "Finishing Up" steps.   ☐ ☐ _____

PROCEDURE 19-3
Assisting a Person With Dressing

	S	U	COMMENTS

Getting Ready

1. Complete the "Getting Ready" steps. ☐ ☐ _____

Procedure

2. Make sure that the bed is positioned at a comfortable working height (to promote good body mechanics) and that the wheels are locked. ☐ ☐ _____

3. Lower the head of the bed so that the bed is flat (as tolerated). If the side rails are in use, lower the side rail on the working side of the bed. The side rail on the opposite side of the bed should remain up. ☐ ☐ _____

4. Put on the gloves if contact with broken skin is likely. ☐ ☐ _____

5. Spread the bath blanket over the top linens (and the person). If the person is able, have him or her hold the bath blanket. If not, tuck the corners under the person's shoulders. Fanfold the top linens to the foot of the bed. ☐ ☐ _____

6. Assist the person with undressing:

    a. **Garments that fasten in the back.** Undo any fasteners, such as buttons, zippers, snaps, or ties. Gently lift the person's head and shoulders and gather the garment around the person's neck. Working with the person's strongest side first, gently remove the arm from the garment by sliding the garment down the arm. Repeat with the other arm. (If it is not possible to lift the person's head and shoulders, roll the person onto his or her side facing away from you. Working with the person's strongest side first, gently remove the arm from the garment. Roll the person onto his or her other side, facing you and remove the other arm from the garment.) Remove the garment completely by lifting it over the person's head. ☐ ☐ _____

b. **Garments that fasten in the front.** Undo any fasteners, such as buttons, zippers, snaps, or ties. To remove the top, gently lift the person's head and shoulders. Working with the person's strongest side first, gently remove the arm from the garment by sliding the garment over the shoulder and down the arm. Gather the garment behind the person and remove the garment completely by sliding the other sleeve over the weak shoulder and arm. To remove the bottoms, undo any fasteners, such as buttons, zippers, or snaps. Ask the person to lift his or her buttocks off the bed and gently slide the pants down to the ankles and over the feet. (If the person cannot raise his or her buttocks off the bed, help the person to roll first to his or her strong side, allowing you to pull the bottoms down on the weak side. Then roll the person to his or her weak side and finish pulling the bottoms down.)

☐ ☐ _____

7. Assist the person with putting on his or her undergarments:

a. **Underpants.** Facing the foot of the bed, gather the underpants together at the leg opening and at the waistband. Working with one foot at a time, slip first one foot and then the other through the waistband and into the leg openings. Slide the underpants up the person's legs as far as they will go, and then ask the person to lift his or her buttocks off the bed. Gently slide the underpants up over the buttocks. (If the person cannot raise his or her buttocks off the bed, help the person to roll first to his or her strong side, allowing you to pull the underpants up on the weak side. Then roll the person to his or her weak side and finish pulling the underpants up.) Adjust the underpants so that they fit comfortably.

☐ ☐ _____

b. **Bra.** Working with the person's weak side first, slip the arms through the straps and position the straps on the shoulders so that the front of the bra is covering the person's chest. Adjust the cups of the bra over the person's breasts. Raise the person's head and shoulders and help the person to lean forward so that you can fasten the bra in the back.

☐ ☐ _____

c. **Undershirt.** Facing the head of the bed, gather the top and the bottom of the undershirt together at the neck opening. Place the undershirt over the person's head. Working with the person's weak side first, slip the arms through the arm openings. Raise the person's head and shoulders and help the person to lean forward so that you can pull the undershirt down, smoothing out any wrinkles.

☐ ☐ _____

8. Assist the person with putting on his or her outerwear:

   a. **Pants.** Assist the person with putting on his or her pants by following the same procedure as that used for putting on underpants (see step 7a). Fasten any buttons, zippers, snaps, or ties.   ☐ ☐ _____

   b. **Shirts and sweaters that fasten in the front.** Facing the head of the bed, place your hand and arm through the wristband of the garment. Working with the person's weak side first, grasp the person's hand and slip the garment off of your hand and arm, gently guiding the person's arm into the sleeve. Pull the sleeve up, adjusting it at the shoulder. Raise the person's head and shoulders and help the person to lean forward so that you can bring the other side of the garment around the back of the person's body. Guide the person's strong arm into the sleeve of the garment. Fasten any buttons, zippers, snaps, or ties.   ☐ ☐ _____

   c. **Sweatshirts and pullover sweaters.** Assist the person with putting on a sweatshirt or pullover sweater by following the same procedure as that used for putting on an undershirt (see step 7c). Fasten any buttons, zippers, snaps, or ties.   ☐ ☐ _____

   d. **Blouses that fasten in the back.** Facing the head of the bed, place your hand and arm through the wristband of the garment. Working with the person's weak side first, grasp the person's hand and slip the garment off of your hand and arm, gently guiding the person's arm into the sleeve. Pull the sleeve up, adjusting it at the shoulder. Repeat for the other side. Raise the person's head and shoulders and help the person to lean forward so that you can bring the sides of the garment around to the back. Fasten any buttons, zippers, snaps, or ties.   ☐ ☐ _____

9. Assist the person with putting on footwear:

   a. **Socks or knee-high stockings.** Gather the sock or stocking, bringing the toe area and the opening together. With the toe area facing up, slip the sock or stocking over the person's foot. Smooth the heel of the sock or stocking over the person's heel, and pull the sock or stocking up into position. Adjust the sock or stocking so that it fits comfortably. Repeat for the other foot.   ☐ ☐ _____

   b. **Shoes or slippers.** If the shoe has laces, loosen them completely to make it easier to slip the shoe onto the foot. Guide the person's foot into the shoe or slipper. A shoehorn may be used to help ease the person's heel into the shoe. Make sure that the foot is seated properly in the shoe. Socks or stockings should not be bunched at the toe. If necessary, tie the shoe or fasten the Velcro™ fasteners securely.   ☐ ☐ _____

10. If the person will be remaining in bed and the side rails are in use, return the side rails to the raised position. Raise the head of the bed as the person requests. □ □ _____

11. Gather the soiled garments and place them in the linen hamper or linen bag. □ □ _____

12. Remove your gloves and dispose of them in a facility-approved waste container. □ □ _____

Finishing Up

13. Complete the "Finishing Up" steps. □ □ _____

PROCEDURE 19-4
Changing a Hospital Gown

	S	U	COMMENTS

Getting Ready

1. Complete the "Getting Ready" steps. ☐ ☐ _____

Procedure

2. Make sure that the bed is positioned at a comfortable working height (to promote good body mechanics) and that the wheels are locked. ☐ ☐ _____

3. Lower the head of the bed so that the bed is flat (as tolerated). If the side rails are in use, lower them on the working side of the bed. The side rails on the opposite side of the bed should remain up. ☐ ☐ _____

4. Put on the gloves if contact with broken skin is likely. ☐ ☐ _____

5. Have the person turn onto his or her side facing away from you so that you can untie the gown at the neck and waist. Assist the person back into the supine position. If the person cannot turn onto his or her side, reach under the person and untie the gown. ☐ ☐ _____

6. Loosen the gown from around the person's body. ☐ ☐ _____

7. Unfold the clean gown and lay it over the person's chest. ☐ ☐ _____

8. Working with the person's strongest side first, remove one sleeve at a time, leaving the old gown draped over the person's body. ☐ ☐ _____

9. Working with the person's weakest side first, slide the arm through the sleeve of the clean gown. Repeat for the other arm. ☐ ☐ _____

10. Remove the soiled gown from underneath the clean gown and place it in the linen hamper or linen bag. ☐ ☐ _____

11. Have the person turn onto his or her side, facing away from you, so that you can tie the gown at the neck and waist (or reach under the person and tie the gown). Adjust the gown so that it fits comfortably. ☐ ☐ _____

12. If the side rails are in use, return the side rails to the raised position. Raise the head of the bed as the person requests. ☐ ☐ _____

13. Remove your gloves and dispose of them in a facility-approved waste container. ☐ ☐ _____

Finishing Up

14. Complete the "Finishing Up" steps. ☐ ☐ _____

PROCEDURE 19-5
Shampooing a Person's Hair in Bed

	S	U	COMMENTS

Getting Ready

1. Complete the "Getting Ready" steps. ☐ ☐ _____

Procedure

2. Make sure that the bed is positioned at a comfortable working height (to promote good body mechanics) and that the wheels are locked. ☐ ☐ _____

3. Fill the water pitcher with warm water (100°F [37.7°C] to 115°F [46.1°C] on the bath thermometer). ☐ ☐ _____

4. Cover the over-bed table with paper towels. Place the hair care supplies and clean linens on the over-bed table. ☐ ☐ _____

5. Raise the head of the bed as tolerated. Comb the person's hair to remove snarls and tangles. ☐ ☐ _____

6. Lower the head of the bed so that the bed is flat (as tolerated). If the side rails are in use, lower the side rail on the working side of the bed. The side rail on the opposite side of the bed should remain up. ☐ ☐ _____

7. Put on the gloves if contact with broken skin is likely. ☐ ☐ _____

8. Gently lift the person's head and shoulders and reposition the pillow under the person's shoulders. Cover the head of the bed and the pillow with the bed protector and place the shampoo trough on the bed protector. Help the person to rest his or her head on the shampoo trough. Place a towel across the person's shoulders and chest. ☐ ☐ _____

9. Place the wash basin on the floor beside the bed to catch the water as it drains from the shampoo trough. ☐ ☐ _____

10. Ask the person to hold the washcloth over his or her eyes. ☐ ☐ _____

11. Holding the water pitcher in one hand, slowly pour water over the person's hair until the hair is completely wet. Use your other hand to help direct the flow of water away from the person's eyes and ears. ☐ ☐ _____

12. Apply a small amount of shampoo to the wet hair. Lather the hair and massage the scalp to help stimulate the circulation. ☐ ☐ _____

13. Using the water pitcher, rinse the hair thoroughly. ☐ ☐ _____

14. Apply conditioner, as the person requests. Rinse the hair thoroughly. ☐ ☐ _____

15. Gently lift the person's head and shoulders and remove the shampoo trough and bed protector. Wrap the person's hair in a towel. ☐ ☐ _____

16. Raise the head of the bed as tolerated. Gently pat the person's face, neck, and ears dry and finish towel drying the hair. □ □ _____

17. Replace any wet or soiled linens. (If the side rails are in use, raise the side rails before leaving the bedside to get the necessary replacement linens.) □ □ _____

18. Comb the person's hair to remove snarls and tangles. □ □ _____

19. Dry and style the hair with the brush and blow dryer, as the person requests. Use the cool setting and take care not to burn the person's scalp or face. □ □ _____

20. Reposition the pillow under the person's head and straighten the bed linens. If the side rails are in use, return the side rails to the raised position. Lower the head of the bed as the person requests. □ □ _____

21. Gather the soiled linens and place them in the linen hamper or linen bag. Dispose of disposable items in a facility-approved waste container. Clean equipment and return it to the storage area. □ □ _____

22. Remove your gloves and dispose of them in a facility-approved waste container. □ □ _____

Finishing Up

23. Complete the "Finishing Up" steps. □ □ _____

PROCEDURE 19-6
Combing a Person's Hair

	S	U	COMMENTS

Getting Ready

1. Complete the "Getting Ready" steps. ☐ ☐ _____

Procedure

2. Make sure that the bed is positioned at a comfortable working height (to promote good body mechanics) and that the wheels are locked. ☐ ☐ _____

3. Cover the over-bed table with paper towels. Place the hair care supplies and clean linens on the over-bed table. ☐ ☐ _____

4. Raise the head of the bed as tolerated. Gently lift the person's head and shoulders and cover the pillow with a towel. Drape another towel across the person's back and shoulders. ☐ ☐ _____

5. If the side rails are in use, lower the side rail on the working side of the bed. The side rail on the opposite side of the bed should remain up. ☐ ☐ _____

6. If the hair is tangled, work on the tangles first. Put a small amount of detangler or leave-in conditioner on the tangled hair. Begin at the ends of the hair and work toward the scalp. Hold the lock of hair just above the tangle (closest to the scalp) and use the wide-tooth comb to gently work through the tangle. ☐ ☐ _____

7. Using the brush and working with one 2-inch section at a time, gently brush the hair, moving from the roots of the hair toward the ends. ☐ ☐ _____

8. Secure the hair using barrettes, clips, or pins or braid the hair, as the person requests. Offer the person the mirror to check his or her appearance when you are finished. ☐ ☐ _____

9. Reposition the pillow under the person's head and straighten the bed linens. If the side rails are in use, return the side rails to the raised position. Lower the head of the bed as the person requests. ☐ ☐ _____

10. Gather the soiled linens and place them in the linen hamper or linen bag. Dispose of disposable items in a facility-approved waste container. Clean equipment and return it to the storage area. ☐ ☐ _____

Finishing Up

11. Complete the "Finishing Up" steps. ☐ ☐ _____

PROCEDURE 19-7
Shaving a Person's Face

	S	U	COMMENTS

Getting Ready

1. Complete the "Getting Ready" steps. □ □ _____

Procedure

2. Make sure that the bed is lowered to its lowest position and that the wheels are locked. □ □ _____

3. Fill the wash basin with warm water (100°F [37.7°C] to 115°F [46.1°C] on the bath thermometer). □ □ _____

4. Cover the over-bed table with paper towels. Place the wash basin, shaving supplies, and clean linens on the over-bed table. □ □ _____

5. If the side rails are in use, lower the side rail on the working side of the bed. The side rail on the opposite side of the bed should remain up. □ □ _____

6. Help the person to transfer from the bed to a bedside chair, assist the person to sit on the edge of the bed, or raise the head of the bed as tolerated. □ □ _____

7. Place a towel across the person's shoulders and chest. □ □ _____

8. Put on the gloves. □ □ _____

9. Wet the washcloth with warm, clean water. Soften the beard by holding the washcloth against the person's face for 2 to 3 minutes. □ □ _____

10. Apply shaving cream, gel, or soap to the beard. □ □ _____

11. Shave the person's cheeks:
    a. Stand facing the person. □ □ _____
    b. Gently pull the skin tight and shave downward, in the direction of hair growth (i.e., toward the chin). Use short, even strokes, rinsing the razor frequently in the wash basin. Repeat until all of the lather on the cheek has been removed. □ □ _____
    c. Repeat for the other cheek. □ □ _____

12. Shave the person's chin:
    a. Ask the person to "tighten the chin" by drawing the lower lip over the teeth. □ □ _____
    b. Shave the chin using short, even, downward strokes. Repeat until all of the lather on the chin has been removed, rinsing the razor frequently in the wash basin. □ □ _____

13. Shave the person's neck:
    a. Ask the person to tip his head back. □ □ _____
    b. Gently pull the skin tight and shave upward, in the direction of hair growth (i.e., toward the chin). Use short, even strokes, rinsing the razor frequently in the wash basin. Repeat until all of the lather on the neck has been removed. □ □ _____

14. Shave the area between the person's nose and upper lip:

    a. Ask the person to "tighten his upper lip" by drawing the upper lip over the teeth. □ □ _____

    b. Shave the area between the nose and the upper lip using short, even downward strokes. Repeat until all of the lather has been removed, rinsing the razor frequently in the wash basin. □ □ _____

15. Change the water in the wash basin. (If the side rails are in use, raise the side rails before leaving the bedside.) Form a mitt around your hand with the washcloth and wet the mitt with warm, clean water. Wash the person's face and neck. Rinse thoroughly and pat the person's face, neck, and ears dry with the face towel. □ □ _____

16. Apply aftershave lotion, as the person requests. □ □ _____

17. If you have accidentally nicked the skin and the person is bleeding, apply direct pressure with a tissue until the bleeding stops. Report the incident to the nurse. □ □ _____

18. If necessary, help the person return to bed. If the side rails are in use, return the side rails to the raised position. □ □ _____

19. Gather the soiled linens and place them in the linen hamper or linen bag. Dispose of disposable items in a facility-approved waste container. Clean equipment and return it to the storage area. □ □ _____

20. Remove your gloves and dispose of them in a facility-approved waste container. □ □ _____

Finishing Up

21. Complete the "Finishing Up" steps. □ □ _____

CHAPTER 20 PROCEDURE CHECKLISTS

PROCEDURE 20-1
Feeding a Dependent Person

	S	U	COMMENTS

Getting Ready

1. Complete the "Getting Ready" steps. ☐ ☐ _____

Procedure

2. Cover the over-bed table with paper towels. Place the oral hygiene supplies on the over-bed table. Fill the wash basin with warm water (1108F [37.78C] to 1158F [46.18C] on the bath thermometer). Place the basin on the over-bed table. ☐ ☐ _____

3. If the side rails are in use, lower the side rail on the working side of the bed. The side rail on the opposite side of the bed should remain up. Raise the head of the bed. Make sure that the bed is positioned at a comfortable working height (to promote good body mechanics) and that the wheels are locked. ☐ ☐ _____

4. Put on the gloves. ☐ ☐ _____

5. Assist the person with oral hygiene. ☐ ☐ _____

6. Offer the bedpan or urinal. If the person uses the bedpan or urinal, empty and clean it before proceeding with the meal. Remove your gloves and dispose of them in a facility-approved waste container. Wash your hands. ☐ ☐ _____

7. Wash the person's hands and face. ☐ ☐ _____

8. Clear the over-bed table and position it over the bed at the proper height for the person. ☐ ☐ _____

9. Get the meal tray from the dietary cart. (If the side rails are in use, raise the side rails before leaving the bedside.) Check the meal tray to make sure that it has the person's name on it and that it contains the correct diet for the person. Place the meal tray on the over-bed table. ☐ ☐ _____

10. Ask the person if he or she would like to use a clothing protector. Put the clothing protector on the person, if desired. ☐ ☐ _____

11. Uncover the meal tray, and prepare the food for eating (for example, cut the meat, butter the bread, open any containers). Tell the person what is on the tray. ☐ ☐ _____

12. Take a seat. ☐ ☐ _____

13. Allow the person to choose what he or she would like to taste first. Using a spoon, offer a small bite to the person (fill the spoon no more than one-third full). Allow the person enough time to swallow the food. ☐ ☐ _____

14. Offer the person something to drink every few bites. Use the napkin to wipe the person's mouth and chin as often as necessary. Allow the person to assist with the eating process to the best of his or her ability. ☐ ☐ _____

15. Continue in this manner until the person is finished. Encourage the person to finish the food on the tray, but do not force the person to eat. ☐ ☐ _____

16. Remove the tray and the clothing protector when the person has finished eating. ☐ ☐ _____

17. Put on a clean pair of gloves. Assist the person with oral hygiene. ☐ ☐ _____

18. If the side rails are in use, return the side rails to the raised position. Lower the head of the bed as the person requests. Make sure that the bed is lowered to its lowest position and that the wheels are locked. ☐ ☐ _____

19. Gather the soiled linens and place them in the linen hamper or linen bag. Dispose of disposable items in a facility-approved waste container. Clean equipment and return it to the storage area. ☐ ☐ _____

20. Remove your gloves and dispose of them in a facility-approved waste container. ☐ ☐ _____

21. Record the percentage of food eaten and the amount of fluid intake in the person's medical record, per your facility's policy. Report an abnormal appetite to the nurse (for example, less than 70% of the total meal consumed). ☐ ☐ _____

Finishing Up

22. Complete the "Finishing Up" steps. ☐ ☐ _____

CHAPTER 21 PROCEDURE CHECKLISTS

PROCEDURE 21-1
Assisting a Person With Using a Bedpan

	S	U	COMMENTS

Getting Ready

1. Complete the "Getting Ready" steps. ☐ ☐ _____

Procedure

2. Make sure that the bed is positioned at a comfortable working height (to promote good body mechanics) and that the wheels are locked. If the side rails are in use, lower the side rail on the working side of the bed. The side rail on the opposite side of the bed should remain up. If necessary, lower the head of the bed so that the bed is flat (as tolerated). ☐ ☐ _____

3. Put on the gloves. ☐ ☐ _____

4. Fanfold the top linens to the foot of the bed. Place the bed protector on the bed. Adjust the person's hospital gown or pajama bottoms as necessary to expose the person's buttocks. ☐ ☐ _____

5. Place the bedpan underneath the person's buttocks. This can be accomplished by either helping the person to lie on her side, facing away from you, or by asking the person to bend her knees, press her heels into the mattress, and lift her buttocks. Slide the bedpan underneath the person (if the person is holding her buttocks away from the bed by bending her knees) or place the bedpan against her buttocks and help her to roll back onto it.

   a. A standard bedpan is positioned like a regular toilet seat. ☐ ☐ _____

   b. A fracture pan is positioned with the narrow end pointed toward the head of the bed. ☐ ☐ _____

6. Raise the head of the bed as tolerated. Draw the top linens over the person for modesty and warmth. ☐ ☐ _____

7. Make sure that the toilet paper and the call-light control are within reach. If the side rails are in use, return the side rails to the raised position. ☐ ☐ _____

8. Remove your gloves and wash your hands. ☐ ☐ _____

9. If safety permits, leave the room and ask the person to call you when she is finished. Remember to close the door on your way out. ☐ ☐ _____

10. Return when the person signals. Remember to knock before entering. ☐ ☐ _____

11. If the side rails are in use, lower the side rail on the working side of the bed. Lower the head of the bed so that the bed is flat (as tolerated). ☐ ☐ _____

12. Put on a clean pair of gloves. ☐ ☐ _____

13. Fanfold the top linens to the foot of the bed. ☐ ☐ _____

14. Ask the person to bend her knees, press her heels into the mattress, and lift her buttocks so that you can remove the bedpan and bed protector. (Or help the person to roll onto her side, facing away from you, while you hold the bedpan securely in place against the mattress to prevent the contents from spilling. Remove the bedpan and bed protector and then help the person to roll back.) If necessary, help the person to use the toilet paper. ☐ ☐ _____

15. Cover the bedpan with the bedpan cover or paper towels. Take the bedpan to the bathroom. (If the side rails are in use, raise them before leaving the bedside.) ☐ ☐ _____

16. Remove your gloves and dispose of them in a facility-approved waste container. Wash your hands. ☐ ☐ _____

17. Return to the bedside. Give the person a wet washcloth and help the person to wash her hands. Make sure the person's perineum is clean and dry. If necessary, provide perineal care. ☐ ☐ _____

18. Adjust the person's hospital gown or pajama bottoms as necessary to cover the buttocks. Help the person back into a comfortable position, straighten the bottom linens, and draw the top linens over the person. Raise the head of the bed, as the person requests. Make sure that the bed is lowered to its lowest position and that the wheels are locked. ☐ ☐ _____

19. Return to the bathroom. Put on a clean pair of gloves. If the person is on intake and output (I&O) status, measure the urine. Note the color, amount, and quality of the urine or feces before emptying the contents of the bedpan into the toilet. (If anything unusual is observed, do not empty the bedpan until a nurse has had a chance to look at its contents.) ☐ ☐ _____

20. Gather the soiled linens and place them in the linen hamper or linen bag. Dispose of disposable items in a facility-approved waste container. Clean equipment and return it to the storage area. ☐ ☐ _____

21. Remove your gloves and dispose of them in a facility-approved waste container. ☐ ☐ _____

Finishing Up

22. Complete the "Finishing Up" steps. ☐ ☐ _____

PROCEDURE 21-2
Assisting a Man With Using a Urinal

	S	U	COMMENTS

Getting Ready

1. Complete the "Getting Ready" steps. □ □ _____

Procedure

2. Ask the man what position he prefers: lying, sitting, or standing. If necessary, raise the head of the bed as tolerated. If the man would prefer to stand, help him to sit on the edge of the bed and then to stand up. □ □ _____

3. Put on the gloves. □ □ _____

4. Hand the man the urinal. If necessary, assist him in positioning it correctly. □ □ _____

5. Make sure that the toilet paper and the call-light control are within reach. □ □ _____

6. Remove your gloves and wash your hands. □ □ _____

7. If safety permits, leave the room and ask the man to call you when he is finished. Remember to close the door on your way out. □ □ _____

8. Return when the man signals. Remember to knock before entering. □ □ _____

9. Put on a clean pair of gloves. Have the man hand you the urinal, or remove it if he is unable to hand it to you. Put the lid on the urinal and hang it on the side rail while you assist the man with handwashing and perineal care as needed. Lower the head of the bed as the man requests. □ □ _____

10. Take the urinal to the bathroom. If the man is on intake and output (I&O) status, measure the urine. Note the color, amount, and quality of the urine before emptying the contents of the urinal into the toilet. (If anything unusual is observed, do not empty the urinal until a nurse has had a chance to look at its contents.) □ □ _____

11. Gather the soiled linens and place them in the linen hamper or linen bag. Dispose of disposable items in a facility-approved waste container. Clean equipment and return it to the storage area. □ □ _____

12. Remove your gloves and dispose of them in a facility-approved waste container. □ □ _____

Finishing Up

13. Complete the "Finishing Up" steps. □ □ _____

Collecting a Routine Urine Specimen

	S	U	COMMENTS

Getting Ready

1. Complete the "Getting Ready" steps. ☐ ☐ _____

Procedure

2. Complete the label with the person's name, room number, and other identifying information. Put the completed label on the specimen container. Take the specimen container to the bathroom. Place a paper towel on the counter. Open the specimen container and place the lid on the paper towel, with the inside of the lid facing up. ☐ ☐ _____

3. If the person will be using a regular toilet or bedside commode, fit the specimen collection device underneath the toilet or commode seat. Otherwise, provide the person with a bedpan or urinal, as applicable. ☐ ☐ _____

4. Assist the person with urination as necessary. Before leaving the room, remind the person not to have a bowel movement or place toilet paper into the specimen collection device, bedpan, or urinal. Provide a plastic bag or waste container for the used toilet paper. ☐ ☐ _____

5. Return when the person signals. Remember to knock before entering. ☐ ☐ _____

6. Put on the gloves. ☐ ☐ _____

7. If the person used a regular toilet or bedside commode, assist the person with handwashing and perineal care as necessary and then help the person to return to bed. If the person used a bedpan or urinal, cover and remove the bedpan or urinal and assist the person with handwashing and perineal care as necessary. ☐ ☐ _____

8. Take the covered bedpan, urinal, or specimen collection device (if the person used a bedside commode) to the bathroom. (If the side rails are in use, raise the side rails before leaving the bedside.) ☐ ☐ _____

9. If the person is on intake and output (I&O) status, measure the urine. Note the color, amount, and quality of the urine. ☐ ☐ _____

10. Raise the toilet seat. While holding the specimen container over the toilet, carefully fill it about three-quarters full with urine from the specimen collection device, bedpan, or urinal. Discard the rest of the urine into the toilet. ☐ ☐ _____

11. Put the lid on the specimen container. Make sure that the lid is tight. Put the specimen container on the paper towel on the counter. ☐ ☐ _____

12. Remove one glove and dispose of it in a facility-approved waste container. Holding the plastic transport bag in your ungloved hand, place the specimen container into the transport bag with your gloved hand. Avoid touching the outside of the transport bag with your glove. ☐ ☐ _____

13. Remove the other glove and dispose of it in a facility-approved waste container. ☐ ☐ _____

14. Gather the soiled linens and place them in the linen hamper or linen bag. Dispose of disposable items in a facility-approved waste container. Clean equipment and return it to the storage area. ☐ ☐ _____

15. Take the specimen container to the designated location. ☐ ☐ _____

Finishing Up

16. Complete the "Finishing Up" steps. ☐ ☐ _____

PROCEDURE 21-4

Collecting a Midstream ("Clean Catch") Urine Specimen

	S	U	COMMENTS

Getting Ready

1. Complete the "Getting Ready" steps. ☐ ☐ _____

Procedure

2. Complete the label with the person's name, room number, and other identifying information. Put the completed label on the specimen container. ☐ ☐ _____

3. If the person will be using a regular toilet or bedside commode, help the person to the bathroom or bedside commode. Otherwise, provide the person with a bedpan or urinal, as applicable. ☐ ☐ _____

4. Put on the gloves. ☐ ☐ _____

5. Place a paper towel on the counter (if the person is in the bathroom) or on the over-bed table (if the person is using a bedside commode, bedpan, or urinal). Open the specimen container and place the lid on the paper towel, with the inside of the lid facing up. ☐ ☐ _____

6. Open the "clean catch" kit. Have the person clean his or her perineum using the wipes in the kit. Assist as necessary:

   a. **If the person is a woman:** Use one hand to separate the labia. Hold the wipe in the other hand. Place your wipe-covered hand at the top of the vulva and stroke downward to the anus. ☐ ☐ _____

   b. **If the person is a circumcised man:** Use one hand to hold the penis slightly away from the body. Hold the wipe in the other hand. Place your wipe-covered hand at the tip of the penis and wash in a circular motion, downward to the base of the penis. ☐ ☐ _____

   c. **If the person is an uncircumcised man:** Retract the foreskin by gently pushing the skin toward the base of the penis. Place your wipe-covered hand at the tip of the penis and wash in a circular motion, downward to the base of the penis. ☐ ☐ _____

7. Assist the person with urination as necessary. Before leaving the room:

   a. Make sure that the toilet paper, call-light control, and specimen container are within reach. ☐ ☐ _____

   b. Remind the person that he or she must start the stream of urine, then stop it, then restart it. The urine sample is to be collected from the restarted flow. If the person is a woman, she must hold the labia open until the specimen is collected. If the person is an uncircumcised man, he must keep the foreskin pulled back until the specimen is collected. ☐ ☐ _____

8. Remove your gloves and dispose of them in a facility-approved waste container.

☐ ☐ _____

9. Return when the person signals. Remember to knock before entering.

☐ ☐ _____

10. Put on a clean pair of gloves.

☐ ☐ _____

11. If the person used a regular toilet or bedside commode, assist the person with handwashing and perineal care as necessary and then help the person to return to bed. If the person used a bedpan or urinal, remove the bedpan or urinal and assist the person with handwashing and perineal care as necessary.

☐ ☐ _____

12. Put the lid on the specimen container, being careful not to touch the inside of the lid or container. Make sure that the lid is tight. Put the specimen container on the paper towel on the counter or over-bed table.

☐ ☐ _____

13. Remove one glove and dispose of it in a facility-approved waste container. Holding the plastic transport bag in your ungloved hand, place the specimen container into the transport bag with your gloved hand. Avoid touching the outside of the transport bag with your glove.

☐ ☐ _____

14. Remove the other glove and dispose of it in a facility-approved waste container.

☐ ☐ _____

15. Gather the soiled linens and place them in the linen hamper or linen bag. Dispose of disposable items in a facility-approved waste container. Clean equipment and return it to the storage area.

☐ ☐ _____

16. Take the specimen container to the designated location.

☐ ☐ _____

Finishing Up

17. Complete the "Finishing Up" steps.

☐ ☐ _____

PROCEDURE 21-5
Collecting a Stool Specimen

	S	U	COMMENTS

Getting Ready

1. Complete the "Getting Ready" steps. ☐ ☐ _____

Procedure

2. Complete the label with the person's name, room number, and other identifying information. Put the completed label on the specimen container. Take the specimen container to the bathroom. Place a paper towel on the counter. Open the specimen container and place the lid on the paper towel with the inside of the lid facing up. ☐ ☐ _____

3. If the person will be using a regular toilet or bedside commode, fit the specimen collection device underneath the toilet or commode seat. Otherwise, provide the person with a bedpan. ☐ ☐ _____

4. Assist the person with defecation as necessary. Before leaving the room, remind the person not to urinate or place toilet paper into the specimen collection device or bedpan. Provide a plastic bag or waste container for the used toilet paper. ☐ ☐ _____

5. Return when the person signals. Remember to knock before entering. ☐ ☐ _____

6. Put on the gloves. ☐ ☐ _____

7. If the person used a regular toilet or bedside commode, assist the person with handwashing and then help the person to return to bed. Provide perineal care as necessary. If the person used a bedpan, cover and remove the bedpan and assist the person with handwashing and perineal care as necessary. ☐ ☐ _____

8. Take the covered bedpan or specimen collection device (if the person used a bedside commode) to the bathroom. (If the side rails are in use, raise the side rails before leaving the bedside.) ☐ ☐ _____

9. Note the color, amount, and quality of the feces. Using the tongue depressor, take two tablespoons of feces from the bedpan or specimen collection device and put them into the specimen container. Dispose of the tongue depressor in a facility-approved waste container. Empty the remaining contents of the bedpan or specimen collection device into the toilet. ☐ ☐ _____

10. Put the lid on the specimen cup. Make sure that the lid is tight. Put the specimen container on the paper towel on the counter. ☐ ☐ _____

11. Remove one glove and dispose of it in a facility-approved waste container. Holding the plastic transport bag in your ungloved hand, place the specimen container into the transport bag with your gloved hand. Avoid touching the outside of the transport bag with your glove.   ☐ ☐ _____

12. Remove the other glove and dispose of it in a facility-approved waste container.   ☐ ☐ _____

13. Gather the soiled linens and place them in the linen hamper or linen bag. Dispose of disposable items in a facility-approved waste container. Clean equipment and return it to the storage area.   ☐ ☐ _____

14. Take the specimen container to the designated location.   ☐ ☐ _____

Finishing Up

15. Complete the "Finishing Up" steps.   ☐ ☐ _____

PROCEDURE 21-6
Providing Catheter Care

	S	U	COMMENTS

Getting Ready

1. Complete the "Getting Ready" steps. ☐ ☐ _____

Procedure

2. Cover the over-bed table with paper towels. ☐ ☐ _____

3. Lower the head of the bed so that the bed is flat (as tolerated). Make sure that the bed is positioned at a comfortable working height (to promote good body mechanics) and that the wheels are locked. ☐ ☐ _____

4. Fill the wash basin with warm water (110°F [43.3°C] to 115°F [46.1°C] on the bath thermometer). Place the wash basin, soap, towels, and washcloths on the over-bed table. ☐ ☐ _____

5. If the side rails are in use, lower the side rail on the working side of the bed. The side rail on the opposite side of the bed should remain up. ☐ ☐ _____

6. Put on the gloves. ☐ ☐ _____

7. Spread the bath blanket over the top linens (and the person). If the person is able, have him or her hold the bath blanket. If not, tuck the corners under the person's shoulders. Fanfold the top linens to the foot of the bed. ☐ ☐ _____

8. Adjust the person's hospital gown or pajama bottoms as necessary to expose the person's perineum. ☐ ☐ _____

9. Ask the person to open his legs and bend his knees, if possible. If the person is not able to bend his knees, help the person to spread his legs as much as possible. ☐ ☐ _____

10. Position the bath blanket over the person so that one corner can be wrapped under and around each leg. ☐ ☐ _____

11. Position a bed protector under the person's buttocks to keep the bed linens dry. ☐ ☐ _____

12. Lift the corner of the bath blanket that is between the person's legs upward, exposing only the perineal area. ☐ ☐ _____

13. Form a mitt around your hand with one of the washcloths. Wet the mitt with warm, clean water and apply soap.

    a. **If the person is a woman:** Using the other hand, separate the labia. Place your washcloth-covered hand at the top of the vulva and stroke downward to the anus. Repeat, using a different part of the washcloth each time, until the area is clean. Rinse and dry the vulva and perineum thoroughly. ☐ ☐ _____

  b. If the person is a circumcised man: Place your washcloth-covered hand at the tip of the penis and wash in a circular motion, downward to the base of the penis. Repeat, using a different part of the washcloth each time, until the area is clean. Rinse and dry the tip and the shaft of the penis thoroughly. □ □ _____

  c. If the person is an uncircumcised man: Retract the foreskin by gently pushing the skin toward the base of the penis. Place your washcloth-covered hand at the tip of the penis and wash in a circular motion, downward to the base of the penis. Repeat, using a different part of the washcloth each time, until the area is clean. Rinse and dry the tip and the shaft of the penis thoroughly before gently pulling the foreskin back into its normal position. □ □ _____

14. Using a clean part of the washcloth, clean the catheter tubing, starting at the body and moving outward from the body about four inches. Hold the catheter near the opening of the urethra. This will help to prevent tugging on the catheter as you clean it. □ □ _____

15. Dry the perineal area thoroughly using a towel. □ □ _____

16. Check that the catheter tubing is free from kinks. Make sure that it is securely taped to the person's leg. □ □ _____

17. Remove your gloves and dispose of them in a facility-approved waste container. □ □ _____

18. Assist the person into the supine position. Remove the bath blanket, and help the person into the clean clothing. □ □ _____

19. If the side rails are in use, return the side rails to the raised position. Raise the head of the bed as the person requests. Make sure that the bed is lowered to its lowest position and that the wheels are locked. □ □ _____

20. Gather the soiled linens and place them in the linen hamper or linen bag. Dispose of disposable items in a facility-approved waste container. Clean equipment and return it to the storage area. □ □ _____

Finishing Up

21. Complete the "Finishing Up" steps. □ □ _____

PROCEDURE 21-7
Emptying a Urine Drainage Bag

	S	U	COMMENTS

Getting Ready

1. Complete the "Getting Ready" steps. ☐ ☐ _____

Procedure

2. Put on the gloves. ☐ ☐ _____

3. Place a paper towel on the floor, underneath the urine drainage bag. Unhook the drainage bag emptying spout from its holder on the urine drainage bag. Position the graduate on the paper towel underneath the emptying spout. ☐ ☐ _____

4. Unclamp the emptying spout on the urine drainage bag and allow all of the urine to drain into the graduate. Avoid touching the tip of the emptying spout with your hands or the side of the graduate. ☐ ☐ _____

5. After the urine has drained into the graduate, wipe the emptying spout with an alcohol wipe (or follow facility policy). Reclamp the emptying spout and return it to its holder. ☐ ☐ _____

6. If the person is on intake and output (I&O) status, measure the urine. Note the color, amount, and quality of the urine before emptying the contents of the graduate into the toilet. (If anything unusual is observed, do not empty the graduate until a nurse has had a chance to look at its contents.) ☐ ☐ _____

7. Dispose of disposable items in a facility-approved waste container. Clean equipment and return it to the storage area. ☐ ☐ _____

8. Remove your gloves and dispose of them in a facility-approved waste container. ☐ ☐ _____

Finishing Up

9. Complete the "Finishing Up" steps. ☐ ☐ _____

PROCEDURE 21-8
Administering a Soapsuds Enema

	S	U	COMMENTS

Getting Ready

1. Complete the "Getting Ready" steps. ☐ ☐ _____

Procedure

2. Make sure that the bed is positioned at a comfortable working height (to promote good body mechanics) and that the wheels are locked. ☐ ☐ _____

3. Prepare the enema solution in the bathroom or utility room. Clamp the tubing and then fill the enema bag with warm water (105°F [40.5°C] on the bath thermometer) in the specified amount (usually from 500 to 1500 mL). Add the castile soap packet and mix by gently rotating the enema bag. Do not shake the solution vigorously. ☐ ☐ _____

4. Release the clamp on the tubing and allow a little water to run through the tubing into the sink or bedpan. This will remove all of the air from the tubing. Reclamp the tubing. ☐ ☐ _____

5. Hang the enema bag on the IV pole and bring it to the person's bedside. Adjust the height of the IV pole so that the enema bag is hanging no more than 18 inches above the person's anus. ☐ ☐ _____

6. If the side rails are in use, lower the side rail on the working side of the bed. The side rail on the opposite side of the bed should remain up. Lower the head of the bed so that the bed is flat (as tolerated). ☐ ☐ _____

7. Spread the bath blanket over the top linens (and the person). If the person is able, have her hold the bath blanket. If not, tuck the corners under her shoulders. Fanfold the top linens to the foot of the bed. ☐ ☐ _____

8. Ask the person to lie on her left side, facing away from you, in Sims' position. Help her into this position, if necessary. ☐ ☐ _____

9. Put on the gloves. ☐ ☐ _____

10. Adjust the bath blanket and the person's hospital gown or pajama bottoms as necessary to expose the person's buttocks. Position the bed protector under the person's buttocks to keep the bed linens dry. ☐ ☐ _____

11. Open the lubricant package and squeeze a small amount of lubricant onto a paper towel. Lubricate the tip of the enema tubing to ease insertion. ☐ ☐ _____

12. Suggest that the person take a deep breath and slowly exhale as the enema tubing is inserted. With one hand, raise the person's upper buttock to expose the anus. Using your other hand, gently and carefully insert the lubricated tip of the tubing into the person's rectum (not more than 3 to 4 inches for adults). Never force the tubing into the rectum. If you are unable to insert the tubing, stop and call the nurse. ☐ ☐ _____

13. Unclamp the tubing and allow the solution to begin running. Hold the enema tubing firmly with one hand so that it does not slip out of the rectum. If the person complains of pain or cramping, slow down the rate of flow by tightening the clamp a bit. If the pain or cramping does not stop after slowing the rate of flow, stop the procedure and call the nurse. ☐ ☐ _____

14. When the fluid level reaches the bottom of the bag, clamp the tubing to avoid injecting air into the person's rectum. ☐ ☐ _____

15. Remove the tubing from the person's rectum and place it inside the enema bag. Gently place several thicknesses of toilet paper against the person's anus to absorb any fluid. ☐ ☐ _____

16. Ask the person to retain the enema solution for the specific amount of time. ☐ ☐ _____

17. Assist the person with expelling the enema as necessary, using the bedpan, bedside commode, or toilet. If the person is using a regular toilet, ask her not to flush the toilet after expelling the enema. ☐ ☐ _____

18. If the person used a regular toilet or bedside commode, assist her with handwashing and then help her to return to bed. Provide perineal care as necessary. If the person used a bedpan, cover and remove the bedpan and assist her with handwashing and perineal care as necessary. ☐ ☐ _____

19. Raise the head of the bed as the person requests. Make sure that the bed is lowered to its lowest position and that the wheels are locked. (If the side rails are in use, raise the side rails before leaving the bedside.) ☐ ☐ _____

20. Take the covered bedpan or commode bucket (if the person used a bedside commode) to the bathroom. ☐ ☐ _____

21. Note the color, amount, and quality of feces before emptying the contents of the bedpan or commode bucket into the toilet. (If anything unusual is observed, do not empty the bedpan or commode bucket until a nurse has had a chance to look at its contents.) ☐ ☐ _____

22. Gather the soiled linens and place them in the linen hamper. Dispose of disposable items in a facility-approved waste container. Clean equipment and return it to the storage area. ☐ ☐ _____

23. Remove your gloves and dispose of them in a facility-approved waste container.

☐ ☐ _____

Finishing Up

24. Complete the "Finishing Up" steps.

☐ ☐ _____

PROCEDURE 21-9

Providing Routine Ostomy Care

	S	U	COMMENTS

Getting Ready

1. Complete the "Getting Ready" steps. ☐ ☐ _____

Procedure

2. Cover the over-bed table with paper towels. Place the ostomy supplies and clean linens on the over-bed table. ☐ ☐ _____

3. Make sure that the bed is positioned at a comfortable working height (to promote good body mechanics) and that the wheels are locked. ☐ ☐ _____

4. If the side rails are in use, lower the side rail on the working side of the bed. The side rail on the opposite side of the bed should remain up. If necessary, lower the head of the bed so that the bed is flat (as tolerated). ☐ ☐ _____

5. Fanfold the top linens to below the person's waist. ☐ ☐ _____

6. Position the bed protector on the bed alongside the person to keep the bed linens dry. Adjust the person's clothing as necessary to expose the person's stoma. ☐ ☐ _____

7. Put on the gloves. ☐ ☐ _____

8. Disconnect the ostomy appliance from the ostomy belt if one is used. Remove the belt. If the ostomy belt is soiled, dispose of it in a facility-approved waste container (if it is disposable), or place it in the linen hamper or linen bag (if it is not disposable). ☐ ☐ _____

9. Remove the ostomy appliance by holding the skin taut and gently pulling the appliance away, starting at the top. If the adhesive is making removal difficult, use warm water or the adhesive solvent to soften the adhesive. Place the ostomy appliance in the bedpan. ☐ ☐ _____

10. Gently wipe the stoma with toilet paper to remove any feces or drainage. Place the toilet paper in the bedpan. Cover the stoma with the gauze pad to absorb any drainage that may occur until the new appliance is in place. ☐ ☐ _____

11. Cover the bedpan with the bedpan cover or paper towels. Take the bedpan to the bathroom. (If the side rails are in use, raise them before leaving the bedside.) ☐ ☐ _____

12. Note the color, amount, and quality of the feces before emptying the contents of the ostomy appliance and the bedpan into the toilet. (If anything unusual is observed, do not empty the ostomy appliance until a nurse has had a chance to look at its contents.) ☐ ☐ _____

13. Dispose of the ostomy appliance in a facility-approved waste container. ☐ ☐ _____

14. Remove your gloves and dispose of them in a facility-approved waste container. Wash your hands. ☐ ☐ _____

15. Fill the wash basin with warm water (110°F [43.3°C] to 115°F [46.1°C] on the bath thermometer). Return to the bedside. Place the basin on the over-bed table. If the side rails are in use, lower the side rail on the working side of the bed. ☐ ☐ _____

16. Put on a clean pair of gloves. ☐ ☐ _____

17. Form a mitt around your hand with one of the wash-cloths. Wet the mitt with warm, clean water and apply soap (or other cleansing agent, per facility policy). Remove the gauze pad from the stoma and dispose of it in a facility-approved waste container. Clean the skin around the stoma. Rinse and dry the skin around the stoma thoroughly. ☐ ☐ _____

18. Apply the skin barrier if needed, according to the manufacturer's directions. ☐ ☐ _____

19. Place the deodorant in the ostomy appliance if deodorant is used. ☐ ☐ _____

20. Put the clean ostomy belt on the person if an ostomy belt is used. ☐ ☐ _____

21. Make sure that the opening on the ostomy appliance is the correct size. Remove the adhesive backing on the ostomy appliance. ☐ ☐ _____

22. Center the appliance over the stoma, making sure that the drain or the end of the bag is pointed down. Gently press around the edges to seal the ostomy appliance to the skin. ☐ ☐ _____

23. Connect the ostomy appliance to the ostomy belt, if one is used. ☐ ☐ _____

24. Remove the bed protector. ☐ ☐ _____

25. Remove your gloves and dispose of them in a facility-approved waste container. ☐ ☐ _____

26. Adjust the person's clothing as necessary to cover the ostomy appliance. If the bedding is wet or soiled, change the bed linens. Help the person back into a comfortable position, straighten the bottom linens, and draw the top linens over the person. Raise the head of the bed, as the person requests. ☐ ☐ _____

27. If the side rails are in use, return the side rail to the raised position. Make sure that the bed is lowered to its lowest position and that the wheels are locked. ☐ ☐ _____

28. Gather the soiled linens and place them in the linen hamper or linen bag. Dispose of disposable items in a facility-approved waste container. Clean equipment and return it to the storage area. ☐ ☐ _____

Finishing Up

29. Complete the "Finishing Up" steps. ☐ ☐ _____

CHAPTER 23 PROCEDURE CHECKLISTS

PROCEDURE 23-1
Providing Postmortem Care

	S	U	COMMENTS

Getting Ready

1. Complete the "Getting Ready" steps. ☐ ☐ _____

Procedure

2. Cover the over-bed table with paper towels. Place your supplies on the over-bed table. ☐ ☐ _____

3. Make sure that the bed is positioned at a comfortable working height (to promote good body mechanics) and that the wheels are locked. Lower the head of the bed so that the bed is flat. Fanfold the top linens to the foot of the bed. ☐ ☐ _____

4. Put on the gloves. ☐ ☐ _____

5. If instructed to by the nurse, remove or turn off any medical equipment. ☐ ☐ _____

6. Place the body in the supine position. Position the pillow under the person's head and shoulders. Undress the body and cover it with the bath blanket. ☐ ☐ _____

7. Close the eyes. Put a moistened cotton ball on each eyelid if the eyes do not stay closed. If the person has an artificial eye, this should be in place, unless you are instructed otherwise. ☐ ☐ _____

8. Replace the person's dentures, unless you are instructed otherwise. Close the mouth and, if necessary, gently support the jaw with the chin strap, a light bandage, or a rolled hand towel. ☐ ☐ _____

9. Remove any jewelry and place it in a plastic bag or envelope for the family. List each piece of jewelry as you remove it. Do not remove engagement or wedding rings, unless it is your facility's policy to do so. ☐ ☐ _____

10. Fill the wash basin with warm water. Place the basin on the over-bed table. Wash the body and comb the hair. ☐ ☐ _____

11. If the family is to view the body, dress the body in a clean gown. If the bedding is wet or soiled, change the bed linens. Draw the top linens over the person, forming a cuff at the shoulders. (Do not cover the person's face.) Straighten the room, lower the lights, and provide for the family's privacy. ☐ ☐ _____

12. After the family leaves, collect all of the person's belongings, noting each item on your list. ☐ ☐ _____

13. Fill out three identification tags:

    a. Attach one to the right great toe or the right ankle. ☐ ☐ _____

    b. Attach one to the person's belongings. ☐ ☐ _____

    c. Save the last to be attached to the outside of the shroud (if used). ☐ ☐ _____

14. If a shroud is to be used, apply it now and attach the third identification tag to the outside of the shroud. ☐ ☐ _____

15. Gather the soiled linens and place them in the linen hamper. Dispose of disposable items in a facility-approved waste container. Clean equipment and return it to the storage area. ☐ ☐ _____

16. Remove your gloves and dispose of them in a facility-approved waste container. ☐ ☐ _____

17. Transfer the body from the bed to a stretcher for transport to the morgue, if appropriate. If the family has made funeral arrangements, leave the body in the room with the door or curtain closed. ☐ ☐ _____

18. Report the time the body was transported and the location of the person's belongings to the nurse. ☐ ☐ _____

Finishing Up

19. Complete the "Finishing Up" steps. ☐ ☐ _____

CHAPTER 25 PROCEDURE CHECKLISTS

PROCEDURE 25-1
Assisting the Nurse With a Dressing Change

	S	U	COMMENTS

Getting Ready

1. Complete the "Getting Ready" steps. ☐ ☐ _____

Procedure

2. Cover the over-bed table with paper towels or the bed protector. Place the dressing supplies on the over-bed table. Fold the top edges of the plastic bag down to make a cuff. Place the cuffed bag on the over-bed table. ☐ ☐ _____

3. Make sure that the bed is positioned at a comfortable working height (to promote good body mechanics) and that the wheels are locked. If the side rails are in use, lower the side rail on the working side of the bed. The side rail on the opposite side of the bed should remain up. ☐ ☐ _____

4. Help the person to a comfortable position that allows access to the wound. ☐ ☐ _____

5. Fanfold the top linens to the foot of the bed. Adjust the person's hospital gown or pajamas as necessary to expose the wound. ☐ ☐ _____

6. Put on the mask, gown, or both, if necessary. Put on the gloves. ☐ ☐ _____

7. The nurse will remove the old dressing. The nurse may ask you to take the old dressing and place it in the cuffed plastic bag. Be careful to keep the soiled side of the dressing out of the person's sight. Do not let the dressing touch the outside of the plastic bag. ☐ ☐ _____

8. Remove your gloves and dispose of them in a facility-approved waste container. ☐ ☐ _____

9. Wait while the nurse inspects the wound and measures it, if necessary. ☐ ☐ _____

10. Put on a clean pair of gloves. ☐ ☐ _____

11. Assist as the nurse applies a new dressing.

   a. Open the wrapper containing the dressing and hold it open so that the nurse can remove the dressing. Do not touch the dressing. Dispose of the wrapper in a facility-approved waste container. ☐ ☐ _____

   b. If the dressing will be secured with tape, cut four pieces of tape for securing the dressing. For a 4 × 4 dressing, each piece of tape should measure 8 inches long. Hang the tape from the edge of the over-bed table. ☐ ☐ _____

    c. If the nurse asks you to, use the tape strips to secure the dressing by placing one piece of tape along each side of the dressing. Center each piece of tape equally over the dressing and the person's skin.

  ☐ ☐ _____

12. Remove your gloves (and gown and mask, if using) and dispose of them in a facility-approved waste container. Wash your hands.

  ☐ ☐ _____

13. Re-cover the wound with the hospital gown or pajamas. Help the person back into a comfortable position, straighten the bottom linens, and draw the top linens over the person.

  ☐ ☐ _____

14. Make sure that the bed is lowered to its lowest position and that the wheels are locked. If the side rails are in use, return the side rail to the raised position on the working side of the bed.

  ☐ ☐ _____

15. Dispose of disposable items in a facility-approved waste container. Clean equipment and return it to the storage area.

  ☐ ☐ _____

Finishing Up

16. Complete the "Finishing Up" steps.

  ☐ ☐ _____

CHAPTER 26 PROCEDURE CHECKLISTS

PROCEDURE 26-1

Assisting a Person With Passive Range-of-Motion Exercises

	S	U	COMMENTS

Getting Ready

1. Complete the "Getting Ready" steps. ☐ ☐ _____

Procedure

2. Make sure that the bed is positioned at a comfortable working height (to promote good body mechanics) and that the wheels are locked. If the side rails are in use, lower the side rail on the working side of the bed. The side rail on the opposite side of the bed should remain up. Raise or lower the head of the bed to a horizontal or semi-Fowler's position. ☐ ☐ _____

3. Assist the person into the supine position. ☐ ☐ _____

4. Spread the bath blanket over the top linens (and the person). If the person is able, have him hold the bath blanket. If not, tuck the corners under his shoulders. Fanfold the top linens to the foot of the bed. ☐ ☐ _____

5. Perform each range-of-motion exercise in steps 6 through 13 according to the person's care plan, being careful to expose only the part of the body that is being exercised. Repeat each exercise three to five times, as written in the care plan. ☐ ☐ _____

6. If your facility permits, exercise the person's neck:

   a. **Forward and backward flexion and extension (neck).** Support the person's head by putting one hand under his chin and the other on the back of the head. Gently bring the head forward, as if to touch the chin to the chest, and then bring it backward, chin pointing to the sky. ☐ ☐ _____

   b. **Side-to-side flexion (neck).** Support the person's head by putting one hand under his chin and the other near the opposite temple. Gently tilt the head toward the right shoulder and then toward the left. ☐ ☐ _____

   c. **Rotation (neck).** Support the person's head by putting one hand under his chin and the other on the back of the head. Gently move the head from side to side, as if the person were shaking his head "no." ☐ ☐ _____

7. Exercise the person's shoulder:

   a. Forward flexion and extension (shoulder). ☐ ☐ _____
Support the person's arm by putting one hand
under his elbow and the other under his wrist.
Keeping the person's arm straight with the palm
facing down, lift the arm up so that it is alongside
his ear and then return it to its original position.

   b. Abduction and adduction (shoulder). Support ☐ ☐ _____
the person's arm by putting one hand under his
elbow and the other under his wrist. Keeping the
person's arm straight with the palm facing up,
move his arm away from the side of his body and
then return it to its original position.

   c. Horizontal abduction and adduction ☐ ☐ _____
(shoulder). Support the person's arm by putting
one hand under his elbow and the other under
his wrist. Keeping the person's arm straight with
the palm facing up, move his arm away from the
side of his body. Gently bending the person's
elbow, touch his hand to the opposite shoulder,
then straighten the elbow and bring the arm back
out to the side.

   d. Rotation (shoulder). Support the person's arm by ☐ ☐ _____
putting one hand under his elbow and the other
under his wrist. Move the person's arm away from
the side of his body and bend his arm at the
elbow. Gently move the person's forearm up so
that it forms a right angle with the mattress and
then back down. This movement is similar to the
motion a police officer makes when he or she is
signaling someone to stop.

8. Exercise the person's elbow.

   a. Flexion and extension (elbow). Support the per- ☐ ☐ _____
son's arm by putting one hand under his elbow
and the other under his wrist. Starting with the
person's arm straight and with the palm facing up,
bend his elbow so that his hand moves toward his
shoulder. Then, straighten out the elbow, returning the person's hand to its original position.

   b. Pronation and supination (elbow). Support the ☐ ☐ _____
person's arm by putting one hand under his elbow
and the other under his wrist. Move the person's
arm away from the side of his body and slightly
bend his arm at the elbow. Gently move the
person's forearm up so that it forms a right angle
with the mattress. Gently turn the person's hand
so that the palm is facing the end of the bed.
Then turn the hand the other way so that the
palm is facing the head of the bed.

9. Exercise the person's wrist.

    a. Flexion and extension (wrist). Support the person's wrist with one hand. Use the other hand to gently bend the person's hand down and then back. ☐ ☐ _____

    b. Radial and ulnar flexion (wrist). Support the person's wrist with one hand. Use the other hand to gently turn the person's hand toward his thumb. Then turn the hand the other way, toward the little finger. ☐ ☐ _____

10. Exercise the person's fingers and thumb.

    a. Flexion and extension (fingers and thumb). Support the person's wrist with one hand. Using your other hand, flex the person's fingers to make a fist, tucking his thumb under the fingers. Then straighten each finger and the thumb, one by one. ☐ ☐ _____

    b. Abduction and adduction (fingers and thumb). With one hand, hold the person's thumb and index finger together. With the other hand, move the middle finger away from the index finger. Then move the middle finger back toward the index finger and hold the middle finger, index finger, and thumb together. Next, move the ring finger away from the other two fingers and thumb, then move it back toward the group. Do the same with the little finger. Finally, reverse the process. Hold the little finger and the ring finger together and move the middle finger away and back. Complete with the index finger and thumb. ☐ ☐ _____

    c. Flexion and extension (thumb). Bend the person's thumb into his palm, then return it to its original position. ☐ ☐ _____

    d. Opposition. Touch each fingertip to the thumb. ☐ ☐ _____

11. Exercise the person's hip and knee.

    a. Forward flexion and extension (hip and knee). Support the person's leg by putting one hand under his knee and the other under his ankle. Gently bend the person's knee, moving it toward his head. Then straighten the person's knee and gently lower the leg to the bed. ☐ ☐ _____

    b. Abduction and adduction (hip). Support the person's leg by putting one hand under his knee and the other under his ankle. Keeping the person's leg straight, move his leg away from the side of his body and then return it to its original position. ☐ ☐ _____

    c. Rotation (hip). Support the person's leg by putting one hand under his knee and the other under his ankle. Keeping the person's leg straight, gently turn the leg inward and then outward. ☐ ☐ _____

12. Exercise the person's ankle and foot.

   a. Dorsiflexion and plantar flexion (ankle and foot). Support the person's ankle with one hand. Use the other hand to gently bend the person's foot up toward the head and then back.

   ☐ ☐ _____

   b. Inversion and eversion (ankle and foot). Support the person's ankle with one hand. Use the other hand to gently turn the inside of the foot inward and then outward.

   ☐ ☐ _____

13. Exercise the person's toes.

   a. Flexion and extension (toes). Put one hand under the person's foot. Put the other hand over the person's toes. Curl the toes downward and then straighten them.

   ☐ ☐ _____

   b. Abduction and adduction (toes). Spread each toe the same way you spread each finger in step 10b.

   ☐ ☐ _____

14. Straighten the bed linens and make sure the person is comfortable and in good body alignment. Draw the top linens over the person and remove the bath blanket.

☐ ☐ _____

15. If the side rails are in use, raise the side rail on the working side of the bed. Make sure that the bed is lowered to its lowest position and that the wheels are locked.

☐ ☐ _____

Finishing Up

16. Complete the "Finishing Up" steps.

☐ ☐ _____

CHAPTER 30 PROCEDURE CHECKLISTS

PROCEDURE 30-1
Assisting a Person With an In-the-Ear Hearing Aid

Inserting an In-the-Ear Hearing Aid

	S	U	COMMENTS
1. Complete the "Getting Ready" steps.	☐	☐	_____
2. Check the hearing aid to make sure the volume is down and the hearing aid is turned off.	☐	☐	_____
3. Help the person to a comfortable position, with his head turned so that the ear needing the hearing aid is closest to you.	☐	☐	_____
4. Inspect the ear canal for excessive cerumen (ear wax). If you see excessive wax build-up in the ear canal, gently wipe the ear canal with a warm, moist washcloth.	☐	☐	_____
5. Gently insert the tapered end of the hearing aid into the external auditory canal. Gently rotate the hearing aid so that it fits into the curve of the ear. With one hand, push up and in. Use your other hand to pull gently down on the person's earlobe. The hearing aid should fit snugly but comfortably, flush with the ear.	☐	☐	_____
6. Turn on the control switch. Adjust the volume by talking to the person as you increase the volume. Stop increasing the volume when the person can hear you.	☐	☐	_____
7. Complete the "Finishing Up" steps.	☐	☐	_____

Removing an In-the-Ear Hearing Aid

	S	U	COMMENTS
1. Complete the "Getting Ready" steps.	☐	☐	_____
2. Turn off the hearing aid.	☐	☐	_____
3. Gently pull up on the person's ear. This will allow you to lift the hearing aid up and out of the person's ear.	☐	☐	_____
4. Remove the batteries before storing the hearing aid in its case. Make sure the case is labeled with the person's name.	☐	☐	_____
5. Complete the "Finishing Up" steps.	☐	☐	_____

CHAPTER 41 PROCEDURE CHECKLISTS

PROCEDURE 41-1
Applying Anti-embolism (TED) Stockings

	S	U	COMMENTS

Getting Ready

1. Complete the "Getting Ready" steps. ☐ ☐ _____

Procedure

2. Make sure that the bed is positioned at a comfortable working height (to promote good body mechanics) and that the wheels are locked. If the side rails are in use, lower the side rail on the working side of the bed. The side rail on the opposite side of the bed should remain up. ☐ ☐ _____

3. Help the person into the supine position. ☐ ☐ _____

4. Fanfold the top linens to the foot of the bed. Adjust the person's hospital gown or pajama bottoms as necessary to expose one leg at a time. ☐ ☐ _____

5. Turn the stocking inside out down to the heel. ☐ ☐ _____

6. Slip the foot of the stocking over the person's toes, foot, and heel. The stocking has an opening in the toe area, which allows the health care team to assess the person's toes to make sure they are receiving enough blood. Depending on the manufacturer, this opening may be on the top or on the bottom of the stocking. ☐ ☐ _____

7. Grasp the top of the stocking and pull it up the person's leg. The stocking will turn itself right-side out as you pull it up the person's leg. ☐ ☐ _____

8. Check to make sure that the stocking is not twisted and that it fits snugly against the person's leg, with no wrinkles. Also make sure that the stocking fits smoothly over the heel and that the opening in the toe area is correctly located in the toe region. ☐ ☐ _____

9. Cover that leg, expose the other leg, and repeat steps 5 through 8. ☐ ☐ _____

10. Help the person back into a comfortable position, straighten the bottom linens, and draw the top linens over the person. Raise the head of the bed as the person requests. Make sure that the bed is lowered to its lowest position and that the wheels are locked. ☐ ☐ _____

Finishing Up

11. Complete the "Finishing Up" steps. ☐ ☐ _____